Get ahead!

specialties

100 EMQs for Finals

Second edition

Get ahead!

specialties

100 EMQs for Finals
Second edition

Peter Cartledge BSc MBChB MRCPCH PCME MSc
Leeds Children's Hospital, Leeds, UK

Fiona Bach MBChB, MRCOG, BSc
Speciality Registrar in Obstetrics and Gynaecology, London, UK

Rebecca Cairns
General Practitioner, Horton Bank Practice, Bradford, UK

Mahesh Jayaram MB BS, DPM, MMedSci, MRCPsych, FRANZCP
Senior Lecturer, Department of Psychiatry,
University of Melbourne, Australia

Mary Watson
General Practitioner, Warwickshire, UK

Series Editor

Saran Shantikumar BA, BSc, MBChB, MRCS
Academic Clinical Fellow in Public Health,
University of Warwick, UK

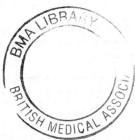

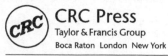
CRC Press
Taylor & Francis Group
Boca Raton London New York

CRC Press is an imprint of the
Taylor & Francis Group, an **informa** business

CRC Press
Taylor & Francis Group
6000 Broken Sound Parkway NW, Suite 300
Boca Raton, FL 33487-2742

© 2016 by Taylor & Francis Group, LLC
CRC Press is an imprint of Taylor & Francis Group, an Informa business

No claim to original U.S. Government works

Printed on acid-free paper
Version Date: 20150904

International Standard Book Number-13: 978-1-4822-5316-0 (Paperback)

Visit the Taylor & Francis Web site at
http://www.taylorandfrancis.com

and the CRC Press Web site at
http://www.crcpress.com

Contents

Preface

Welcome to *Get ahead! Specialties*. This book contains 100 extended matching questions (EMQs) covering various topics within obstetrics, gynaecology, paediatrics and psychiatry. These are arranged by specialty as ten practice papers, each containing ten themes. Allow yourself 90 minutes for each paper. You can either work through the practice papers systematically or dip in and out of the book using the EMQ contents pages as a guide to where questions on a specific topic can be found. We have tried to include all the main conditions about which you can be expected to know, as well as some more detailed knowledge suitable for candidates aiming towards distinction. As in the real exam, these papers have no preset pass mark. Whether you pass or fail depends on the distribution of scores across the whole year group, but around 60% should be sufficient.

We would like to acknowledge the help of Stephen Clausard, Editor at CRC Press, for his patience and proactivity in commissioning and supporting this edition and others in the *Get ahead!* series.

Peter Cartledge
Fiona Bach
Rebecca Cairns
Mahesh Jayaram
Mary Watson

Introduction to *Get ahead!*

GET AHEAD!

Extended matching questions (EMQs) are becoming more popular as a method of assessment in summative medical school examinations. EMQs have the advantage of testing candidates' knowledge of clinical scenarios rather than their ability at detailed factual recall. However, they do not always parallel real-life situations and are not always comparable to clinical decision making. Either way, the EMQ is here to stay.

The *Get ahead!* series is aimed primarily at undergraduate finalists. Much like the real exam, we have endeavoured to include commonly asked questions as well as a generous proportion of harder stems, appropriate for the more ambitious student aiming for honours. The Medical Schools Council Assessment Alliance (MSCAA) is a partnership aiming to improve assessment practice between all undergraduate medical schools in the UK. The questions in the *Get ahead!* series are written to follow the style of the MSCAA EMQs, and hence are of a similar format to what many of you can expect in your exams. All the questions in the *Get ahead!* series are accompanied by explanatory answers, including a succinct summary of the key features of each condition. Even when you get an answer right, I strongly suggest you read these – I guarantee you will learn something. For added interest, we have included details of eponymous persons ('eponymous' from Greek *epi* = upon + *onyma* = name; 'giving name'), and, as you have just seen, some etymological derivations.

HOW TO PASS YOUR EXAMS

Exam EMQs are intended to be based on 'house officer knowledge'. Sadly, this is not always the case, and you shouldn't be surprised when you get a question concerning the management of various stages of prostate cancer (as I was). So start revising early and don't restrict yourself to the given syllabus if you can avoid it. If your exam is only two weeks away, then cram, cram, cram – you will be surprised at how much you can learn in a fortnight.

During the exam...

1. Try to answer the questions without looking at the responses first – the questions are often written such that this should be possible.
2. Take your time to read the questions fully. There are no bonus marks for finishing the paper early.

3. If you get stuck on a question, then make sure you mark down your best guess before you move on. You may not have time to return to it at the end.
4. Answer all the questions – there is no negative marking. If you are unsure, go with your instinct – it's probably going to be your best guess.
5. Never think that the examiner is trying to catch you out. Red herrings are not allowed, so don't assume there is one. If a question looks easy, it probably is!

But all this is obvious and there is no substitute for learning the material thoroughly and practising as many questions as you can. With this book, you're off to a good start!

A final word...

The *Get ahead!* series is written by doctors who have recently finished finals and/or who have experience teaching students. As such, I hope the books cover information that is valuable and relevant to you as undergraduates who are about to sit finals.

I wish you the best of luck in your exams!

Saran Shantikumar
Series Editor, Get ahead!

Practice Paper 1: Questions

THEME 1: ANTENATAL SCREENING

Options

A. Amniocentesis
B. Antenatal fetal blood sampling
C. Cardiotocography
D. Chorionic villus sampling
E. Combined screening
F. Fetal echocardiography
G. Fetal tissue sampling
H. First-trimester ultrasound scan
I. Nuchal translucency test
J. Routine anomaly scan
K. Serum 'triple test'
L. Uterine artery Doppler

For each of the following scenarios, select the most appropriate screening test. Each option may be used once, more than once or not at all.

1. A 42-year-old woman and a 51-year-old man have conceived their first child together and currently the gestation is 13 weeks. They are concerned about the possibility of Down's syndrome after receiving a high-risk screening result. They would like a test that would give them the definitive diagnosis as to whether their baby has Down's syndrome.

2. A 24-year-old woman is 12 weeks pregnant. She would like to know whether there are any gross anatomical deformities of the fetus. Also, her sister has twins, and she would like to know if her current pregnancy involves more than one baby.

3. A 35-year-old woman and a 45-year-old man have been given a high-risk result for Down's syndrome after screening performed at 17 weeks' gestation. They would like definite clarification as to whether or not the baby will be born with Down's syndrome.

4. A 25-year-old woman would like a screening test for Down's syndrome at 16 weeks' gestation.

5. A 34-year-old pregnant woman had operations for a congenital heart disease as a child. She would like to have her baby's heart investigated for a similar problem.

THEME 2: CHRONIC PELVIC PAIN

Options

A. Adhesions from surgery
B. Chronic pelvic inflammatory disease
C. Constipation
D. Endometriosis
E. Fibroid degeneration
F. Functional pain
G. Irritable bowel syndrome
H. Ovarian cysts
I. Primary dysmenorrhoea
J. Primary menorrhagia
K. Renal calculus
L. Secondary dysmenorrhoea

For each of the following scenarios, select the most likely underlying cause. Each option may be used once, more than once or not at all.

1. A 35-year-old woman presents with heavy, painful periods and deep pelvic pain on intercourse. She reports occasional rectal bleeding. She had a caesarean section 3 years ago for fetal distress after having difficulty conceiving.

2. A 31-year-old woman complains of feeling generally unwell, with constant lower abdominal pain and pain on intercourse. She and her current partner have been trying to conceive for 2 years without success. She complains of irregular bleeding and postcoital bleeding. Her observations include heart rate 82 beats/minute, blood pressure 124/88 mmHg and a normal temperature. She had a previous laparoscopy which showed Fitz-Hugh–Curtis adhesions around the liver.

3. A 33-year-old woman presents with colicky lower abdominal pain, loin pain and pain on passing water. She also describes passing blood-stained urine. Her observations are pulse 68 beats/minute, blood pressure 128/92 mmHg and temperature 36.8°C. She has never been in hospital before.

4. A 37-year-old woman complains of very painful periods since a large loop excision of the transformation zone procedure. The pain generally starts on the day of or the day before menstruation, and lasts for 2 days.

5. A 42-year-old woman has been attending the gynaecology clinic for 7 years complaining of pelvic pain and dyspareunia, which has not improved despite various medications. She has had a laparoscopy, hysteroscopy and multiple ultrasound scans, all of which revealed no pathology. She was reviewed by the surgeons who also performed a colonoscopy and cystoscopy. She is convinced that her partner is unfaithful and she has contracted an infection because of this, but multiple swabs have revealed no evidence of infection.

THEME 3: CARDIOTOCOGRAPHY

Options

A Accelerations
B. Baseline bradycardia
C. Early decelerations
D. Late decelerations
E. Normal baseline fetal heart rate
F. Normal variability
G. Pseudosinusoidal pattern
H. Reduced variability
 I. Sinusoidal pattern
 J. Sustained tachycardia
K. Variable decelerations

For each of the following scenarios, select the most appropriate description of a cardiotocogram. Each option may be used once, more than once or not at all.

1. A pattern that is associated with maternal pyrexia.
2. This feature is associated with fetal sleep.
3. On a cardiotocogram tracing, a dip in the fetal heart rate of 20 beats/minute is seen. It starts at the same time as contractions and recovers to normal by the end of the contraction.
4. This reassuring sign, although not always present, occurs in a healthy fetus particularly with an increase in activity.
5. This pattern is often seen in cord compression.

THEME 4: SEXUALLY TRANSMITTED INFECTIONS

Options

A. Bacterial vaginosis
B. Cervical cancer
C. Chancroid
D. Chlamydia
E. Epstein–Barr virus
F. Genital candidiasis
G. Genital herpes
H. Genital warts
I. Gonorrhoea
J. Granuloma inguinale (Donovanosis)

K. HIV
L. Lymphogranuloma venereum
M. Molluscum contagiosum
N. Phthiriasis
O. Reiter's syndrome
P. Scabies
Q. Syphilis
R. Trichomoniasis

For each of the following scenarios, select the most likely diagnosis. Each option may be used once, more than once or not at all.

1. A 35-year-old man presents with a 3-day history of left knee pain and dysuria. On examination, his temperature is 37.2°C and you notice that his eyes are red.
2. A 45-year-old woman who is HIV positive presents with multiple lesions on her face. The lesions are raised and shiny, non-tender, non-erythematous and around 3 mm in diameter. They have an umbilicated centre.
3. A 34-year-old woman presents to her GP with pain on passing urine and increased frequency. She is started on a course of trimethoprim and a urine sample is sent to the laboratory. She returns 4 days later complaining of an 'itching down there' and pain when having sexual intercourse. On speculum examination, there is redness of the vulva and a thick white discharge is seen within the vagina.
4. A 30-year-old man presents with a single ulcer on his penis which he says developed from a spot. He denies any pain in the area. On examination, lymphadenopathy is palpable in the left groin, with evidence of a discharging sinus. A culture of the discharge reveals *Chlamydia trachomatis* (serovars L1/L2/L3).
5. A 45-year-old woman attends the GP with fever, general malaise, arthralgia and severe headaches. She has recently finished a round-the-world expedition. On examination, she has several ulcers in her mouth and genitals and lymphadenopathy in her axilla and groin. On further questioning, she tells you that 2 months ago she had a painless ulcer on her labia.

THEME 5: HORMONES OF MENSTRUATION

Options

A. Activin
B. Follicle-stimulating hormone
C. Inhibin
D. Luteinizing hormone
E. Luteinizing hormone and follicle-stimulating hormone
F. Estradiol
G. Progesterone
H. Progesterone and estradiol

For each of the following descriptions, select the most appropriate hormone(s). Each option may be used once, more than once or not at all.

1. It is the surge in this hormone(s) that stimulates ovulation.
2. This hormone(s) would continue to rise to maintain pregnancy if the ovum was fertilized.
3. This hormone(s) stimulates the growth of 6–12 primary follicles each month.
4. This steroid hormone(s) stimulates proliferation of glandular and stromal elements of the endometrium. It also encourages production of thin cervical mucus that is easily penetrable by sperm.
5. Hormone(s) released by the pituitary gland.

THEME 6: PAIN IN PREGNANCY

Options
A. Acute fatty liver of pregnancy
B. Acute pyelonephritis
C. Braxton Hicks contractions
D. Cholecystitis
E. Chorioamnionitis
F. HELLP syndrome
G. Labour
H. Obstetric cholestasis
 I. Placental abruption
 J. Round ligament stretching
K. Symphysis pubis dysfunction
L. Urinary tract infection
M. Uterine rupture

For each of the following scenarios, select the most likely diagnosis. Each option may be used once, more than once or not at all.

1. A 32-year-old woman of 39 + 6 gestation attends the antenatal day unit feeling unwell with sudden-onset epigastric pain associated with nausea and vomiting. Her temperature is 36.7°C and blood pressure is 165/104 mmHg. On examination, she is found to be tender over the right upper quadrant. Her blood results show mild anaemia, haemolysis, elevated liver enzymes and low platelets.

2. A 32-year-old woman of 38 + 2 gestation complains of feeling unwell with fever, rigors and abdominal pains. The pain was initially located in her lower abdomen and was associated with urinary frequency and dysuria. The pain has now become more generalized, specifically radiating to her right loin. She says that she has felt occasional 'uterine tightenings'. A CTG is reassuring.

3. A 32-year-old woman para 3 of 39 + 3 gestation reports having had spontaneous rupture of membranes 4 days ago. She did not attend the delivery suite, as she knew what would happen and had already decided on a home birth. Today, she feels very hot and sweaty. She thought that she was starting to have labour pains, but she describes the pain as more constant. On examination, her uterus is tender throughout. Blood tests show a raised CRP and white cell count.

4. A 32-year-old woman of 40 + 3 gestation attends the antenatal day unit with sudden-onset epigastric pain with nausea and vomiting. She is clinically jaundiced. Her biochemistry results show a raised bilirubin, abnormal liver enzymes, high uric acid and hypoglycaemia.

5. A 32-year-old woman of 38 + 4 gestation attends the antenatal day unit with pain in the suprapubic area that radiates to the upper thighs and perineum. It is worse on walking. Her urine dipstick showed a trace of protein, but no white cells, nitrites or blood.

THEME 7: FETAL PRESENTATION

Options
A. Brow
B. Extended breech
C. Face
D. Footling breech
E. Left occipitoposterior
F. Left occipitotransverse
G. Occipitoanterior
H. Occipitoposterior

For each of the following descriptions, select the most likely fetal presentation. Each option may be used once, more than once or not at all.

As part of your obstetrics end-of-firm assessment, your tutor asks you to examine someone and comment on the likely fetal presentation.

1. On vaginal examination, the cervix is fully dilated and with cephalic presentation. Anteriorly, you can feel a Y-shaped dip in the bones of the skull, with a straight suture leading to a diamond-shaped dip posteriorly.
2. On abdominal examination, you palpate a 37-week fetus with a longitudinal lie. The fundus is filled with a round ballotable fetal part. The fetal heart is heard above the umbilicus. The mother has just received a scan and counselling from the consultant and they have agreed that she is going to have a normal delivery.
3. On vaginal examination, the head is high. Anteriorly, the sagittal suture is palpable leading to the anterior fontanelle. The supraorbital ridges and bridge of the nose are also palpable.
4. On abdominal palpation, the lie is longitudinal, although the back is not easily felt. The contour of the uterus is irregular. The head is two-fifths palpable. The anterior fontanelle is easily palpable on vaginal examination.
5. On abdominal examination, you palpate a 40-week fetus with a longitudinal lie. The presenting part at the lower uterine pole is difficult to assess for engagement. At the fundus is a hard ballotable fetal part to the left of the midline, and the fetal heart is heard above the umbilicus. After a scan, the mother is told that it is not appropriate for her to have a vaginal delivery and she has a high risk of cord prolapse if her membranes rupture.

THEME 8: DIABETES IN PREGNANCY

Options

A. Angiotensin II receptor antagonist
B. Diet and exercise
C. Folic acid 400 µg/day
D. Folic acid 5 mg/day
E. Gliclazide
F. Insulin
G. Intravenous (IV) dextrose and insulin infusion
H. IV dextrose alone
I. Metformin
J. Ramipril
K. Statin

The following questions concern the management of diabetes in pregnancy. For each, select the most appropriate response. Each option may be used once, more than once or not at all.

1. This is the first-line treatment for gestational diabetes.
2. Medication recommended for a type 1 diabetic preconceptually up to 12 weeks.
3. This oral hypoglycaemic should be stopped preconceptually.
4. This is used in labour for a gestational diabetic if the blood glucose is over 7 mmol/L.
5. This is used in babies of diabetic mothers if the blood glucose is persistently under 2 mmol/L despite good feeding support.

THEME 9: HORMONE REPLACEMENT THERAPY

Options

A. Bisphosphonates
B. Continuous combined hormone replacement therapy
C. Cyclical combined hormone replacement therapy
D. Not suitable for hormone replacement
E. Oestrogen cream/pessary
F. Oestrogen-only hormone replacement therapy
G. Specialist referral

For each of the following scenarios, select the most appropriate choice for hormone replacement therapy. Each option may be used once, more than once or not at all.

1. A 52-year-old postmenopausal woman presents to her GP with symptoms of atrophic vaginitis. She denies any other symptoms related to her menopause.
2. A 51-year-old woman presents to the GP with irregular, infrequent light periods. She complains of debilitating hot flushes and night sweats. Her last menstrual period was 4 months ago.
3. A 52-year-old woman attends her primary care clinic complaining of bouts of hot flushes and a low mood. She had her last menstrual period 2 years ago. She has no medical or surgical history.
4. A 55-year-old woman is requesting treatment for hot flushes and irritability – symptoms she attributes to menopause. She says she is still getting periods and describes her menstrual cycle as heavy and irregular. She has bled continuously for the last 2 months.
5. A 64-year-old woman, who is postmenopausal, attends the emergency department following a fall on an outstretched hand. An X-ray confirms a Colles' fracture and a subsequent DXA scan shows evidence of osteoporosis. She has no menopausal symptoms.

THEME 10: PREMATURE LABOUR

Options

A. Atosiban
B. Betamethasone
C. Co-amoxiclav
D. Erythromycin
E. Gentamicin
 F. Indomethacin
G. Nifedipine
H. Ritodrine
 I. Magnesium sulphate

For each of the following descriptions, select the most appropriate drug. Each option may be used once, more than once or not at all.

1. An infusion used for cerebral protection under 32 weeks' gestation.
2. An oxytocin receptor agonist licensed for tocolysis.
3. A drug that is proven to reduce the risk of respiratory distress syndrome when given prior to preterm labour.
4. Clinical evidence recommends this to be used for infection prophylaxis in preterm rupture of membranes.
5. Use of this drug in preterm labour is associated with necrotizing enterocolitis.

Practice Paper 1: Answers

THEME 1: ANTENATAL SCREENING

1. D – Chorionic villus sampling

Chorionic villus sampling (CVS) means taking a biopsy of the placenta. It is done either transabdominally or transcervically under ultrasound guidance, and the cells are analysed for chromosomal abnormalities. It is performed between 11 and 14 weeks and therefore a decision regarding possible termination can be made as early as possible before a pregnancy becomes easily visible 'under the clothes'. It is not performed before 10 weeks, as there is a risk of fetal limb abnormalities. The risk of miscarriage is around 1%.

CVS is a diagnostic test which means it will give a definite answer rather than the 'risk' of a condition being present. Indications include a high-risk screening test, such as in this case, or an abnormality on first-trimester ultrasound scan.

Results of CVS can be ready in 48 hours using quantitative fluorescence polymerase chain reaction (a laboratory technique). In a few cases, inconclusive results occur due to placental mosaicism (a variation in the chromosomal complements of the placenta that is not a reflection of the true genetics of the fetus); this would mean that amniocentesis would have to be performed later. There is also a possibility of maternal contamination, which would lead to false-negative results. Rhesus D-negative women must receive anti-D when undergoing CVS.

> Mosaic, from Greek *mouseios* = artistic.
> Chorionic villus, from Greek *khorion* = placenta + Latin *villus* = hair.

2. H – First-trimester ultrasound scan

The first-trimester ultrasound scan establishes fetal number, viability and gestation. It detects defects in gross anatomy and determines the chorionicity and amnionicity of multiple pregnancies. Nuchal translucency (NT) can be measured at this stage and used in the combined screening test.

The routine anomaly scan (second-trimester scan), which should be performed between 18 and 21 weeks, examines fetal anatomy, locates the site of the placenta and fetal sex can be determined if requested. Accuracy is limited by fetal position and maternal obesity. A fetal medicine referral would be required if there were fetal abnormalities.

3. A – Amniocentesis

Amniocentesis is a diagnostic test that is used at a later gestation than CVS and is appropriate for the couple in this scenario, as they have already had a screening test and the pregnancy is at too great a gestation to have CVS. Amniocentesis can be used for chromosomal analysis (either for diagnosis following a positive Down's syndrome screening test or for pregnancies that are known to be at high risk of chromosomal disorders), DNA analysis for genetic diseases, enzyme assays for inborn errors of metabolism, diagnosis of fetal infection and information about rhesus isoimmunization. Amniocentesis is performed from 15 weeks' gestation, as there is increased risk of miscarriage and talipes if performed earlier. The risk of miscarriage is 0.5%–1%.

A needle is inserted abdominally, under ultrasound guidance, into the uterus. Amniotic fluid, containing fetal cells shed from the gut and skin, is extracted and cultured for chromosome analysis. It takes up to 3 weeks for a full karyotype; however, laboratory techniques such as polymerase chain reaction and fluorescence *in situ* hybridization can provide a more rapid result for a number of conditions, including trisomies, triploidy and Turner's syndrome. Anti-D is given to rhesus D-negative women undergoing amniocentesis.

Amniocentesis, from Greek *amnion* = bowl + *kentesis* = puncture.

4. K – Serum 'triple test'

This patient is too late in her pregnancy for the combined test so she should be offered the triple or quadruple test, which are both available from 15 to 20 weeks. A blood test is taken from the woman, at a known gestation, and certain serum markers are measured to give a 'risk' of Down's syndrome. The serum markers used are α-fetoprotein (AFP), oestriol and the human chorionic gonadotropin β-subunit (βhCG), hence 'triple', with the addition of inhibin for the 'quadruple' test. A high βhCG, low AFP and low oestriol are associated with Down's syndrome. The false-positive rate is around 5%. Most units now offer the quadruple test. A 'risk' of the fetus having Down's syndrome is presented to the parents with a counsellor present so that the appropriate course of action can be taken. A 'positive' result is said to be anything above a risk of 1 in 150. In these cases, amniocentesis or CVS is offered.

The incidental finding of a raised AFP alone is associated with a break in fetal skin, often indicating neural tube defects such as spina bifida and anencephaly. As there is a large overlap with the normal and abnormal levels of AFP, further testing (imaging) is needed to confirm a diagnosis of spina bifida.

5. F – Fetal echocardiography

Echocardiography is used to examine the fetal heart in greater detail in cases with a high risk of fetal cardiac abnormalities and is performed in the second trimester. Indications for fetal echocardiography are mothers with congenital heart disease, type 1 diabetes or epilepsy on certain medications, a previous child with congenital heart disease that required surgery, abnormal or inadequate views of the heart at routine second-trimester scans or a high-risk NT result.

The NT test is a screening tool for Down's syndrome and other abnormalities. It is offered at the ultrasound scan between 11 and 14 weeks. A measurement is made of the thickness of the skinfold over the back of the neck of the fetus. A greater NT measurement (i.e. oedema of the fetal neck) is associated with a higher risk of Down's syndrome, cardiac defects and other chromosomal abnormalities such as trisomies 18 and 13 and Turner's syndrome. The patient should be referred to a fetal medicine specialist and a diagnostic test such as CVS or amniocentesis may be offered to assess the chromosomes. Where there is increased NT but no chromosomal abnormality, an association with multiple structural abnormalities is seen (congenital heart disease, exomphalos, diaphragmatic hernia and skeletal defects). This measurement can be used in conjunction with certain serum markers (βhCG and pregnancy-associated plasma protein A) in the combined screening test, which is performed between 11 + 0 and 13 + 6 weeks to give a 'risk' of Down's syndrome.

Uterine artery Doppler ultrasound is an analysis of the uterine artery waveform (N.B. not of the umbilical artery) to measure the resistance in the maternal uterine arteries. If high resistance with notching is seen between 20 and 24 weeks, there is an increased chance of preeclampsia and growth restriction; such mothers require increased antenatal surveillance.

Antenatal fetal blood sampling (FBS) is a diagnostic test performed transabdominally under ultrasound guidance (not to be confused with FBS in labour). The target is blood from the umbilical cord (cordocentesis), fetal intrahepatic vessels or fetal heart. The risk of miscarriage is much greater than that with the other invasive diagnostic tests, so it is used only where blood is the only source of the information required (prior to *in utero* transfusion in haemolytic disease or alloimmune thrombocytopenia, investigation of fetal infection such as parvovirus and investigation of fetal hydrops). Anti-D must be given to rhesus D-negative women undergoing antenatal FBS.

Fetal tissue sampling is rarely performed to diagnose uncommon conditions that specifically require histological examination of the skin or assay of the enzymes restricted to the liver. It is performed under ultrasound guidance.

Cardiotocography (CTG) is where the fetal heart and maternal contractions are recorded after 24 weeks to assess the well-being of the fetus.

Non-invasive prenatal testing is not currently widely available but it is likely to significantly change the way fetal chromosomal abnormalities are detected, so it is vital you have knowledge of it. Fetal DNA is found in maternal plasma and therefore it is possible to gain information about fetal conditions using a blood test from the mother. It can be used for assessing a fetus at risk of haemolytic disease of the newborn, determining sex in cases where high-risk sex-linked conditions may be present and to test for aneuploidy, especially Down's syndrome. It is much more accurate than existing screening strategies but it is not yet regarded as a diagnostic assay, and at present, a 'diagnostic test' such as CVS or amniocentesis would still be used to confirm the diagnosis.

THEME 2: CHRONIC PELVIC PAIN

1. D – Endometriosis

Endometriosis is a painful inflammatory condition where functioning endometrial tissue is found outside the uterine cavity. This tissue responds to the cyclical hormonal changes and can bleed during menstruation, leading to pelvic and abdominal scarring. Common sites of deposition are the ovaries, uterosacral ligaments and ovarian fossae, although endometriosis may be found further afield (bladder, rectum or lung). It is most common in 30–40-year-olds, with a prevalence of between 1.5% and 6.2%. The aetiology is unclear and likely to be multifactorial.

Women present with cyclical abdominal pain due to bleeding at the affected sites during menstruation, dyspareunia, secondary dysmenorrhoea and subfertility. Bimanual palpation may reveal uterosacral nodules, endometriomas leading to ovarian enlargement or adnexal tenderness. In advanced cases, the uterus is retroverted, retroflexed and immobile, with thickening of the cardinal or uterosacral ligaments. Ultrasound is useful to exclude other pathologies, but is not diagnostic of endometriosis. Diagnosis is made at laparoscopy when brown spots on the peritoneum ('powder burn'), adhesions and endometriomas ('chocolate cysts') can be directly visualized.

The management plan is individualized to each patient and is dependent upon their fertility wishes. Medical treatments include analgesia, combined oral contraceptive pill (COCP), progestogens, gonadotropin-releasing hormone (GnRH) analogues and anti-androgens, and are useful for symptomatic relief but will not improve fertility (indeed, some are actually contraceptives). Surgical treatment involves burning the endometriotic lesions at laparoscopy and removing endometriomas. This can be useful to reduce pain but also improves fertility. Total abdominal hysterectomy with bilateral salpingoophorectomy is reserved for those who have untreatable pain and have completed their family.

2. B – Chronic pelvic inflammatory disease

Chronic pelvic inflammatory disease (PID) is where there are recurrent or untreated episodes of acute pelvic infection (see 'Acute pelvic pain' – Paper 4 Answers, Themes 5 and 7), which result in chronic inflammation of the pelvic organs and multiple adhesions, causing abdominal pain, dyspareunia and subfertility.

3. K – Renal calculus
This woman presents with spasmodic 'loin-to-groin' pain and haematuria, suggestive of underlying renal calculi. Calculi can be identified using ultrasound or an intravenous (IV) urogram and management should be coordinated by a urologist. Haematuria must be investigated and malignancy ruled out.

4. L – Secondary dysmenorrhoea
Dysmenorrhoea describes a cyclical cramping pain that occurs before or during menstruation. It may be associated with malaise and gastrointestinal symptoms. A total of 50% of women have some pain during periods, with 10% describing it as severe. Primary dysmenorrhoea begins at menarche and there is often no cause found. Secondary dysmenorrhoea by definition occurs later in a woman's life and is often associated with pathology such as endometriosis and PID, or with iatrogenic causes (copper intrauterine contraceptive device or cervical stenosis after large loop excision of the transformation zone). Treatments include analgesia such as paracetamol or non-steroidal anti-inflammatory drugs (NSAIDs – especially mefenamic acid) or hormonal options such as the COCP, oral or depot progestogens and the Mirena coil.

Menorrhagia
This refers to heavy menstrual bleeding causing an impact upon a woman's physical or psychological well-being. There was a definition of monthly menstrual blood loss greater than 80 mL but this is very difficult to quantify, so now it is diagnosed based on the history from the woman. Menorrhagia may be associated with other symptoms, such as dysmenorrhea, and can lead to anaemia, particularly if caused by fibroids.

5. F – Functional pain
Women must be informed at the beginning of investigations for pelvic pain that no cause may be found. This can reassure women and causes resolution of symptoms in some cases. If no pathology is found, then questions about sexual and social circumstances must be asked, as there may be an underlying problem, such as relationship difficulties, sexual abuse or other fears around sexuality or fertility.

Adhesions
Pain can be caused by adhesions from previous surgery or infection. Adhesiolysis (surgical removal of adhesions) is not proven, but is more likely to be effective if there are large adhesions and if it is done laparoscopically. However, there is significant risk of visceral damage and there is a chance of further adhesions developing.

Ovarian cysts

These vary greatly with regard to symptoms and investigation findings. An ovarian cyst could be benign or it could be cancerous. The Risk of Malignancy Index (RMI) is used to establish the possibility of malignancy which involves ultrasound scanning (U), menopausal status (M) and serum CA125 level.

$$RMI = U \times M \times CA125$$

The ultrasound score depends on the presence of five features: multiloculation, solid areas, metastases, ascites and bilateral lesions. If none of these are seen, $U = 0$; if one is seen, $U = 1$; but if two or more are seen, $U = 3$. If a woman is premenopausal, she scores $M = 1$, and if postmenopausal, she scores $M = 3$. CA125 is a blood test. If there is a high risk of malignancy, patients may need referral to a gynae-oncologist for their treatment. If a simple, unilateral, unilocular cyst with a normal CA125 is found in a premenopausal woman, it is exceptionally unlikely to be cancer so can be managed conservatively if the patient is asymptomatic. A follow-up ultrasound scan can be performed in 3–4 months, and 50% resolve spontaneously. Ovarian cysts can undergo torsion and women should be informed about the symptoms of this.

Fibroids

Fibroids are common, affecting 20% of women by 40 years. They rarely cause pain if uncomplicated, but are often associated with menorrhagia. Torsion of a pedunculated fibroid can occur, would present with lower abdominal pain and may require surgery to remove the necrotic fibroid. If the blood supply to a fibroid is compromised, fibroid degeneration can occur and again this would present with pain. Degeneration is initially managed conservatively with analgesia, fluids and antibiotics, but may need surgery if pain is persistent or recurrent.

Constipation

Constipation is seen in many women with pelvic pain. A palpable loaded colon can be felt on examination. Diet modification is the first-line treatment of constipation, with the use of laxatives and suppositories/enemas. Irritable bowel syndrome affects 10%–15% of people in the UK. It is a diagnosis made clinically after exclusion of other pathologies. Symptoms include constipation or diarrhoea, pelvic pain, passage of mucus with the stool and bloating. Symptoms are worse with eating, defecation, stress and in the premenstrual period. Treatment is symptomatic.

THEME 3: CARDIOTOCOGRAPHY

CTG measures the fetal heart rate and uterine activity. It can be used confidently after 32 weeks' gestation to monitor the condition of a fetus in correlation with the clinical situation. Prior to this gestation, the autonomic nervous system is not sufficiently developed to produce the predictable responses of the more mature fetus. A normal CTG is reassuring, but an abnormal CTG does not always mean that the baby is struggling.

Indications for CTG monitoring can be maternal (pain, preeclampsia, diabetes or antepartum haemorrhage), fetal (intrauterine growth restriction, prematurity, oligohydramnios, multiple pregnancy or breech) or intrapartum (oxytocin use or induction of labour).

The use of CTG does not appear to improve long-term neonatal outcome.

1. **J – Sustained tachycardia**
2. **H – Reduced variability**
3. **C – Early decelerations**
4. **A – Accelerations**
5. **K – Variable decelerations**

A CTG tracing should be categorized into normal, suspicious or pathological depending on how many of the features are reassuring/non-reassuring/abnormal. It is also helpful to think about the risk factors for the pregnancy before reading any CTG.

Baseline

The baseline rate is the mean fetal heart rate over 5–10 minutes. The normal range is 110–160 beats/minute. This represents a balance between sympathetic and parasympathetic systems. Sustained tachycardia may be due to prematurity, with the rate slowing physiologically with advancing gestational age. It is also seen in hypoxia, fetal distress and maternal pyrexia and with the use of exogenous β-agonists (e.g. salbutamol). Baseline bradycardia may suggest severe fetal distress, possibly due to placental abruption or uterine rupture, but occurs more commonly with hypotension, maternal sedation, postmaturity and hypoxia. A sustained baseline rate under 90 beats/minute is known as a prolonged deceleration or bradycardia and usually indicates impending fetal demise and should be acted on without delay.

Baseline variability

This describes the fluctuations in the fetal heart rate from one beat to the next. Variability is produced by the balance between the parasympathetic and sympathetic nervous systems. Minor fluctuations in the baseline fetal heart rate occur at 3–5 cycles/minutes. Baseline variability can be calculated by measuring the distance between the highest peak and the lowest trough in a 1-minute segment of a CTG trace. Normal variability is over 5 beats/minute and is a good indicator of fetal well-being. Reduced variability can be seen most commonly during phases of fetal sleep, which may safely last up to 40 minutes. After this time it becomes non-reassuring, and if it remains for >90 minutes, this feature is said to be abnormal. It is also seen in early gestation (as the nervous system develops only later in pregnancy) and with certain drugs, particularly opiates or benzodiazepines. A prolonged reduced variability suggests acute fetal distress.

Accelerations and decelerations

Accelerations are defined as a rise in the fetal heart rate of at least 15 beats/minute, for at least 15 seconds. Antenatally, you should expect at least two accelerations every 15 minutes. They are reassuring, although their absence in advanced labour is not uncommon and of uncertain significance. Decelerations are a fall in the fetal heart rate of at least 15 beats/minute for more than 15 seconds. Early decelerations occur with contractions and return to normal by the end of the contraction. They are probably physiological and are thought to reflect increased vagal tone when fetal intracranial pressure increases during a contraction. They are uniform in depth, length and shape. Typical variable decelerations vary in timing and shape in relation to uterine contraction. They suggest cord compression, especially in oligohydramnios. 'Shouldering' is a sign that the fetus is coping well with the compression: this is when there is a small acceleration before and after the deceleration. These may resolve if the mother's position is changed. If present with over 50% of contractions for over 90 minutes, they become a non-reassuring feature. Atypical variable or late decelerations occur during a contraction and return to baseline only after the contraction. If present with over 50% of the contractions for over 30 minutes, they are an abnormal feature and suggest fetal distress.

Sinusoidal trace

A sinusoidal trace is a smooth undulating sine wave-like baseline with no variability. The pattern lasts over 10 minutes with an amplitude of 5–15 beats/minute. A sinusoidal pattern may be physiological or can represent fetal anaemia/hypoxia, but must be considered serious until proven otherwise. Sinusoidal patterns should be distinguished from pseudosinusoidal traces, which are benign, uniform, long-term patterns. They are less regular in shape and amplitude when compared with sinusoidal traces.

Sinusoidal, from Latin *sinus* = curve or hollow space.

If there is a pathological CTG, a fetal blood sample should be performed to confirm fetal distress. Here, an amnioscope is used to visualize the fetal scalp, a small cut is made and the resulting blood is collected in a microtube. The following results give a pH and are a guide to management:

- Normal (pH >7.25): labour can continue
- Borderline (pH 7.20–7.25): repeat pH is needed in 30–60 minutes
- Abnormal (pH <7.20): confirms fetal compromise – needs delivery

THEME 4: SEXUALLY TRANSMITTED INFECTIONS

The presence of a sexually transmitted infection (STI) points towards the possibility of the affected person having further STIs; therefore, all patients should be fully examined and investigated.

1. O – Reiter's syndrome

Reiter's syndrome, or reactive arthritis, is a triad of urethritis, seronegative (rheumatoid factor-negative) arthritis and conjunctivitis resulting from a pathological immune response to an infectious agent ('can't see, can't pee, can't climb a tree!'). There are two main subtypes of Reiter's syndrome: genitourinary infection (chlamydial infection or gonorrhoea) or gastrointestinal infection (*Salmonella*, *Shigella*, *Yersinia* or *Campylobacter* spp.). Reiter's syndrome is much more common in males than females (20:1). Diagnosis is normally clinical, although the erythrocyte sedimentation rate is raised and HLA-B27 is often present. Two other associated features of Reiter's syndrome are circinate balanitis (erythematous lesions on the penis) and keratoderma blenorrhagicum (hard nodules on the soles of the feet that are clinically and histologically indistinguishable from plantar psoriasis).

> Hans Conrad Reiter, German military physician (1881–1969). Reiter was convicted of war crimes for his medical experiments on concentration camp detainees. Because of this association, it is becoming more preferable to use the term 'reactive arthritis'.

2. M – Molluscum contagiosum

Molluscum contagiosum is caused by a DNA poxvirus. Spread is by sexual contact, personal contact and fomites (an inanimate object that is contaminated with disease-causing microorganisms, such as a used towel). Hemispherical papules of 2–5 mm diameter that are pearly, raised and firm develop on the face, abdomen, buttocks and genitals. There is a latent period of 3–12 weeks. Spontaneous regression generally occurs, but lesions can be present for several months. Lesions can be extensive and persistent in immunocompromised patients, including those with HIV.

3. F – Genital candidiasis

Candidiasis (thrush) is caused by yeasts, particularly *Candida albicans* and *C. glabrata*, and produces vulval pruritus, burning, swelling and dyspareunia. White discharge and plaques are seen in the vagina, with redness of the vulva and labia minora. Candidiasis is seen more commonly with pregnancy, diabetes mellitus, HIV infection and use of antimicrobial agents and immunosuppressive drugs. Diagnosis is confirmed by culture, and treatment is with antifungals (e.g. topical imidazole [Canesten] or oral fluconazole).

> *Candida*, from Latin *candidus* = clear and white.

4. L – Lymphogranuloma venereum

Lymphogranuloma venereum is a STI caused by serovars L1, L2 and L3 of *Chlamydia trachomatis*. It is mainly found in the tropics. Between 3 and 21 days after infection, one-third of people develop a small painless papule, which ulcerates and heals after days. The patients then develop lymphadenopathy, which is unilateral in two-thirds of cases. Inguinal abscesses (buboes) may form and develop a sinus. Acute ulcerative proctitis may develop when infection takes place via the rectal mucosa. Treatment is with appropriate antibiotics.

Bubo, from Greek *boubon* = groin or swollen groin. Also gives rise to the 'bubonic plague' and, allegedly, the American colloquial 'boo boo', used to describe little cuts and scrapes.

Venereal, from Latin *venereus* = desire (derived from Venus, the goddess of love).

Chlamydia trachomatis

- Serovars Ab, B, Ba, C – lead to infection of the eye (trachoma), which can cause blindness
- Serovars D–K – genital infection
- Serovars L1, L2, L3 – lymphogranuloma venereum

5. Q – Syphilis (specifically neurosyphilis)

Syphilis is caused by the bacterium *Treponema pallidum* and is spread by sexual contact (it can also be acquired congenitally). There are many stages of syphilis infection:

- Primary syphilis: occurs 10–90 days postinfection. A dull, red papule develops on the external genitalia and forms a single, well-demarcated, painless ulcer associated with bilateral inguinal lymph node enlargement. This lesion heals within 3–10 weeks.
- Secondary syphilis: develops 6–8 weeks after primary infection and involves malaise, mild fever, headache, a pruritic skin rash, hoarseness, swollen lymph nodes, patchy or diffuse hair loss, bone pain and arthralgia.
- Latent syphilis: there is no clinical evidence of disease, but it is still detectable by serological testing.
- Gummatous syphilis: a late stage of infection when the host resistance to the infection begins to fail. Areas of syphilitic granulation tissue develop on the scalp, upper aspect of the leg or sternoclavicular region. These so-called 'gummatous' lesions are copper in colour. Granulation can also occur internally (e.g. on heart valves and bone). At this stage, there is still a good response to treatment.
- Neurosyphilis: disease is detectable in the cerebrospinal fluid. Patients complain of headache, cranial nerve palsies, general paralysis of the insane (psychosis with muscular reflex abnormality, dementia and seizures), tabes dorsalis (degeneration of the dorsal column of the spinal cord, resulting in poor coordination), trophic ulcers, Charcot's joints (a

peripheral neuropathy resulting in excessive trauma to distal joints, with subsequent bony destruction) and Argyll Robertson pupils (bilateral small, irregular pupils that do accommodate but do not react to light).

Jean-Martin Charcot, French neurologist (1825–1893).
Douglas Argyll Robertson, Scottish ophthalmologist (1837–1909).

Trichomoniasis

This is a STI caused by the flagellated protozoan *Trichomonas vaginalis*, which invades superficial epithelial cells of the vagina, urethra, glans penis, prostate and seminal vesicles. Affected females present with an offensive greenish-grey discharge, vulval soreness, dyspareunia, dysuria, vaginitis and vulvitis. On examination, the cervix may have a punctate erythematous (strawberry) appearance. 15%–50% of males are asymptomatic, or they may complain of a mild discharge and dysuria. Treatment is with metronidazole.

Granuloma inguinale (Donovanosis)

This is caused by the bacterium *Klebsiella granulomatis*. A flat-topped papule develops on the genitalia days to months postinfection, and then degenerates into a painless ulcer. The ulcer spreads along skinfolds and heals with scarring.

Gonorrhoea

This is caused by the Gram-negative diplococcus *Neisseria gonorrhoeae*. 50% of females are asymptomatic, but some complain of vaginal discharge, lower abdominal pain and urethritis. Complications include Bartholin's abscess, PID and gonococcal salpingitis with irreversible tube damage. Infected males present with dysuria, frequency and/or a mucopurulent discharge after 3–5 days, coupled with urethritis and meatal oedema. Epididymo-orchitis or prostatitis can develop. Disseminated gonococcal infection occurs in <1% of cases and causes pyrexia, a vasculitic rash and polyarthritis.

'Crabs'

These are caused by the crab-louse *Phthirus pubis*, which mainly lives in the hairs of the pubic and perianal areas. Most are transmitted by sexual contact, but any close contact with an infected person can transmit the crabs. Clinically, there is itching in the affected areas. The lice feed on blood and can leave spots on the skin (pediculosis pubis).

Phthirus, from Greek *phtheir* = louse.

THEME 5: HORMONES OF MENSTRUATION

1. D – Luteinizing hormone

Luteinizing hormone (LH) is a glycoprotein produced by the anterior pituitary gland. LH causes ovulation to occur and peaks 18 hours prior to release of the ovum. It is regulated by GnRH from the hypothalamus.

LH is initially inhibited by oestrogen from the ovary until the level of circulating oestrogen becomes so high that it induces the preovulatory surge. Concentrations of LH are low in childhood, higher during puberty and much higher in menopause.

Luteinizing, from Latin *luteus* = yellow (so called because this hormone stimulates growth of the corpus luteum, or 'yellow body').

2. G – Progesterone
Progesterone is a steroid hormone produced by the corpus luteum (and by the placenta during pregnancy). It creates secretory changes in the endometrium. It stimulates the production of thick cervical mucus, which is less penetrable by sperm. Progesterone also decreases the contractility of uterine smooth muscle and inhibits lactation during pregnancy (hence a drop in progesterone facilitates the onset of labour and the production of breast milk).

Progesterone, from PROGEstational STERoidal ketONE.

3. B – Follicle-stimulating hormone
Follicle-stimulating hormone (FSH) is a glycoprotein that is produced by the anterior pituitary gland. Its function is to stimulate the growth of 6–12 primary follicles each month; therefore, it is low during childhood, increases with puberty and is very high after the menopause (as there are no follicles left to be released, so there is no negative-feedback mechanism). It is variable through the menstrual cycle – at the onset of menstruation, there is a rise in FSH, which eventually falls as oestrogen levels increase. GnRH from the hypothalamus stimulates FSH production. The ovary is involved in the control of FSH via oestrogen and inhibin (which both inhibit FSH production) and activin (which stimulates FSH production). FSH production is also inhibited by high levels of progesterone.

4. F – Estradiol
Estradiol is a steroid hormone that is mainly secreted by the ovary. It is maximal just before day 14 of menstruation. It stimulates proliferation of glandular and stromal elements of the endometrium and increases progesterone receptors in endometrial cells. It stimulates the production of thin cervical mucus that is easily penetrable by sperm.

5. E – Luteinizing hormone and follicle-stimulating hormone
As mentioned above, LH and FSH are secreted by the anterior pituitary gland. Other hormones released by the anterior pituitary are growth hormone, prolactin, thyroid-stimulating hormone and adrenocorticotrophic hormone. The posterior pituitary gland secretes oxytocin and antidiuretic hormone.

THEME 6: PAIN IN PREGNANCY

1. F – HELLP syndrome

HELLP syndrome is a variant of preeclampsia but it can develop without any previous indication of preeclampsia. The name is derived from the biochemical findings: Haemolysis, Elevated Liver enzymes and Low Platelets (HELLP). It can be found without any preceding symptoms or patients can present with nausea and vomiting, feeling generally unwell or epigastric/right upper quadrant pain due to haemorrhage which stretches the liver capsule. It has a high mortality and morbidity, and can progress to acute renal failure, disseminated intravascular coagulation and an increased risk of abruption; therefore, a multidisciplinary approach may be required. Management includes haematological and biochemical monitoring and treatment of hypertension but ultimately, like preeclampsia, delivery is the only cure. Deterioration can still occur 48 hours after delivery and patients should be managed in an obstetric high-dependency unit.

Cholecystitis

The biliary stasis (due to high progesterone) and increased lithogenicity of bile (due to high oestrogen) seen in pregnancy means that gallstones are more common at this time. The patient presents with right upper quadrant pain, which is colicky in nature, coupled with nausea, vomiting and fever (jaundice is rare). Differential diagnoses include severe preeclampsia, acute fatty liver, appendicitis and HELLP. Biochemical tests and an ultrasound scan are needed to confirm the diagnosis. Treatment includes antibiotics, analgesia and fluids. Surgery can be performed during pregnancy as delaying it may lead to high recurrence, increased risk of pancreatitis and preterm labour. Endoscopic retrograde cholangiopancreatography can also be used with techniques to reduce the radiation to the fetus.

2. B – Acute pyelonephritis

Ascending urinary tract infections (UTIs) are more common in pregnancy, thanks to dilatation of the urinary system by progesterone and obstructive uropathy with urinary stasis. Patients typically present with fever and rigours, nausea and vomiting, abdominal and loin pain and urinary frequency with dysuria. Assessment of the patient includes urine dipstick, culture from midstream urine (MSU) and blood and an ultrasound scan to exclude renal abnormalities including hydronephrosis. Management includes analgesia, antipyretics, IV fluids and IV antibiotics. Uterine tightenings may be reported – do not confuse these with contractions; however, there is a risk of preterm labour with severe UTI and bacteraemia.

The incidence of UTIs in pregnancy is high and 1%–2% of pregnancies have pyelonephritis. A short female urethra and a gravid uterus are predisposing features. Clinically, there is increased frequency, dysuria, offensive urine, suprapubic pain, fever, tachycardia and suprapubic tenderness. A dipstick and MSU culture should be performed, with the most likely organism being *Escherichia coli*. Treatment is with oral cephradine or amoxicillin, which are both safe and effective in pregnancy. Recurrent UTIs need further investigations. All women should have a MSU culture in early pregnancy to screen for asymptomatic bacteriuria and, if positive, treatment should be offered to reduce the risk of pyelonephritis.

Labour is the most common cause of physiological pain in pregnancy. Pains are intermittent with uterine contractions. There is associated cervical dilatation and downward progression of the presenting part. It is important to remember that pathological causes of abdominal pain may also precipitate labour. Braxton Hicks' contractions ('false labour') describe when the uterus contracts intermittently from early pregnancy. As labour approaches, the frequency and amplitude of these contractions increase.

John Braxton Hicks, English obstetrician (1823–1897).

3. E – Chorioamnionitis

Chorioamnionitis (inflammation of the chorion and amnion) presents with abdominal pain, uterine tenderness and maternal pyrexia with a raised CRP and white cell count, meconium-stained or foul-smelling liquor and often a fetal tachycardia. It is usually preceded by prelabour rupture of the membranes, but it can be present without membrane rupture. Chorioamnionitis is more likely if there is proven UTI or vaginal infection. It can result in overwhelming neonatal and maternal infection. As with all severe infections, a multidisciplinary team approach and 'sepsis bundle' should be initiated as soon as possible. This includes taking blood cultures, administering broad-spectrum antibiotics, measuring serum lactate and fluid resuscitation with consideration of vasopressors to maintain blood pressure. Delivery may be required for maternal or fetal well-being regardless of the gestation.

4. A – Acute fatty liver of pregnancy

Acute fatty liver of pregnancy is rare and occurs in only 1 in 10,000–15,000 pregnancies in the third trimester. It presents similarly to cholecystitis, with sudden-onset epigastric abdominal pain, anorexia, malaise, nausea, vomiting and diarrhoea, with the distinguishing features of jaundice, mild hypertension, proteinuria and fulminant liver failure. On biochemical testing, there is raised bilirubin with abnormal liver enzymes, leukocytosis, thrombocytopenia, hypoglycaemia and coagulation defects. Acute fatty liver of pregnancy is biochemically distinguished from HELLP syndrome by the hypoglycaemia and high uric acid. Diagnosis is clinical (computed tomography or magnetic resonance imaging may help), but a liver biopsy may be needed. Management is by correction of fluid balance, coagulation, electrolyte disturbances and hypoglycaemia, with hasty delivery. Women may need admission to a specialist liver unit or intensive care unit. Maternal mortality rate is 20%.

Obstetric cholestasis generally only occurs in the third trimester. Women present with pruritus primarily of the palms and feet but it can affect any part of the body. There is no abdominal pain or rash. It is more common in women with a personal or family history of the condition. Liver function tests should be taken and a raised ALT, AST, γ-GT or bile acids may be seen. It is a diagnosis of exclusion so other causes of itching and abnormal liver function should be investigated with full liver screen, infection screen and liver ultrasound scan. There is an increased risk of post-partum haemorrhage (PPH), preterm labour, fetal distress and intrauterine fetal death. There are no long-term maternal risks. Delivery used to be advised at 37–38 weeks to reduce the risk of intrauterine death; however, the evidence for this is lacking and now decisions are made on a case-by-case basis. Chlorphenamine is used for symptomatic relief of itching. Ursodeoxycholic acid can be used to reduce serum bile acids and vitamin K is offered from 36 weeks to reduce the risks of bleeding if there are clotting abnormalities. LFTs must be checked postnatally to ensure they have normalized.

5. K – Symphysis pubis dysfunction

This common condition occurs in many pregnancies. Women describe pain and discomfort in the pelvic area, which can radiate to the upper thighs or perineum. Pain is worse on walking and may be severe enough to limit mobility. Diagnosis is clinical, and can be confirmed by increased pain on pressure over the symphysis pubis or compression of the pelvis. Treatment is supportive, with analgesia, pelvic support braces and crutches.

The round ligaments are prone to stretching during pregnancy with the increasing size of the uterus. This presents with non-specific abdominal pain.

A placental abruption occurs when the placenta detaches from the uterus prior to delivery of the baby. Presentation is with severe, constant lower abdominal pain. Delivery is usually indicated.

Uterine rupture can occur in labour in patients with previous uterine surgery. Bleeding can be very heavy and significant abnormalities in the fetal heart beat are usually seen. Laparotomy to deliver the baby and repair the damage should be expedited.

THEME 7: FETAL PRESENTATION

It is important to be proficient in abdominal and vaginal examination, as they can provide important information that affects the progress of labour. Do not forget the labour triad of the 'powers' of the uterus (contractions), the 'passages' (the birth canal) and the 'passenger' (the fetus).

Abdominal examination

First inspect for previous scars. The pregnant uterus is palpable from 12 weeks. By 20–22 weeks, it reaches the umbilicus and, by 36 weeks, it lies under the ribs. Your aim is to determine the number of fetuses, the lie (longitudinal, oblique or transverse), the presentation (cephalic or breech) and the engagement. Engagement involves passage of the maximum presenting part through the pelvic inlet. 'Fifths palpable' states the proportion of the head palpable abdominally if the head was divided into fifths. Always watch the patient's face, as the examination can be uncomfortable. Measure the symphysis–fundal height (SFH) from the symphysis pubis to the fundus in centimetres (from 16 weeks, the SFH increases by approximately 1 cm/week). Finally, auscultate the fetal heart (with a Doppler ultrasound or a Pinard stethoscope).

Vaginal examination

This can be uncomfortable and may be embarrassing, so a full explanation should be given and consent obtained. Speculum examination is used to assess the vagina and cervix. A speculum examination alone is appropriate in spontaneous rupture of membranes (SROM) or suspected SROM to avoid infection. Placenta praevia is a contraindication to manual vaginal examination. The Bishop score is used to assess the favourability of the cervix (see 'Induction of labour' – Paper 2 Answers, Theme 10). An assessment of the presenting part is important for gaining information regarding the position of the fetal head and to rule out malpresentation. Malpresentation includes breech, shoulder, face and brow presentations, in decreasing order of incidence.

Adolphe Pinard, French obstetrician (1844–1934).

1. G – Occipitoanterior

Occipitoanterior is the most preferable position of presentation. The 'attitude' of the fetal head refers to the degree of flexion/extension. In this case, the head is well flexed, allowing the smallest diameter to pass through the outlet first. The fontanelles are junctions between the sutures of the skull bones. The anterior fontanelle is diamond shaped, and the posterior fontanelle is Y-shaped or triangular. They allow the bones to 'mould' without affecting the brain in order to facilitate labour.

2. B – Extended breech

Breech presentation is where the head is at the fundus and the lower half of the baby is presenting. The indicators of breech presentation are the ballotable head at the fundus and the fetal heart heard above the umbilicus.

There are three types of breech presentation, from most to least common: extended/frank (feet extended near head), flexed (feet next to bottom) and footling (foot presents at cervix). The incidence of breech presentation at term is 3%–4% of singleton pregnancies. Risk factors for breech presentation include grand multiparity, bony pelvic abnormalities, uterine abnormalities, fetal prematurity (insufficient time to rotate), multiple pregnancy, fetal abnormality, extended legs, oligo-/poly-hydramnios and placenta praevia.

If a breech presentation is found after 36 weeks' gestation, a management plan will be formulated which involves the wishes of the woman. External cephalic version (ECV) is offered, in which the fetus is manually rotated to a cephalic presentation under ultrasound guidance provided there are no contraindications (e.g. previous caesarean section, history of antepartum haemorrhage, multiple pregnancy, oligo-/poly-hydramnios and placenta praevia). It is more difficult in primips with firm abdominal muscles and in overweight women. ECV is successful in two-thirds of attempted cases when performed by a senior obstetrician. Complications of ECV include placental abruption, transplacental haemorrhage (possibly requiring anti-D in rhesus-negative women), fetal bradycardia and prelabour rupture of membranes (PROM). If ECV is declined, contraindicated or unsuccessful, a mode of delivery must be discussed. Many women will opt for an elective caesarean section and certainly this would be recommended for a footling breech, but for an extended breech, vaginal delivery can be discussed.

3. A – Brow
This is the least common presentation, occurring in 1 in 2000 labours. For the brow to present, the neck is extended, which results in the largest diameter of the fetal head presenting (chin to occiput). This is often too large to pass through the pelvis, and if it persists can cause delay in the second stage of labour. Do not forget that the pelvic brim (inlet) is widest in transverse diameter, but the outlet is widest in anterior–posterior diameter, which requires the head to rotate.

Face presentation occurs in 1 in 500 cases and occurs with full extension of the head. It can delay engagement and progress, possibly because the facial bones do not mould. These babies are at risk of facial oedema. This case is not a face presentation, as the sagittal suture and anterior fontanelle are palpable, as well as some of the face.

4. H – Occipitoposterior
In the occipitoposterior position, the limbs are anterior, which may visibly affect the contour of the abdomen. An occipitoposterior position can result in relative cephalopelvic disproportion of the fetal head to the maternal pelvis (i.e. the diameter of the head in that particular position may be too big to fit through the mother's pelvis), particularly if the head becomes partially extended.

5. D – Footling breech
There is a higher risk of cord prolapse in this case, as the presenting part (the feet) does not fill the pelvis like a head or buttocks would, leaving more space for the cord to come down and out of the cervix. In this case, an elective caesarean should be offered at 39 weeks.

THEME 8: DIABETES IN PREGNANCY

1. B – Diet and exercise

Gestational diabetes mellitus (GDM) is where impaired carbohydrate intolerance is diagnosed in pregnancy. People with previous GDM, body mass index >30, a previous macrosomic baby >4.5 kg, family history of diabetes or family origin with a high prevalence of diabetes have a higher risk and should therefore be offered screening for GDM. This is done with an oral glucose tolerance test. First-line treatment should be diet and exercise for 2 weeks, and if successful, this can be an excellent way to treat GDM and introduce a healthy lifestyle to the woman and potentially the whole family. If diet alone does not reduce the blood glucose, then metformin and then insulin can be added. Scans should be performed throughout the pregnancy to ensure correct fetal growth. A further glucose tolerance test should be performed 6 weeks postnatally to ensure a diagnosis of type 2 diabetes has not been missed.

2. D – Folic acid 5 mg/day

Women with preexisting diabetes should use a higher dose of folic acid (of 5 mg/day compared to the normal dose of 400 µg/day) to reduce the incidence of neural tube defects. Other conditions in which a higher dose may be recommended include previous or family history of neural tube defects, epilepsy, coeliac disease, diabetes, sickle cell anaemia and if the woman is taking medication to treat epilepsy.

3. E – Gliclazide

All oral hypoglycaemic medications, apart from metformin, should be stopped preconceptually and only metformin and insulin should be used to control diabetes. Of note, ACE inhibitors and angiotensin II receptor antagonists should also be stopped and swapped for more appropriate antihypertensives. Statins should be stopped preconceptually.

4. G – Intravenous (IV) dextrose and insulin infusion

This is commonly known as a sliding scale. This is appropriate as labour is a period of time in which it is difficult to regulate sugars due to the many stresses occurring. A target of between 4–7 mmol/L should be sought.

5. H – IV dextrose alone

Babies born from diabetic mothers are used to the hyperglycaemia of the mother and are therefore constantly trying to reduce their own glucose levels. They will continue to do this when they are born, so they can easily become hypoglycaemic and this must be monitored. Women should be encouraged to feed their babies as soon as possible and then regularly every 2–3 hours. Ideally, a prefeed glucose level should not fall below 2 mmol/L. If the capillary glucose reading is persistently below 2 mmol/L, IV dextrose can be given. NG tube feeding with milk is another option that may allow sugars to normalize without needing to resort to IV feeding. It is, of course, important in all cases to keep babies warm, as a cold baby is more likely to have hypoglycaemia.

THEME 9: HORMONE REPLACEMENT THERAPY

The majority of symptoms associated with the menopause come from oestrogen-sensitive tissue, such as the skin, bladder, brain and uterus (see 'Perimenopausal hormones' – Paper 4 Answers, Theme 4). Symptoms that women describe include hot flushes, night sweats, palpitations, headaches, mood changes, sleeping problems, loss of libido, vaginal dryness, menstrual disturbances and UTIs. Hormone replacement therapy (HRT) can be used to improve these symptoms and dramatically improve quality of life.

Additional benefits of HRT include a reduction in the risk of developing osteoporosis and cancer of the rectum and colon; however, HRT should not be used solely for this reason. HRT may also delay the onset of Alzheimer's disease (although it has no effect on established disease). The downsides of HRT include increased risks of breast cancer, endometrial cancer, ovarian cancer, stroke and venous thromboembolism, and these risks increase with increasing duration of treatment. Contraindications to oestrogen-containing HRT are carcinoma of the endometrium, liver disease (e.g. active hepatitis), suspected pregnancy and inherited thrombophilias. Relative contraindications to HRT are uncontrolled hypertension and a personal or family history of thromboembolism or breast cancer. High blood pressure should be controlled prior to treatment.

All women who are considered for HRT should be assessed to determine the extent of their symptoms, the consequences on their daily life, the desired effect of treatment and their personal risk of using HRT. Screening for contraindications in their past medical and family history is very important. The patient should be fully counselled on risks, benefits and side effects. The date of the last period must be established, as this will affect the HRT used.

1. E – Oestrogen cream/pessary

The woman in this scenario has no global menopausal symptoms and so is not in need of systemic hormone replacement. Systemic therapies should be limited to avoid the risks as described above. A preferable option would be topical oestrogen administration in the form of a cream or a pessary, which is used in a reducing dose for 3 months initially, after which symptoms can be reviewed.

2. C – Cyclical combined hormone replacement therapy

There are a huge number of hormone replacement options available on the market. Overall, the minimum effective dose should be used, and for the shortest possible duration.

For the purposes of treatment, women should be divided into those with a uterus still *in situ* and those who have had a hysterectomy. In women with a uterus who have bled within the last year (perimenopausal), low-dose cyclical HRT is recommended, which gives continuous oestrogen with added progesterone on the last 12 out of 28 days. This results in a regular postprogesterone withdrawal bleed, which protects the endometrium. Prolonged use of cyclical HRT can increase the risk of endometrial cancer, so should be given for a maximum of 5 years. A patch or tablet can be used. Once the patient has been amenorrhoeic for 1 year or reaches 54 years of age (whichever is sooner), she should be transferred to continuous combined therapy.

3. B – Continuous combined hormone replacement therapy

In women with a uterus who have not bled for 1 year (postmenopausal), low-dose continuous combined HRT is the first-line option. This means that they are given continuous oestrogen and progesterone. Around 90% of women will experience symptomatic relief on a low dose. The combined preparation causes endometrial atrophy, so treated women should have no bleeding. The progesterone protects the endometrium from hyperplasia and reduces the risk of endometrial cancer.

There is evidence of a small increased risk of cardiovascular disease with combined HRT preparations. This is influenced by dose, patient age and other risk factors for atherosclerosis.

Women taking HRT should be followed up 6-monthly to assess symptomatic improvement and adverse effects and to review risk factors. Blood pressure, weight and smoking status should be checked, and lifestyle discussed if necessary. Regular breast self-examination should be advised.

Oestrogen-only hormone replacement therapy

Women who have had a hysterectomy can be given oestrogen-only preparations in doses titrated to their symptoms. This is available as a patch, topical gel or tablet. Estradiol implants are also available. They do not require progesterone, as they are not at risk of unopposed oestrogen-induced endometrial hyperplasia. The risk of breast cancer is reduced compared to combined HRT.

Testosterone implants are sometimes offered by gynaecologists to improve libido.

4. G – Specialist referral

This patient has undiagnosed irregular vaginal bleeding and requires gynaecological assessment with an ultrasound scan and a hysteroscopy before HRT can be considered.

Patients who have a history of thromboembolism or breast cancer should probably be referred to a specialist for close consideration of the risk–benefit analysis. Other indications for specialist referral are menopause before the age of 40, a confirmed risk of osteoporosis and a high risk or a personal history of oestrogen-dependent cancers, such as those of the breast or endometrium. Women should also be referred for specialist assessment if they have abnormal bleeding while using cyclical HRT or for more than 6 months after the start of continuous combined HRT.

5. A – Bisphosphonates

Bisphosphonates are drugs that inhibit osteoclast-mediated bone resorption, and consequently prevent osteoporosis. Examples include risedronate and alendronate. Oral calcium and vitamin D supplements are often given in addition to bisphosphonates for the prevention of osteoporosis.

Tibolone is a synthetic steroid that has oestrogenic, progestogenic and some androgenic effects. It does not cause endometrial proliferation, but can still cause irregular bleeding within the first few months. Raloxifene is the first of the new class of selective oestrogen receptor modulators (SERMs). They selectively stimulate oestrogen receptors, so can prevent osteoporosis and have a beneficial effect upon the lipid profile. However, SERMs do not relieve the menopausal symptoms of oestrogen deficiency.

THEME 10: PREMATURE LABOUR

Prematurity is defined as delivery before 37 weeks' gestation, but the morbidity and mortality rates are much greater at the earlier gestations. Preterm labour complicates 5%–10% of pregnancies and is responsible for 75% of all perinatal deaths. Survival rates are improving with advances in maternal and neonatal management; however, the long-term consequences of prematurity for the individual and family can be dramatic. The management of each case must be adjusted to the individual. Although there is national evidence-based guidance, as with much of obstetrics, there are always local protocols with which you must be familiar.

The biggest risk factor for preterm delivery is a previous preterm delivery. Other risk factors include maternal age <20 years, low socioeconomic class, multiparity, smoking and multiple pregnancy. Certain features of the current pregnancy can also increase the risk of preterm delivery, including antepartum haemorrhage, preeclampsia, polyhydramnios and infection (e.g. chorioamnionitis).

Premature labour may be preceded by premature PROM (PPROM) or can occur with intact membranes, with subsequent rupture of membranes and delivery. In reality, the diagnosis of premature labour can be difficult. A clear history and examination are required, as well as discussion with a registrar or consultant. A good history includes noting the strength, intensity and frequency of contractions, evidence of a 'show' (characteristic cervical mucus) or rupture of membranes, presence of fetal movements and additional symptoms, such as urinary symptoms, vaginal bleeding, discharge or systemic symptoms (fever, cough or shortness of breath).

Examination includes observations (temperature, blood pressure, pulse rate and urine testing for protein, leucocytes and nitrites) and abdominal palpation (for tenderness, SFH, fetal lie and position, as well as palpation for contractions). A sterile speculum examination will help assess the cervix and detect SROM by looking for pooling of liquor in the speculum or leakage on coughing. Investigations include vaginal swabs, blood tests for inflammatory markers, a CTG (if >26 weeks) and a pelvic ultrasound (can provide information about fetal growth/presentation and an estimate of liquor volume, low amounts of which suggest rupture of membranes).

Do not perform a digital examination if rupture of membranes is suspected. There is a risk of transmission of infection from the vagina into the cervix, which can cause intrauterine infection, prostaglandin release and preterm labour.

1. I – Magnesium sulphate

An infusion of magnesium sulphate given to mothers prior to delivery of a preterm infant has been found to protect gross motor function and reduce the risk of cerebral palsy in the baby. It is thought to have greater benefit for the most preterm gestations and is effective just prior to delivery.

2. A – Atosiban

Atosiban is a tocolytic drug. Tocolytics act by inhibiting smooth muscle contraction in the uterus in an attempt to delay labour. They are generally used to delay labour for enough time to allow steroids to be given to benefit the fetal lungs or for transfer to a unit that could care for a preterm infant. There is, however, no evidence that tocolytic drugs alone improve outcome. Atosiban is an oxytocin receptor agonist that is licensed as a tocolytic and has a preferable side-effect profile compared with ritodrine. Ritodrine, a β-agonist, is the most widely evaluated tocolytic, but it is being overtaken by other drugs due to its poor side-effect profile. Side effects include tachycardia, headache, palpitations and impaired glucose tolerance. Because of these effects, it is avoided in cardiac disease and diabetes.

Nifedipine, a calcium channel blocker that is often used as a tocolytic, is easier and cheaper to administer than atosiban. It is not, however, licensed for this use in the UK. Another less widely used tocolytic is indomethacin, a NSAID. Tocolytics should not be used when there are contraindications to continuing the pregnancy, such as bleeding, fetal distress and chorioamnionitis, and should be used in caution in rupture of membranes.

3. B – Betamethasone

Corticosteroids such as betamethasone and dexamethasone are indicated in preterm labour, from 24 to 34 + 6 weeks, to promote pulmonary maturity and stimulate surfactant production. They have been proven to reduce the incidence of neonatal death, respiratory distress syndrome and intraventricular haemorrhage in the premature infant. One commonly used dosing regimen is two intramuscular injections of betamethasone 12 mg given 24 hours apart. The steroids take 24 hours to become effective but some effect is seen within the first 24 hours. Delivery can be delayed, by tocolysis if necessary, to allow steroids to take effect. Steroids should also be considered if an elective caesarean section is going to be performed prior to 39 weeks, as they have been shown to reduce the need for admission to the neonatal care unit.

4. D – Erythromycin
5. C – Co-amoxiclav

Antibiotics are indicated as infection prophylaxis in preterm rupture of membranes. Erythromycin is the antibiotic of choice following the diagnosis of PPROM. It is given as a 10-day course and has been found to reduce the incidence of delivery within 48 hours, and has a positive impact upon neonatal and maternal morbidity. Co-amoxiclav (Augmentin) is not recommended, as it has been associated with an increased incidence of fetal necrotizing colitis. Gentamicin is not advised in pregnancy, as it has been associated with auditory or vestibular damage in the second and third trimesters.

Women with PPROM should be observed for signs of chorioamnionitis (infection of the chorion and amnion affecting fetal and maternal blood vessels), which include maternal pyrexia, offensive vaginal discharge and fetal tachycardia. If there is evidence of sepsis, then delivery should be expedited and broad-spectrum antibiotics given IV after blood cultures and swabs are taken. The neonatologists should be informed of any suspicion of maternal infection as the baby may also be affected.

The ORACLE trial showed that short-term respiratory function, chronic lung disease and major neonatal cerebral abnormality were reduced with the use of erythromycin following preterm prelabour rupture of membranes.

Practice Paper 2: Questions

THEME 1: ANTEPARTUM HAEMORRHAGE

Options

A. Bloody show
B. Cervical ectropion
C. Cervical polyp
D. Placental abruption
E. Placenta praevia
F. Uterine rupture
G. Vasa praevia

For each of the following scenarios, select the most likely cause of ante-partum haemorrhage. Each option may be used once, more than once or not at all.

1. A 34-year-old woman is labouring well at term with an epidural *in situ*. She has reached 8 cm of cervical dilatation with good progression. Since insertion of the epidural, she has felt no contractions. Suddenly, she experiences severe lower abdominal pain associated with vaginal bleeding and tachycardia. The cardiotocograph (CTG) does not detect any contractions and shows signs of significant fetal distress. She has had three previous pregnancies, including two spontaneous vaginal births and one caesarean section for failure to progress.

2. A 42-year-old woman, who is at 39 weeks' gestation with five previous normal deliveries, calls an ambulance as she is having heavy, unprovoked, painless vaginal bleeding. The midwife had mentioned on her previous visit that the baby was still high and free on abdominal palpation. She decided to have no scans in this pregnancy as she felt that there were no problems with her previous children.

3. A 32-year-old primigravida woman is being induced at term +14 days and has an artificial rupture of membranes performed. The midwife confirms that there is no cord in the cervix, although she does note heavily blood-stained liquor. The mother is not complaining of pain, but the CTG demonstrates significant abnormalities.

4. A 33-year-old primigravida woman attends the antenatal day unit. She is concerned as she had a mucus-like blood-stained loss vaginally earlier in the day, and this was associated with gradual-onset abdominal cramps approximately every 15–20 minutes.

5. A 24-year-old low-risk primip at 38 weeks' gestation presents to the antenatal day unit with significant lower abdominal pain and back pain. She also admits to having some *per vagina* blood loss. On examination, the uterus is tender and hard. Maternal observations are pulse rate 115 beats/minute and blood pressure 95/68 mmHg. The CTG shows fetal distress.

THEME 2: MENSTRUAL DYSFUNCTION

Options

A. Antifibrinolytics (tranexamic acid)
B. Combined oral contraceptive pill
C. Danazol
D. Endometrial ablation
E. Gonadotropin-releasing hormone analogues
F. Hysterectomy
G. Hysteroscopic laser/resection of fibroids
H. Intrauterine or systemic progestogens
I. Myomectomy
J. Polypectomy
K. Non-steroidal anti-inflammatory drugs
L. Uterine artery embolization

For each of the following scenarios, select the most appropriate management option. Each option may be used once, more than once or not at all.

1. A 16-year-old girl, who is normally fit and well, sees her GP complaining of heavy and painful periods. She is requesting treatment for these complaints. She denies being sexually active and would prefer not to receive hormone treatment.

2. A 43-year-old woman has suffered with heavy periods for many years and has tried many medical and surgical treatments without success. She is constantly flooding and at times cannot leave her house due to heavy bleeding. She has completed her family of five children and her last blood test showed a haemoglobin level of 7.8 g/dL despite taking regular ferrous sulphate. She feels that she cannot cope with the bleeding anymore, and is asking for a hysterectomy.

3. A 29-year-old woman presents to the gynaecology clinic with troublesome heavy periods. The medical treatments that she has tried have made little difference. She is known to have large uterine intramural fibroids. You confirm that she would like more children in the future.

4. A 38-year-old overweight smoker attends with heavy periods. She would like a long-term treatment with minimal side effects that would offer treatment for the menorrhagia and provide contraception. She is unsure whether she would like more children. She is adamant that she does not want surgery, as she is terrified of the prospect.

5. A 41-year-old woman, who has completed her family, has suffered from extremely heavy periods for many years. An ultrasound scan showed a couple of large fibroids. No medical treatments have worked. She says she would rather avoid surgery. After discussion, you collectively decide on a procedure that would not require open surgery or a general anaesthetic.

THEME 3: PHYSIOLOGICAL CHANGES IN PREGNANCY

Options

A. Decreases
B. Increases
C. Increases only with twins
D. Increases only with female fetuses
E. Increases only with male fetuses
F. Stays the same

For each of the following, select the correct answer for what happens physiologically in pregnancy. Each option may be used once, more than once or not at all.

1. Respiratory rate
2. Haemoglobin concentration
3. Renal blood flow
4. Albumin
5. Heart rate

THEME 4: VAGINAL BLEEDING

Options
A. Cervical cancer
B. Cervical ectropion
C. Chlamydial infection
D. Endometrial carcinoma
E. Endometrial polyps
F. Perimenopausal symptoms
G. Pregnancy
H. Uterine fibroids (leiomyoma)

For each of the following scenarios, select the most likely diagnosis. Each option may be used once, more than once or not at all.

1. A 59-year-old overweight woman says that she has had some irregular vaginal bleeding. Her regular menstrual periods stopped 7 years ago. She has suffered from an offensive discharge for the last 3 months. She has never had sexual intercourse.

2. A 38-year-old woman presents to you complaining of postcoital bleeding for 3 years and significant weight loss. She has a constant dull ache in the pelvis. She has now sought help as she has blood in her urine. She is a smoker. She admits to having a number of sexual partners from a young age. She has not seen a healthcare professional for the last 10 years, as she feels that she has previously been healthy.

3. A 51-year-old woman presents to the clinic with light vaginal bleeding every 3–4 months, unrelated to sexual intercourse. Her last period was 3 months ago. She has night sweats and discomfort during intercourse.

4. A 35-year-old woman presents with a long history of very heavy periods. She has visited you now as she cannot cope with the bleeding. On examination, you feel a bulky uterus equivalent to a pregnancy at 18 weeks; however, the patient states that she has not been sexually active for over 3 years.

5. A 25-year-old student attends your surgery concerned about postcoital bleeding. She has recently had a genitourinary medicine (GUM) clinic appointment, and she was told her smears and swabs were normal. She mentions that the doctor said her examination was 'reassuring'. She has been taking the combined oral contraceptive pill (COCP) for several years.

THEME 5: CONTRAINDICATIONS TO CONTRACEPTION

Options

A. An insulin-dependent diabetic
B. A smoker
C. Body mass index 39 kg/m²
D. Thromboembolism
E. Hypertension
F. A wheelchair-bound patient
G. Migraine with a typical focal aura
H. Migraine without focal aura
 I. Pelvic inflammatory disease

For each of the following descriptions, select the appropriate contraindication. Each option may be used once, more than once or not at all.

1. This type of headache is an absolute contraindication to using combined hormonal contraception.
2. The risk of venous thromboembolism for this patient becomes unacceptably high once they reach 35 years of age.
3. It is advised that other contraceptive options may be more suitable for patients with this chronic disease, even if it is well controlled.
4. This is neither a caution nor a contraindication to using combined oral contraception.
5. A family history of this condition in a relative under 45 years of age is a relative contraindication to the combined pill.

THEME 6: RHESUS DISEASE

Options

A. Give antenatal anti-D prophylaxis 250 IU and perform Kleihauer test
B. Give antenatal anti-D prophylaxis 500 IU and perform Kleihauer test
C. Give postnatal anti-D 500 IU and perform Kleihauer test
D. Give routine antenatal anti-D prophylaxis at 28 weeks
E. Give routine antenatal anti-D prophylaxis at 34 weeks
F. No action needed

For each of the following scenarios, select the most appropriate course of action you would take on that day. Each option may be used once, more than once or not at all.

1. A 28-year-old rhesus D (RhD)-negative pregnant woman attends the emergency department with a small vaginal bleed at 7 weeks' gestation.
2. A 34-year-old RhD-negative woman, in her second pregnancy at 23 weeks' gestation, attends the antenatal day unit with a story that her son pushed his play trolley hard into her abdomen (accidentally). The baby has been moving well since and there has been no bleeding *per vagina*. The fetal heart is heard and is regular.
3. A 41-year-old woman who is RhD positive attends the emergency department with a vaginal bleed at 25 weeks' gestation. She says she does not want any more children and the baby's father is known to be RhD negative.
4. A 30-year-old woman attends the antenatal clinic to have her routine antenatal anti-D prophylaxis at 28 weeks. She tells you that she has already had an anti-D injection due to bleeding earlier on in her pregnancy.
5. A 31-year-old RhD-negative woman has had routine antenatal anti-D prophylaxis, as well as an antenatal anti-D prophylaxis injection for some bleeding prior to this. She has just delivered an RhD-positive infant and is asking you what needs to be done.

THEME 7: CLASSIFICATION OF OVARIAN TUMOURS

Options

A. Brenner's tumour
B. Clear cell tumour
C. Dysgerminoma
D. Fibroma
E. Krukenberg's tumour
F. Mucinous tumour
G. Non-gestational choriocarcinoma
H. Serous tumour
 I. Sex cord tumour
 J. Teratoma

For each of the following descriptions, select the most appropriate ovarian tumour. Each option may be used once, more than once or not at all.

1. Metastatic cancer of the ovaries with 'signet-ring' cells on microscopy.
2. This is the commonest of the epithelial ovarian tumours.
3. This ovarian tumour is associated with Meigs' syndrome.
4. Rupture of these large tumours can lead to pseudomyxoma peritonei.
5. These arise from germ cells and can contain hair and teeth.

THEME 8: MANAGEMENT OF ENDOMETRIAL AND CERVICAL CANCER

Options

A. Chemotherapy and radiotherapy
B. Cone biopsy
C. Cryocautery
D. Radical hysterectomy and bilateral salpingo-oophorectomy
E. Radical trachelectomy
F. Radiotherapy
G. Reassurance

For each of the following scenarios, select the most appropriate management plan. Each option may be used once, more than once or not at all.

1. A 34-year-old woman with cervical cancer stage Ia1. She would like to retain her fertility.
2. A 68-year-old woman undergoes staging magnetic resonance imaging after being found to have an invasive cervical tumour. The cancer extends into the pelvic wall.
3. A 32-year-old woman has a 2 cm tumour that is confined to the cervix. She says that she still wishes to conceive.
4. A 41-year-old woman, who was admitted under gynaecology with abdominal pain and heavy periods, is found to have a myometrial leiomyosarcoma confined to the uterus.
5. A 65-year-old woman has a diagnosis of endometrial adenocarcinoma given following a pipelle biopsy for postmenopausal bleeding. Magnetic resonance imaging is performed and the lesion extends to <50% through the myometrium.

Options
A. Betamethasone
B. Furosemide
C. Hydralazine
D. Labetalol
E. Magnesium sulphate
F. Methyldopa
G. Misoprostol
H. Nifedipine
I. Phenytoin
J. Ramipril

For each of the following descriptions, select the most appropriate drug. Each option may be used once, more than once or not at all.

1. An α-1-adrenergic and ß-adrenergic blocker, which is the first-line treatment for moderate/severe gestational hypertension and moderate/severe hypertension in preeclampsia.
2. A calcium channel blocker used as second- or third-line antihypertensive in pregnancy.
3. The most effective infusion used in preeclampsia for preventing eclamptic convulsions.
4. This long-acting antihypertensive, also used in pregnancy, is contraindicated in depression.
5. An antihypertensive agent that is avoided in women with asthma.

THEME 10: INDUCTION AND AUGMENTATION OF LABOUR

Options

A. Artificial rupture of membranes
B. Caesarean section
C. Observation alone
D. Prostaglandin
E. Twice-weekly cardiotocography and ultrasound of liquor volume
F. Twice-weekly ultrasound
G. Oxytocin infusion

For each of the following scenarios, select the most appropriate management. Each option may be used once, more than once or not at all.

1. A 30-year-old woman at 41 weeks and 6 days attends the antenatal clinic and is keen for induction of labour. On vaginal examination, she has a 1–2 cm dilated, posterior, firm cervix that is 2 cm in length and 2 cm above the ischial spines (Bishop score 3).
2. A 26-year-old woman who has had two previous caesarean sections attends the antenatal clinic when she is 1 week overdue. She did not attend her previous appointments as she wanted to await spontaneous onset of labour. She is now requesting induction of labour.
3. A 24-year-old woman at 42 weeks attends the clinic. She declines induction of labour despite appropriate counselling.
4. A 27-year-old low-risk primip with cephalic presentation is in spontaneous labour after her membranes ruptured. Her initial cervical assessment was 5 cm, and after 4 hours it is 6 cm.
5. You are called to see a 25-year-old primigravida woman 6 hours after her third dose of prostaglandin gel who is being induced for mild preeclampsia. She is having irregular mild contractions. Her cardiotocography is reassuring. The midwife tells you that her Bishop score is 8, and that she is now 3 cm dilated.

Practice Paper 2: Answers

THEME 1: ANTEPARTUM HAEMORRHAGE

Antepartum haemorrhage is bleeding from the genital tract between 24 weeks' gestation and delivery. Around 3% of women suffer antepartum haemorrhage. Bleeding can be maternal, fetal or placental. The patient with antepartum haemorrhage is at increased risk of postpartum haemorrhage.

1. F – Uterine rupture

Uterine rupture, where the uterine wall tears, is very rare. It generally occurs only in patients who have had previous surgery to the uterus, such as myomectomy or caesarean section, but can occur with excessive oxytocin use, obstructed labour and in women of high parity. Pain is the principal feature (although a good epidural can mask this pain), with associated maternal shock, sudden termination of contractions and cardiotocography (CTG) abnormalities. The fetus may be particularly easy to feel on abdominal examination as it is no longer contained in the uterus and the head may ascend into the abdomen so it cannot be reached on vaginal examination. A laparotomy must be performed immediately to deliver the baby and control maternal haemorrhage.

2. E – Placenta praevia

Placenta praevia is where the placenta lies close to or covers the internal os of the cervix. It occurs in 1% of pregnancies and is more common in older women, smokers and women who have undergone previous uterine surgery including myomectomy, curettage and caesarean section. It is usually detected on the ultrasound scan performed at around 20 weeks of gestation but a repeat scan should be performed at around 34 weeks as the placenta will often move away from the internal os with uterine growth as the pregnancy progresses. Placenta praevia is classified according to its proximity to the internal os as minor (placenta in lower segment, but not covering the os) or major (placenta partially or completely covering the os).

Clinically, there is unprovoked (or postcoital) intermittent, fresh, painless vaginal bleeding. The lack of pain makes placental abruption much less likely. On abdominal examination, there is a soft, non-tender uterus with a high head or malpresentation (as the placenta blocks passage of the presenting part into the pelvis). Vaginal examination is contraindicated in suspected placenta praevia, as it can precipitate massive bleeding.

The clinical condition of the mother correlates with the visible blood loss (unlike placental abruption – see below). Because the blood is maternal blood, there is little risk to the fetus unless the mother becomes extremely hypovolaemic (compare to vasa praevia). Women with bleeding placenta praevia should be admitted and the baby delivered by elective caesarean section at 39 weeks. Massive haemorrhage requires maternal resuscitation and immediate delivery.

> Placenta, from Greek *plakous* = flat cake.
> Praevia, from Latin *prae* = ahead of + *via* = road (i.e. 'in the way').

3. G – Vasa praevia

In vasa praevia, fetal vessels traverse the membranes and overlie the internal cervical os. Presentation includes a small amount (<500 mL) of painless blood loss with associated CTG abnormalities, caused by tearing of the vessels due to cervical dilatation and rupture of membranes. The blood lost in vasa praevia is fetal. This means the fetal mortality rate is very high (35%–95%), whereas there is little physical risk to the mother. A caesarean section must be performed immediately and the neonate may need a blood transfusion. Screening using an ultrasound scan is not commonly practised due to limited evidence of benefit and the rarity of the condition (1 in 3000).

> Vasa, plural of Latin *vas* = vessel.

4. A – Bloody show

The 'show' is a bloody, mucus-like vaginal loss that is associated with contractions and the initial stages of early labour.

5. D – Placental abruption

In placental abruption, the placental bed bleeds and a haematoma forms behind it, lifting the placenta away from the uterus. Abruption is associated with hypertension, preeclampsia, sudden decompression after membrane rupture in polyhydramnios or multiple pregnancies, previous or family history of abruption (10% recurrence), trauma to the abdomen and tobacco or cocaine abuse (although the cause is unknown in many cases). The incidence is up to 5%; however, mild abruption presents with only a small amount of pain or bleeding with little effect on the fetus or mother, and may only be diagnosed postnatally after studying the placenta. Major abruptions present with vaginal bleeding coupled with constant, severe abdominal pains, and maternal shock may be seen. The uterus is irritable and tender and may become 'woody' hard due to tonic contraction. It is therefore difficult to palpate the fetal parts. There is often loss of fetal movements with fetal distress. The volume of vaginal bleeding is a poor indicator of the amount of maternal blood loss (unlike placenta praevia), as bleeding can be contained behind the placenta (concealed abruption).

Intrauterine death from hypoxia is common, as there is a sudden reduction in the blood available for placental gas exchange. Delivery should be expedited, often by caesarean section.

The cervical ectropion is the most common cervical lesion that accounts for antepartum haemorrhage. It is diagnosed by appearance on speculum examination. The ectropion can resolve during the puerperium, and cauterization should be avoided in pregnancy. Cervical polyps are occasionally found in pregnancy and should be managed expectantly. Avulsion should be avoided, as haemostasis is much harder to maintain due to the greater cervical vascularity in pregnancy.

THEME 2: MENSTRUAL DYSFUNCTION

Menorrhagia means heavy periods and should not be confused with dysmenorrhoea (painful periods), although both often occur simultaneously. Menorrhagia is defined as menstrual blood loss >80 mL per period. This value represents two standard deviations above the mean period blood loss (40 mL). However, in reality there is no requirement for measurement – only a good history is needed to reveal heavy cyclical menstrual bleeding over several consecutive cycles.

Menorrhagia, from Greek *meniaios* = monthly + *rhoia* = flowing.

1. K – Non-steroidal anti-inflammatory drugs

This girl is suffering from subjective menorrhagia and dysmenorrhea, and non-steroidal anti-inflammatory drugs (NSAIDs) will help with both of these complaints. They are commonly used for pain, but can reduce blood loss by 25%. The benefit they have over tranexamic acid is that they also are helpful with dysmenorrhoea. Side effects of NSAIDs are mainly gastrointestinal. The NICE guidelines suggest using a levonorgestrel-releasing intrauterine system as the first-line treatment of menorrhagia; however, this is not suitable, as she does not want hormones and fitting would be difficult as she has never been sexually active.

Tranexamic acid is an antifibrinolytic which reduces fibrinolytic activity by inhibiting plasminogen activator (i.e. they stop activation of plasminogen to plasmin). Clot formation is subsequently increased in the spiral arteries, which reduces menstrual loss. Antifibrinolytics must not be used by women with a predisposition to thromboembolism. These drugs can reduce blood loss by 50%. Tranexamic acid does not reduce pain.

2. F – Hysterectomy

This woman is clearly at the end of her tether and requires definitive treatment. A hysterectomy is the best option, as this is the only treatment that will ensure amenorrhoea, and the patient has finished her family. The surgical approach is either vaginal or abdominal and it is likely that a vaginal hysterectomy would be possible in this woman, as she has had five children. Risks of this procedure are bleeding, infection, pain, damage to the bowel/urinary tracts, postoperative thromboembolism and vaginal prolapse in later life.

3. I – Myomectomy

Myomectomy allows conservation of a patient's fertility. This is either an open abdominal or a laparoscopic procedure. The pseudocapsules of the fibroids are incised, allowing removal of the fibroid, and the resulting defect is sealed. Risks of this procedure include uncontrolled bleeding requiring hysterectomy, adhesion formation (leading to reduced fertility) and recurrence of fibroids. Hysteroscopic resection is not an option in this case, as this woman's fibroids are too large and are intramural. Hysteroscopic resection is possible only with small, submucosal fibroids.

Gonadotropin-releasing hormone analogues will treat menorrhagia but would only be considered prior to surgery or when all other treatments for fibroids are contraindicated. These cause amenorrhoea by downregulation of pituitary function, which leads to an inhibition of ovarian activity. There are consequences of the hypo-oestrogenic state, including hot flushes and vaginal dryness, and add-back hormone-replacement therapy should be considered in these cases or if treatment length is above 6 months.

4. H – Intrauterine or systemic progestogens

Progestogen administration is the most appropriate treatment in this woman, who does not wish to have surgery. This treatment offers her both contraception and a reduction in bleeding. She can use either a systemic formulation (progesterone-only pill) or a Mirena coil (an intrauterine device impregnated with progestogen, licensed for 5 years' use in the treatment of menorrhagia). Mirena is the first line in the NICE guidance, but this would be her personal choice. Because of the risk of thromboembolism (weight, age and smoking habits), she is not suitable for the combined oral contraceptive pill. It may be advisable to give some opportunistic lifestyle advice.

5. L – Uterine artery embolization

Uterine artery embolization is performed by radiologists and aims to reduce blood flow to the fibroids, leading to symptomatic relief in the short and medium term. A catheter is inserted via the femoral artery and is fed up to the uterine artery, where a coil or piece of foam is deposited to occlude the blood supply to the fibroid. This can cause fibroids to shrink by up to 50%. Healthy myometrium is unaffected, as there is collateral circulation via the ovarian and vaginal vessels. Risks of this procedure include pain, bleeding, infection, fibroid expulsion and damage to the ovaries secondary to ionizing radiation. The effects of the procedure on pregnancy are uncertain.

Endometrial ablation can improve menorrhagia by destroying the endometrium. Hysteroscopic procedures include laser ablation, resection or coagulation using an electric roller-ball, microwave ablation, heat ablation or electrocautery. Pregnancy is contraindicated after ablation.

THEME 3: PHYSIOLOGICAL CHANGES IN PREGNANCY

1. F – Stays the same
2. A – Decreases
3. B – Increases
4. A – Decreases
5. B – Increases

The physiological changes in pregnancy are summarized as follows:

	Increase	Unchanged	Decrease
Respiratory	Tidal volume: +200 mL Inspiratory capacity: +100 mL Oxygen consumption (+20%–33%)	Respiratory rate Peak flow	Total lung capacity: −200 mL Residual volume: −200 mL Expiratory reserve: −100 mL Inspiratory reserve: −100 mL Functional residual capacity: −300 mL
Cardiovascular system	Plasma volume: 45% by 32 weeks Cardiac output: 40% Heart rate: 10% Stroke volume: 30% Uterus blood flow: 400 mL Renal blood flow: 300 mL	Mean arterial pressure Central venous pressure Pulmonary wedge pressure	Mid-trimester blood pressure Systemic and pulmonary vascular resistance
Haematology	Mean cell volume White cell count Total iron-binding capacity Red cell mass: 25%	Mean cell haemoglobin concentration Serum ferritin, iron – however, often reduced in anaemia	Haemoglobin concentration Haematocrit (dilutional) Platelet count
Gastrointestinal	Weight: 10 kg (variable) Nutritional requirements Gastric reflux Gallstones	Amylase	Gastrointestinal tract motility Stomach pH
Liver	Alkaline phosphatase (placental)	Bilirubin	Albumin Aspartate transaminase and alanine transaminase
Immunology	Erythrocyte sedimentation rate	C-reactive protein	

(Continued)

	Increase	Unchanged	Decrease

Endocrinology	Insulin
	Total tri-iodothyronine
	  (T_3) + thyroxine (T_4)
	Thyroid-binding globulin
	Adrenocorticotropic
	  hormone, corticotrophin-
	  releasing hormone,
	  cortisol
	Prolactin
	1,25-dihydroxyvitamin-D_3
		Free T_3 +T_4
		Adrenaline,
		  noradrenaline
		Calcitonin, free
		  ionized
		  calcium
			Fasting glucose
			Glucose tolerance
			Thyroid-stimulating
			  hormone
			Total serum calcium,
			  parathyroid
			  hormone

Renal	Renal blood flow: 25%
	Creatinine clearance: 40%
	Kidney length: 1–1.5 cm
	Renin–angiotensin system
	Aldosterone
		Daily voided
		  volume
		Plasma
		  Na^+, K^+, Cl^-
			Plasma urea,
			  creatinine

THEME 4: VAGINAL BLEEDING

1. D – Endometrial carcinoma

Presentation of endometrial carcinoma is often with postmenopausal bleeding but can also present with discharge or irregularities of the menstrual cycle in older women, or pyometra (pus in the uterus). Endometrial tumours are generally oestrogen dependent and are therefore linked with long-term unopposed oestrogen due to a number of reasons. There is a higher risk in obese women (as adiposity increases oestrogen levels) and in nulliparous women with a late menopause. Investigations include urgent ultrasound or magnetic resonance imaging for endometrial thickness, then hysteroscopy and endometrial sampling for tissue diagnosis. Prior to surgery, imaging of the chest, abdomen and pelvis should be performed to check for metastases. Endometrial tumours are locally invasive, spreading through the endometrial cavity and cervix, along the fallopian tubes to the ovaries and peritoneal cavity.

2. A – Cervical cancer

Cervical cancer is the sixth most common malignancy in women, accounting for 4% of female malignancies. There is an association with early sexual activity, multiple partners and smoking. Other risk factors include immunosuppression, and there is a small increase in those who have taken the contraceptive pill for over 5 years, which reduces once the pill is stopped. There are 15 types of human papillomaviruses considered to be high risk for the cervix, with types 16 and 18 being associated with 70% of tumours. 60% of women with invasive carcinoma have not had screening, and there are small numbers of women who are diagnosed with early cervical cancer from cervical screening. Most (80%) are symptomatic, complaining of abnormal *per vagina* bleeding (postcoital, intermenstrual or postmenopausal) or a chronic vaginal discharge. Pain, haematuria, malaise and weight loss may occur in advanced disease.

This patient has the signs and symptoms of invasive disease and has not had smear tests.

3. F – Perimenopausal symptoms

The average age of the menopause is 51 years. This is the cessation of periods due to ovarian failure following the depletion of oocytes. As oestrogen production falls, the production of follicle-stimulating hormone rises. Irregular bleeding often precedes absolute cessation of periods. Any bleeding experienced after 1 year following the menopause warrants immediate investigation for endometrial carcinoma.

4. H – Uterine fibroids (leiomyoma)

Fibroids are whorls of smooth muscle cells interspersed with collagen. They are benign tumours of the myometrium. Fibroids are present in 20% of women of reproductive age and are largely asymptomatic. They are more common in nulliparous and African–Caribbean women. Fibroids can be intramural (within the uterine wall), subserous (beneath the serosal surface of the uterus) or submucosal (beneath the mucosal surface of the uterus). They can be multiple and vary widely in size. Presentation depends on the size and location of fibroids, as some are microscopic and others have been as large as 10 kg. The most common presentation is menorrhagia, but pressure symptoms are also described. Pressure on the bladder can lead to frequency of micturition or hydronephrosis, due to ureteric compression. Other presenting features include abdominal bloating, infertility, miscarriage and pelvic discomfort. Treatment is not required if fibroids are asymptomatic. Medical treatments include gonadotropin-releasing hormone analogues or a low dose of ulipristal acetate (a selective progesterone receptor modulator). If menorrhagia is the main complaint, a Mirena coil may be used, providing the fibroids do not obstruct the uterine cavity. Surgical options include myomectomy (abdominally, laparoscopically or hysteroscopically), uterine artery embolization and hysterectomy.

Leiomyoma, from Greek *leios* = smooth + *myos* = muscle + *oma* = tumour.

5. B – Cervical ectropion

Cervical ectropion describes a florid appearance of the lower cervical canal. It is caused by hormonal changes during puberty, pregnancy and oral contraceptive pill use. Ectropion is usually asymptomatic, but may cause persistent vaginal discharge or postcoital bleeding. If the patient has had a normal smear test, it can be treated by diathermy or cryocautery.

Cervical polyps are the most common benign growth of the cervix. They are usually pedunculated and arise from the endocervical mucosa.

Cervical polyps often protrude through the external cervical os and look like bright-red growths. They can be up to a few centimetres in diameter.

Endometrial polyps

These are very common and may present with menstrual irregularities. They are found in the body of the uterus and are adenomatous. They can cause dysmenorrhoea or postcoital bleeding if they protrude through the cervix. If found, they should be excised and the tissue sent for histology.

THEME 5: CONTRAINDICATIONS TO CONTRACEPTION

1. **G – Migraine with a typical focal aura**
2. **B – A smoker**
3. **E – Hypertension**
4. **I – Pelvic inflammatory disease**
5. **D – Thromboembolism**

The combined hormonal contraceptive pill (COCP) contains the hormones oestrogen and progesterone. These prevent ovulation, thicken cervical mucus to prevent sperm reaching the ovum and thin the lining of the uterus to prevent implantation. They are over 99% effective if taken perfectly, but the estimated failure rate with typical use is up to 9% in the first year. Advantages are a reduction in bleeding, period pains and premenstrual symptoms. They protect against cancer of the ovary, uterus and colon, as well as some pelvic infections. Fertility quickly returns to normal when the medication is discontinued. The disadvantages include temporary minor side effects such as headaches, mood changes and breast tenderness. Women should be screened for additional risk factors such as a family history of venous thrombosis and breast cancer, which may make other contraceptive options more suitable. Missed pills, some enzyme-inducing drugs, vomiting or severe long-lasting diarrhoea can make the COCP less effective.

Prescribers should be aware of conditions in which combined oral contraceptives should not be used. These are detailed in UK Medical Eligibility Criteria (UKMEC), in which conditions are divided into being

1. Unrestricted for use
2. Advantages outweigh risks
3. Risks outweigh advantages
4. Unacceptable risk

If the patient falls into category 3 or 4, they should be fully counselled and other forms of contraception offered.

Diabetes: The COCP is contraindicated only if neuropathy/retinopathy/nephropathy or other vascular disease is present.

Smokers over the age of 35 years should be advised not to use the COCP.

Women with a body mass index (BMI) >35 should be advised that the risks outweigh the benefits and ideally to lose weight or use another form of contraception.

Venous thromboembolism (VTE): Women should not be prescribed the COCP if they have a personal history of VTE or are undergoing major surgery with prolonged immobilization. They should be advised that the risk outweighs the benefit if they are immobile or have a first-degree relative who developed a VTE under the age of 45 years. Those with known thrombogenic mutations should not be prescribed the COCP.

Hypertension: Uncontrolled hypertension is a complete contraindication to the COCP and it should be avoided in controlled hypertension, as the risks outweigh the benefits.

Other contraindications include migraine with aura, ischaemic heart disease (IHD), stroke, complicated valvular and congenital heart disease, liver tumours (malignant or hepatocellular adenoma), Raynaud's with lupus anticoagulant and systemic lupus erythematosus (SLE) with positive antiphospholipid antibodies.

Breast cancer: Avoid in current breast cancer, and risks outweigh benefits in previous breast cancer and in carriers of known gene mutations associated with breast cancer.

Postpartum: Women should not use the COCP if they are breastfeeding and are within 6 weeks of delivery, and it is thought that the risks outweigh the benefits even up to 6 months after delivery.

THEME 6: RHESUS DISEASE

1. **F – No action needed**
2. **B – Give antenatal anti-D prophylaxis 500 IU and perform Kleihauer test**
3. **F – No action needed**
4. **D – Give routine antenatal anti-D prophylaxis 500 IU at 28 weeks**
5. **C – Give postnatal anti-D and perform Kleihauer test**

At booking, all women have their bloods taken to screen for infection and to determine maternal blood group. Around 15% of women are rhesus negative (RhD–ve), which means that their red blood cells do not carry the inherited RhD antigen. Women who are rhesus positive (RhD + ve) do carry the D antigen on their red blood cells. Rhesus status should be clearly documented, as it can have serious consequences for future pregnancies if there is fetomaternal haemorrhage (where fetal blood enters the maternal circulation).

RhD–ve women are at risk of developing anti-D antibodies to a RhD+ve fetus. If a RhD–ve woman is carrying a RhD+ve fetus and any fetal blood cells cross into the maternal circulation (a sensitizing event), she will react to the 'foreign' D antigens on the red blood cells of the fetus and produce antibodies against them. This will not cause a problem in the current pregnancy, but in later pregnancies, the antibodies from the mother can cross the placenta and destroy the blood cells of a subsequent RhD+ve fetus. This is known as haemolytic disease of the newborn. Haemolytic disease of the newborn can vary from very mild disease, which is detectable only by laboratory testing, to severe disability or stillbirth. Anti-D prophylaxis prevents women producing antibodies against RhD+ve blood cells by providing anti-D immunoglobulins routinely and following sensitizing events. A Kleihauer test is used after 20 weeks' gestation to detect and quantify the level of fetomaternal haemorrhage, and this can alter the amount of anti-D that is required for each woman.

Royal College of Obstetrics and Gynaecology guidelines: Use of anti-D immunoglobulin for RhD prophylaxis

All women who are RhD–ve are offered routine antenatal anti-D prophylaxis during their pregnancy regardless of any sensitizing events which may have meant they previously received a dose of anti-D. Depending on local protocol, a large dose is given at 28 weeks or two smaller doses are given at 28 and 34 weeks.

Early pregnancy

Spontaneous miscarriage: anti-D prophylaxis should be given to all non-sensitized RhD–ve women who have spontaneous complete or incomplete miscarriage after 12 weeks' gestation. In RhD–ve women with spontaneous complete or incomplete miscarriage of less than 12 weeks' gestation, anti-D prophylaxis is not required unless uterine evacuation is performed. Threatened miscarriage: anti-D prophylaxis should be given to all RhD–ve women after 12 weeks' gestation, but not before. Termination of pregnancy: anti-D prophylaxis should be offered to all non-sensitized RhD–ve women having termination of pregnancy, whether it is medical or surgical, regardless of gestational age. Ectopic pregnancy: anti-D prophylaxis should be given to all non-sensitized RhD–ve women who have ectopic pregnancy.

Prophylaxis following sensitizing events before delivery

A sensitizing event is defined as an event in which fetal blood could pass into the maternal circulation, such as antepartum haemorrhage, blunt abdominal injury, external cephalic version of fetus, invasive prenatal diagnosis (amniocentesis, villus sampling or fetal blood sampling), other intrauterine procedures (insertion of shunts or embryo reduction) or intrauterine death. Following a sensitizing event, anti-D should be given to prevent the production of antibodies.

The minimum doses of anti-D are 250 IU before 20 weeks' gestation and 500 IU after 20 weeks' gestation, but more may be required following the results of the Kleihauer test. The anti-D immunoglobulin is given as soon after the sensitizing event as possible (ideally within 72 hours).

However, there is some evidence that it still provides some protection if given within 10 days.

Postnatal prophylaxis

If, on testing the baby's cord blood after birth, it is found to be RhD+ve, the mother is offered postnatal anti-D prophylaxis even if she has received antenatal anti-D. A dose of 500 IU should be administered and a Kleihauer blood test should be taken as more anti-D may be required if there is a large amount of fetomaternal haemorrhage.

The patient in question 3 is RhD+ve so would never require anti-D, but if she had been RhD–ve, she would also not have required anti-D as long as she was factually correct. If both parents are RhD–ve, the baby must also be RhD–ve and she does not want any further children, and as explained above, the risk is not in this pregnancy but in the next. The difficulty in this situation is that women may change their mind about wanting further pregnancies and there may be misidentification of the father.

The rhesus system is named after the rhesus macaque (the 'rhesus monkey'), which was first shown to possess the antigens. The five main rhesus antigens are C, c, D, E and e.

THEME 7: CLASSIFICATION OF OVARIAN TUMOURS

Ovarian cancer is the most common cause of death from gynaecological cancer in England and Wales (whereas endometrial cancer is the most prevalent). The incidence of ovarian cancer is around 1 in 2500 women aged over 55 years, and it is seven-times more common in western countries. 1% of those affected have familial disease, and having two close relatives affected (i.e. mother or sister) increases the risk by up to 40%. Other risk factors include early menarche, late menopause and nulliparity, as continuous ovulation is thought to be contributory. The COCP is thought to be protective. Lynch II syndrome, an autosomal dominant condition, predisposes to ovarian, endometrial, breast and colon cancer. Most (70%) women with ovarian tumours have no presenting symptoms, but those who do describe vague abdominal discomfort and distension, a 'dragging' sensation, urinary frequency (due to pressure effects), weight loss and occasionally menstrual changes such as bleeding. Because of the chance of spread, workup of these patients includes abdominal examination, palpation for enlarged supraclavicular lymph nodes, examination of the breast and chest, and rectal and vaginal examination. Features suggestive of malignancy include rapid growth, size >5 cm and ascites.

Staging of ovarian tumours is as follows:

- Stage I: disease is macroscopically confined to the ovaries
- Stage II: disease is beyond the ovaries, but confined to the pelvis
- Stage III: disease is beyond the pelvis, but confined to the abdomen
- Stage IV: disease is beyond the abdomen

Because of a lack of specific symptoms, ovarian tumours tend to present as advanced disease (stage III or stage IV). Sites of spread include the breast, stomach, colon and lung.

Ovarian cancer is staged at the time of laparotomy. Serum CA125 is a useful tumour marker in 80% of cases, which can be used to assess response to treatment. Pelvic and abdominal ultrasound and computed tomography scans may also be useful. Staging laparotomy includes pelvic washings, total abdominal hysterectomy with bilateral salpingo-oophorectomy and omentectomy for tissue diagnosis and lymph node sampling. Radiotherapy may be used for remaining disease not removed in theatre, and may be useful for palliative symptom control to reduce tumour bulk or metastases. Adjuvant chemotherapy is given more commonly than radiotherapy, and is used when the disease has spread further than stage I.

Henry Lynch, American physician (born 1928).
Lynch I syndrome describes a familial predisposition to colorectal carcinoma alone.

1. E – Krukenberg's tumour
This is actually a metastatic deposit, which is growing in the ovary and often found to be bilateral. The primary is gastric or colon cancer. The signet cells are mucin secreting and are generally also found in the primary cancer. Optimal treatment remains unclear.

2. H – Serous tumour
These are the most common type of epithelial ovarian tumour (40%–50%). Other epithelial tumours include mucinous, endometrioid, clear cell, transitional cell, mixed epithelial and undifferentiated.

3. D – Fibroma
Meigs' syndrome describes the simultaneous presence of an ovarian fibroma, ascites and a transudative pleural effusion (more commonly on the right side). The effusions are benign, and often resolve after removal of the offending tumour.

Joe Vincent Meigs, American gynaecologist (1892–1963).

4. F – Mucinous tumour
Pseudomyxoma peritonei (also known as 'jelly belly') is the rupture and dissemination of jelly-like mucus in the pelvis from mucinous ovarian tumours or, rarely, mucinous appendiceal tumours. If left untreated, the mucus can eventually build up enough to cause compression damage to the surrounding organs.

5. J – Teratoma
Teratomas arise from primitive germ cells. Over 95% of germ cell tumours are benign dermoid cysts, which can contain well-differentiated

ectodermal tissue including hair and teeth. Teratomas are the most common benign tumours, especially in premenopausal females. Dysgerminomas are also germ cell tumours, the equivalent of testicular seminomas, which usually occur in adolescence and early adulthood.

Other ovarian tumours include non-gestational choriocarcinomas, a rare form of germ cell tumour that secretes the β-subunit of human chorionic gonadotropin and can therefore mimic pregnancy. Yolk sac tumours and malignant teratomas secrete α-fetoprotein. Sex cord carcinomas are rare and arise from the gonadal stroma. Granulosa cell tumours and thecomas are both examples of sex cord tumours. They both secrete oestrogen and can result in precocious puberty, endometrial hyperplasia and endometrial carcinoma.

Brenner's tumours are rare, small, benign ovarian tumours of uroepithelial origin.

Fritz Brenner, German physician (1877–1969).
Friedrich Ernst Krukenberg, German physician (1871–1946).

THEME 8: MANAGEMENT OF ENDOMETRIAL AND CERVICAL CANCER

1. B – Cone biopsy

Stage Ia is where the disease is only identified microscopically, and if it has a depth of less than 3 mm and a width of less than 7 mm, it is classified as stage Ia1. These can be fully treated with a knife cone biopsy, and provided no disease (or cervical intraepithelial neoplasia (CIN)) is seen at the margins, no further treatment is required. If disease or CIN is seen at the margins, further excision or hysterectomy should be performed. Lymph node sampling is not required because it is exceptionally rare for this stage of cervical cancer to have lymph node involvement.

2. A – Chemotherapy and radiotherapy

Cervical tumours are staged as follows:

- Stage 0: carcinoma *in situ*
- Stage I: lesions confined to cervix
- Stage II: invasion into upper vagina but not pelvic wall
- Stage III: invasion of lower vagina/pelvic wall, or causing ureteric obstruction
- Stage IV: invasion of bladder or rectal mucosa and/or distant metastases

Stage I is further divided into Ia1 (tumour <3 mm deep and <7 mm across), Ia2 (tumour <5 mm deep and <7 mm across), Ib1 (tumour <4 cm) and Ib2 (tumour >4 cm). Stage II is divided into IIa (invasion of upper two-thirds of vagina but not parametrium) and IIb (invasion of parametrium).

Management depends on the stage of the tumour. Stage Ia1 can be treated with cone biopsy or simple hysterectomy. All other stage I and stage 2a diseases require radical abdominal hysterectomy (Wertheim's procedure). This operation involves a hysterectomy with the additional removal of the upper third of the vagina, parametrium and pelvic lymph nodes (and the ovaries if the patient is not a young woman). Adjuvant radiotherapy is often used in these cases. Cervical tumours that are stage IIb and beyond, and less invasive tumours in women who are unfit for surgery, are treated with radiotherapy and chemotherapy, without hysterectomy. The cervical malignancy in this scenario invades the pelvic wall, and is thus a stage III tumour. Management is therefore by chemotherapy and radiotherapy.

Ernst Wertheim, Austrian gynaecologist (1864–1920).
Parametrium, from Greek *para* = beside + *metra* = womb. This term describes the connective tissue found immediately alongside the body of the uterus.

3. E – Radical trachelectomy
This young woman has a stage I cervical tumour, specifically stage Ib1. Although this is normally managed with radical hysterectomy, a radical trachelectomy provides a less invasive alternative for women who wish to remain fertile. Radical trachelectomy involves removal of the cervix, part of the vagina and the parametrial tissue, including pelvic lymph nodes. It aims to allow women to retain their fertility, but this cannot be guaranteed and there is a risk of late miscarriage.

Trachelectomy, from Greek *trachelos* = neck, the cervix essentially being the neck of the uterus.

4. D – Radical hysterectomy and bilateral salpingo-oophorectomy
Uterine sarcomas are rare tumours and account for <4% of uterine tumours. A recognized risk factor is pelvic irradiation. There are three types: leiomyosarcoma, endometrial stromal tumours and mixed müllerian tumours (derived from embryological remnants of the uterus). Management is by radical hysterectomy, with or without lymphadenectomy. Surgery can be curative if the tumour is confined to the uterus; however, sarcomas are highly malignant and have a poor response to chemoradiotherapy. Less than 0.1% of fibroids become malignant, but leiomyosarcoma should be considered if a uterus with the scan appearance of a fibroid rapidly increases in size.

5. D – Radical hysterectomy and bilateral salpingo-oophorectomy
Endometrial cancer is the most common cancer of the female genital tract, occurring most frequently in the over-65s. The majority of tumours are adenocarcinomas (>90%). Risk factors include those related to unopposed oestrogen exposure (e.g. oestrogen-only hormone-replacement therapy, nulliparity and late menopause). The COCP and pregnancy are

protective. Affected women usually present with postmenopausal bleeding (in postmenopausals) and irregular/intermenstrual bleeding or menorrhagia (in premenopausals).

Endometrial tumours spread directly through the myometrium to the cervix and upper vagina. Staging is as follows:

- Stage I: lesion confined to uterus
- Stage II: lesion confined to uterus and cervix
- Stage III: tumour invades through cervix/uterus
- Stage IV: bowel/bladder involvement or distant metastases

Endometrial biopsy (e.g. using a pipelle) helps confirm a diagnosis. Stage I and II tumours are treated with radical hysterectomy and bilateral salpingo-oophorectomy, with or without lymphadenectomy. Adjuvant radiotherapy is used in addition if there is a high risk of recurrence. Stage III disease may require surgical debulking before proceeding with radiotherapy and chemotherapy. Stage IV tumour treatment depends on the site and the symptoms and is often palliative radiotherapy.

Radiotherapy has many side effects, which are easily divided into acute and chronic problems. Acute issues include skin irradiation, dysuria and diarrhoea. More chronic side effects are urinary frequency, vaginal dryness and dyspareunia.

THEME 9: DRUG MANAGEMENT OF PREECLAMPSIA

Preeclampsia is a pregnancy-specific condition, characterized by high blood pressure and proteinuria, which occurs after the 20th week of pregnancy and, in rare cases, can progress to eclampsia. Eclampsia describes convulsions due to brain hypoxia, which occurs as a result of oedema and vasospasm. If hypertension develops after 20 weeks without proteinuria, it is known as gestational hypertension. Significant proteinuria is defined as a urinary protein:creatinine ratio >30 mg/mmol or 24-hour urine protein of >300 mg protein. Once proteinuria has been established, there is no need to repeat for further quantification.

Preeclampsia occurs in 5%–7% of pregnancies. It is the most important cause of intrauterine growth restriction in singletons without congenital malformations. It has two peaks of incidence: mothers under 20 years of age and those over 35 years of age. Risk factors include nulliparity, twins/triplets, BMI >35, chronic hypertension, renal disease and a family or previous history of preeclampsia. The aetiology of preeclampsia is unknown.

Symptoms of preeclampsia include headache, blurred vision and epigastric pain (although most cases are asymptomatic). Clinical signs are high blood pressure, hyper-reflexia, proteinuria, vomiting, hepatic tenderness, oliguria and spontaneous bleeding. Clinical indicators of severe disease are cerebral or visual disturbances, abdominal pain, fetal growth restriction, oliguria (urine output <500 mL in 24 hours), impaired liver function tests and thrombocytopenia.

In pregnancy, classification (NICE) of hypertension is as follows:

	Diastolic blood pressure (mmHg)	Systolic blood pressure (mmHg)
Mild	90–99	140–149
Moderate	100–109	150–159
Severe	>110	>160

1. D – Labetalol

The ultimate treatment of preeclampsia for the mother is delivery. This obviously may not be in the best interests of the fetus, so safe measures are used to prolong pregnancy. The decision to induce labour or consider emergency caesarean section should be made with consultant input. Factors to consider include severity of disease, fetal maturity, maternal and fetal condition and cervical status.

All patients who develop preeclampsia should be admitted to hospital, yet only those with moderate/severe hypertension require treatment. First-line medication is labetalol to keep the diastolic blood pressure between 80 and 100 mmHg and the systolic blood pressure less than 150 mmHg. Other medications used are nifedipine and methyldopa.

There are no known adverse effects of labetalol on babies who are breastfed by mothers using this medication.

2. H – Nifedipine

Nifedipine is a calcium channel blocker and vasodilator. This can be used if labetalol is contraindicated or can be added to labetalol if this alone does not control blood pressure.

3. E – Magnesium sulphate

An intravenous infusion of magnesium sulphate is indicated in those at high risk of an eclamptic seizure. Such patients include those with very high, uncontrolled blood pressure, abnormal blood results or symptoms such as headache/epigastric pain, abnormal vision, clonus or hyper-reflexia. This should be done while delivery is planned, as that is the only thing that will 'cure' the preeclampsia. Regular assessment is required of patients on magnesium sulphate, including details of urine output, respiratory rate and reflexes, as rarely toxicity can occur. Infusions must be continued for at least 24 hours after delivery, as women are still at high risk of seizures at this time.

Convulsions in pregnancy require an ABC approach and multidisciplinary coordination. Fits are prevented and also terminated with intravenous magnesium sulphate. Blood pressure is controlled with intravenous antihypertensives. If the fetus is still *in utero*, the mother is stabilized and delivery is expedited with emergency caesarean section. Intensive monitoring is required and a HDU or ICU setting is appropriate.

4. F – Methyldopa

Methyldopa is a centrally acting antihypertensive that stimulates β-adrenergic receptors and decreases total peripheral vascular resistance.

5. D – Labetalol

Labetalol should be avoided in asthmatics as it can cause bronchospasm. Hydralazine acts through an unknown mechanism to vasodilate arterioles and reduce blood pressure. Angiotensin-converting enzyme inhibitors (e.g. ramipril) are avoided in pregnancy and diuretics (e.g. furosemide) are generally not needed in preeclampsia.

THEME 10: INDUCTION AND AUGMENTATION OF LABOUR

1. D – Prostaglandin

Induction of labour (IOL) describes the artificial initiation of labour before its spontaneous onset. Around 15%–25% of pregnancies in the UK require IOL. IOL is considered when the risks to the baby/mother in continuing the pregnancy outweigh the risks of induction. The most common indication is prolonged pregnancy. Research has shown that the risk of stillbirth trebles between 37 and 42 weeks' gestation, to 1 in 1000 pregnancies (so still thankfully quite low). Other risks of prolonged pregnancy are fetal compromise in labour, meconium aspiration and mechanical problems during delivery.

Women are seen in clinic postterm to discuss and offer induction when they progress beyond 41 weeks. They are also offered a 'stretch and sweep' at this time, in which a midwife/doctor does a vaginal examination to gently stretch the cervix and release the membranes manually from the lower segment of the uterus. This is thought to release prostaglandins which cause spontaneous onset of labour.

Bishop observed a natural change in the cervix at the time of labour. In 1964, he devised a scoring system to assess the 'favourability' of the cervix, to assist in predicting whether IOL would be required. A higher score is associated with an easier, shorter induction that is less likely to fail.

Bishop score	0	1	2	3
Dilatation (cm)	0	1 or 2	3 or 4	≥5
Consistency	Firm	Medium	Soft	–
Length of canal (cm)	>2	1–2	0.5–1	<0.5
Position	Posterior	Central	Anterior	–
Station of presenting part (related to ischial spines)	–3	–2	–1 or 0	Below spines

Total score (out of 13): 0–5 unfavourable; 6–13 favourable.

Induction is performed using prostaglandin (gel or tablets) inserted vaginally into the posterior fornix, 6 hours apart, or a small tampon-like device with the prostaglandin embedded into it can be used (the benefit of this method is that if hyperstimulation occurs it can be removed). Induction can be done whether or not membranes have ruptured. Fetal well-being must always be confirmed with CTG before induction, and periodically throughout induction.

NB: augmentation of labour is when a patient is already in labour but progress is slow and requires intervention to increase the speed.

2. B – Caesarean section

Most obstetricians would advise that she should have a further caesarean section, as the risk of uterine rupture with two previous caesarean sections, although currently unknown, is thought to be higher than that for one previous caesarean section (approximately 1:200). The use of prostaglandin and syntocinon is known to increase the risk of uterine rupture by two- to three-fold in those with one previous lower segment caesarean section (LSCS), so with two previous caesarean sections, she would be advised against IOL. Of course, a large part of obstetrics is ensuring maternal choice, so it is important to tell the patient about all the risks involved so she can make an informed decision. We do see people who have a normal delivery following two previous caesarean sections, but it is not routine. After a decision has been made, it might be an idea to discuss with this patient her thoughts for contraception, as a bilateral tubal ligation could be performed at caesarean section.

3. E – Twice-weekly Cardiotocography and ultrasound of liquor volume

These patients must be counselled thoroughly about the risks of postterm pregnancies and labour (see above). Beyond 42 weeks, they are advised to return to the antenatal day unit for twice-weekly CTG and weekly ultrasound scans to check that liquor (amniotic fluid) volume is over 3 cm at the deepest pool and that the Doppler of umbilical arteries is normal. A reduced liquor volume is indicative of placental insufficiency.

4. G – Oxytocin infusion

'Normal' progress of labour is cervical dilatation of at least 2 cm every 4 hours, and if this does not occur, a 'delay in the first stage' can be diagnosed. The first course of action is to perform an amniotomy (i.e. 'break the waters') which means you pop the bag of membranes around the baby using a small hook on vaginal examination. If this has already been done or the membranes have already ruptured, an oxytocin infusion can be started (which is a synthetic version of the natural oxytocin produced by the body).

5. A – Artificial rupture of membranes

This patient should be transferred to the delivery suite for artificial rupture of membranes (ARM), as she has now required a third dose of prostaglandin but is still not in labour. ARM is considered when patients have a favourable cervix (Bishop score >5) and some uterine activity. ARM is performed under aseptic conditions with an amnihook or Kocher's forceps, and the membranes should be swept back to induce prostaglandin release. After ARM, some women will spontaneously commence labour, but most require augmentation with an oxytocin infusion, on the instruction of medical staff. High-risk patients, such as those with previous caesarean sections, should be discussed with the registrar or consultant.

Complications of induction and augmentation of labour include the following:

- Failure – this requires operative delivery.
- Uterine hyperstimulation (>7 contractions/15 minutes) – this can cause maternal and fetal distress. An oxytocin infusion must be stopped, and continuous monitoring is needed. Tocolysis (suppression of contractions) can be used, but if there is suspicion of fetal compromise, delivery maybe considered.
- Nausea, vomiting and diarrhoea – these are systemic side effects of prostaglandins.
- Uterine rupture.

Toco-, from Greek *tokos* = childbirth.

Midwives complete a partogram, which must be kept accurately to assess progress in labour. Data include demographics (name and date of birth), fetal heart rate, liquor colour, dilatation of the cervix, descent of the head, oxytocin infusion rate, contractions per minute, drugs and intravenous fluids, blood pressure and pulse, urinalysis and temperature. CTG is also recorded to assess fetal well-being. This documentation can quickly illustrate poor progress in labour, primary dysfunctional labour (poor progress in the active phase of labour with slow cervical dilatation) and secondary arrest (when the active phase stops or slows). Early recognition of these events and their complications are crucial. Presumed fetal compromise in labour is the most common reason for medical intervention, and may be indicated by meconium liquor or an abnormal CTG.

Practice Paper 3: Questions

THEME 1: INFECTION IN PREGNANCY

Options

A. Bacterial vaginosis
B. Chickenpox
C. Cytomegalovirus
D. Group B streptococci
E. *Listeria* spp.
F. Parvovirus
G. Rubella
H. *Salmonella* spp.
 I. Toxoplasmosis

For each of the following scenarios, select the most likely underlying infection. Each option may be used once, more than once or not at all.

1. A 34-year-old woman tells you that she had a flu-like illness with a macular rash at around 20 weeks' gestation. She has a child with learning difficulties who is deaf. When he was a baby, he underwent a heart operation.
2. A 24-year-old woman is very concerned that she had severe gastroenteritis in the 28th week of her pregnancy, which she attributed to poorly cooked eggs. She has delivered what appears to be a healthy baby.
3. A 27-year-old woman of 32 weeks' gestation was admitted to hospital 4 weeks ago with fever, headache and abdominal pain. She has just delivered a stillborn baby. On further questioning, she admitted to eating unpasteurized French cheese 6 weeks ago.
4. A 32-year-old woman is in labour. She is receiving antibiotics to treat an infection that was picked up on swabs she had taken during an admission 4 weeks previously. The antibiotics, she has been told, are for the benefit of the baby.
5. A baby is in special care with dermatomal skin scarring, neurological defects, limb hypoplasia and eye defects. The mother reports having had a vesicular rash over her trunk and legs at 16 weeks' gestation.

THEME 2: FEMALE ANATOMY

Options
A. Ampulla
B. Ascending colon
C. Bladder
D. Broad ligament
E. Cervix
F. Fimbriae
G. Hepatic vein
H. Inferior vena cava
I. Infundibulum
J. Ligament of the ovary
K. Pouch of Douglas
L. Right renal vein
M. Round ligament of the uterus
N. Suspensory ligament of the ovary
O. Uterine vein

For each of the following descriptions, select the most appropriate anatomical structure. Each option may be used once, more than once or not at all.

1. The venous drainage of the right ovary.
2. A relation of the posterior vagina.
3. This is made up of, in part, the mesovarium.
4. This is the longest and broadest part of the fallopian tube.
5. This ligament attaches to the medial side of the ovary and passes to the lateral side of the uterus posteroinferior to the uterotubular junction.

THEME 3: OBSTETRIC EMERGENCIES

Options

A. Cervical shock
B. Cord prolapse
C. Deep vein thrombosis
D. Disseminated intravascular coagulation
E. Shoulder dystocia
F. Uterine inversion
G. Uterine rupture

For each of the following scenarios, select the most appropriate obstetric emergency that the mother is at risk of. Each option may be used once, more than once or not at all.

1. A 32-year-old primigravida woman, who is 34 weeks pregnant, presents to the emergency department with severe, constant lower abdominal pain associated with heavy vaginal bleeding. On examination, the uterus is rigid. Maternal observations are pulse 120 beats/minute, blood pressure 90/60 mmHg. The mother looks pale and feels dizzy.
2. A 28-year-old woman, who has had five children, attends the antenatal clinic for a routine ultrasound scan which finds a normally grown baby with cephalic presentation. The midwife informs her that she has a fundal placenta.
3. A 35-year-old woman, who has gestational diabetes, attends the antenatal clinic for a routine ultrasound scan. She is told that her baby is large for its gestational age.
4. A 24-year-old woman has an artificial rupture of membranes for failure of progression of labour.
5. A 25-year-old woman is having her labour induced using prostaglandin and oxytocin infusion as she is term + 12. She has a previous child born by caesarean section.

THEME 4: CONTRACEPTION

Options

A. Doxycycline
B. Cerazette (desogestrel)
C. Depo-Provera (medroxyprogesterone acetate)
D. Nexplanon
E. Levonelle (levonorgestrel)
F. Lisinopril
G. Microgynon (levonorgestrel, ethinylestradiol)
H. Mirena
I. EllaOne (ulipristal acetate)
J. Rifampicin

For each of the following scenarios, select the most appropriate medication. Each option may be used once, more than once or not at all.

1. A 25-year-old woman attends the early morning GP clinic. She had unprotected intercourse the night before last and is requesting a tablet to stop her from becoming pregnant. She was taking the progesterone-only pill but ran out 1 week ago, and would like to continue this afterwards.

2. A 29-year-old woman is requesting long-term contraception but she does not like the idea of having anything 'left inside her body'. She thinks she will forget to take the pill. She works full-time and finds it hard to get to the clinic.

3. A 37-year-old smoker is requesting oral contraception. She has no significant past medical history.

4. When counselling patients on using combined oral contraception, you must inform them that this drug decreases the effectiveness of both combined and progesterone-only oral contraceptives by hepatic enzyme induction.

5. A 41-year-old wishes for a reliable long-acting reversible contraception. She has a body mass index (BMI) of 35 and has heavy and painful periods. She is requesting a method that will reduce the bleeding during her periods.

THEME 5: POSTPARTUM HAEMORRHAGE

Options

A. Atonic uterus
B. Cervical tear
C. Disseminated intravascular coagulation
D. High vaginal spiral tear
E. Infection
F. Perineal trauma
G. Retained placenta

For each of the following descriptions, select the most appropriate answer. Each option may be used once, more than once or not at all.

1. This is the most common cause of primary postpartum haemorrhage.
2. This is the most common cause of secondary postpartum haemorrhage.
3. Carboprost can be used in the management of this condition.
4. A B-lynch brace suture can be used in the management of this condition.
5. Non-rotational forceps delivery increases the likelihood of this complication.

Options

A. Colposcopy
B. Hysterectomy
C. Repeat in 6 months
D. Repeat in 4 months
E. Repeat in 1 year
F. Repeat in 3 years
G. Repeat in 5 years
H. Urgent colposcopy

For each of the following scenarios, select the most appropriate management plan. Each option may be used once, more than once or not at all.

1. A 30-year-old woman attends her GP clinic for a smear test. Cytology returns showing borderline changes and is negative for human papillomavirus.
2. A 30-year-old woman attends her GP clinic for a smear test. Cytology returns showing moderate dyskaryosis.
3. A 32-year-old woman, who is HIV positive, attends her GP clinic for a smear test. Cytology confirms a normal smear.
4. A 35-year-old woman was found to have grade 3 cervical intraepithelial neoplasia, and has a large loop excision of the transformation zone.
5. A 35-year-old woman presents to her GP with 3 months of postcoital bleeding after starting a new relationship. On speculum examination, she has an abnormal cervix. She has never had a smear test performed.

THEME 7: MECHANISMS OF LABOUR

Options

A. Descent
B. Effacement
C. Engagement
D. Extension
E. External rotation (restitution)
F. Flexion
G. Internal rotation
H. Resolution

For each of the following descriptions, select the most appropriate term. Each option may be used once, more than once or not at all.

1. This term refers to when the maximum diameter of the head has passed through the pelvic brim.
2. This is required for easy passage into the mid-cavity of the pelvis.
3. The levator ani muscle helps the head move into an occipitoanterior position by this movement.
4. This movement occurs with delivery of the head.
5. This term describes the way that the head moves into alignment with the shoulders before they are delivered.

THEME 8: COMPLICATIONS OF CAESAREAN SECTION

Options

A. Aspiration pneumonia
B. Aspiration pneumonitis
C. Endometritis
D. Fetal head compression
E. Pleurisy
F. Pulmonary embolism

G. Retained products of conception
H. Spontaneous pneumothorax
I. Urinary tract infection
J. Urinary tract injury
K. Uterine rupture

For each of the following scenarios, select the most appropriate diagnosis. Each option may be used once, more than once or not at all.

1. A 37-year-old woman had an elective lower segment caesarean section (LSCS) 1 day ago. You are called to see her as she has become short of breath with left-sided chest pain and a cough. She has had three other children, two of these born by LSCS. She has a BMI of 37. On examination, she has reduced air entry at both lung bases. Her observations include saturations 92% in air, blood pressure 105/84 mmHg, pulse 120 beats/minute and temperature 37.4°C.

2. You are called to see a 30-year-old woman 24 hours after a LSCS as she has had two previous caesarean sections. She has continued to pass only very small amounts of blood-stained urine since her operation and has increasing lower abdominal pain. She denies any urinary symptoms preoperatively. On examination, she appears well, with a temperature of 37.0°C, blood pressure 115/73 mmHg, pulse 86 beats/minute and saturations 97% in air. Her abdomen is distended with lower abdominal pain. Bowel sounds are not audible. She has normal urea and electrolytes.

3. A 25-year-old woman had an LSCS 24 hours ago for fetal distress. She now complains of vaginal bleeding that is becoming heavier and increasing lower abdominal discomfort. Observations include saturations 98% in air, blood pressure 124/82 mmHg, pulse 84 beats/minute and temperature 38.8°C. The midwife tells you the patient had spontaneous rupture of membranes for 36 hours prior to delivery.

4. A 28-year-old woman at 39 + 4 gestation is in labour. She develops abdominal pain and a heart rate of 125 beats/minute. Blood pressure is 100/42 mmHg, temperature 37.2°C and saturations 99% in air. On examination, her lower abdomen is exquisitely tender. The cardiotocography, which was previously normal, now shows a prolonged deceleration. She has had one previous LSCS for a breech baby.

5. The woman in Case 4 becomes acutely short of breath in the recovery bay and is coughing after a general anaesthetic. On auscultation, she has reduced air entry at the right lung base and diffuse wheeze. Observations include a heart rate of 88 beats/minute, blood pressure 112/76 mmHg, temperature 37.8°C and saturations 91% in air.

THEME 9: GYNAECOLOGICAL MALIGNANCIES

Options
A. Cervix
B. Endometrium
C. Fallopian tube
D. Ovary
E. Vagina
F. Vulva

For each of the following descriptions, select the most appropriate site of the malignancy. Each option may be used once, more than once or not at all.

1. Lichen sclerosus is a predisposing factor of this malignancy.
2. This is the most common cause of gynaecological cancer death in the UK.
3. There is an effective screening programme for the precursor of this cancer.
4. Type 2 diabetes is a risk factor for this malignancy.
5. Presentation of this tumour can include intermittent abdominal pain, which is relieved following a sudden watery discharge.

THEME 10: THE INFERTILITY CLINIC

Options

A. Anorexia nervosa
B. Asherman's syndrome
C. Hyperprolactinaemia
D. Hypogonadotropic hypogonadism
E. Iatrogenic amenorrhoea
F. Mayer–Rokitansky–Küster–Hauser syndrome
G. Polycystic ovary syndrome
H. Premature ovarian failure
 I. Primary ovarian failure
 J. Sheehan's syndrome
K. Turner's syndrome

For each of the following presentations at the infertility clinic, select the most appropriate underlying diagnosis. Each option may be used once, more than once or not at all.

For reference ranges, see Answers.

1. A 35-year-old woman with a BMI of 26 presents with subfertility. Previously, she had a 28-day menstrual cycle, but her last period was 1 year ago. She has had no recent change in weight and no previous surgery, and is having regular intercourse. Her blood tests show follicle-stimulating hormone (FSH) 35 U/L, luteinizing hormone (LH) 15.1 U/L, estradiol 102 pmol/L, prolactin 100 U/L, sex hormone-binding globulin (SHBG) 42 nmol/L and thyroid-stimulating hormone (TSH) 3.2 mU/L. An ultrasound scan is normal with small ovaries. A pregnancy test is negative. A further FSH test done 6 weeks prior to these tests showed a result of 34 U/L.

2. A 34-year-old woman is referred with secondary infertility. She has been trying to have another baby for 2 years. She has a menstrual cycle of 35–50 days. Her BMI is 39. She has no other symptoms. She has had one normal delivery. Blood tests (day 3) show FSH 6 U/L, LH 20 U/L, testosterone 5 nmol/L, estradiol 358 pmol/L, SHBG 15 nmol/L and TSH 3.2 mU/L.

3. A 36-year-old woman attends the infertility clinic with her partner. She complains of 'deep' pelvic pain on intercourse and a failure to conceive in the last 2 years. She has had one previous miscarriage which required a suction evacuation under anaesthetic and she says she developed a severe uterine infection following this. Since this procedure, she only gets very scanty amounts of bleeding during her periods. Her last smear was normal. Blood tests (day 3) show FSH 3.1 U/L, LH 7 U/L, estradiol 305 pmol/L and day 21 progesterone 40 nmol/L.

4. A 32-year-old woman attends a follow-up appointment for oligomenor-rhoea. She is obviously hirsute, with scarring from acne on her face. She

has a 7-year-old son, delivered with forceps following a induction for gestational diabetes. Her BMI is 30. Her ultrasound scan shows increased ovarian volume and the presence of multiple small follicles.

5. A 23-year-old nulliparous woman is concerned about her periods and her lack of ability to conceive. She previously had regular periods and her BMI was 22. She is now training for a marathon and her weight has dramatically reduced. She is struggling with work and is always stressed out. She now says her last period was 8 months ago. Her pregnancy test is negative. She informs you she has no interest in sexual intercourse. Blood tests show FSH 1.2 U/L, LH 3 U/L and estradiol 94 pmol/L.

Practical Paper 3: Answers

THEME 1: INFECTION IN PREGNANCY

1. G – Rubella

Rubella is a viral infection spread by person-to-person contact. It has an incubation period of 14–21 days. Rubella is now rare thanks to the MMR vaccine. Women develop a non-specific, flu-like illness with a macular rash covering their trunk (20%–50% of infections are asymptomatic). Viral culture or serological antibody testing confirms diagnosis. There is an 80% risk of infection to the fetus if rubella develops in the first trimester, dropping to 25% at the end of the second trimester. Teratogenic effects are worse at earlier gestations. The characteristic abnormalities from congenital rubella syndrome include sensorineural deafness, cataracts, congenital heart disease, learning difficulties, hepatosplenomegaly and microcephaly.

Rubella is also known as German measles because the first three reported cases were described by German physicians, who all thought that the condition was a variant of measles.

2. H – *Salmonella* spp.

This Gram-negative bacterium is found in raw or partially cooked eggs, raw meat and chicken. Incubation time is 12–72 hours. Pregnancy increases the incidence and severity of symptoms of gastroenteritis. There are no adverse effects of maternal gastroenteritis on the fetus as long as the mother remains well hydrated.

3. E – *Listeria* spp.

The Gram-positive coccus *Listeria monocytogenes* is found in soil, animal faeces and certain contaminated foods, including soft cheese, ice cream, unpasteurized milk, raw meat and vegetables. The incubation period is 3–70 days. The incidence and severity of infection are increased in pregnancy. Symptoms include fever, headache, malaise, backache, abdominal pain, pharyngitis and conjunctivitis. Diagnosis is by blood cultures or placental/neonatal swabs. Treatment is with high-dose penicillin. *Listeria* infection during pregnancy can lead to miscarriage, stillbirth, preterm delivery and neonatal listeriosis, which carries a 50% mortality rate.

4. D – Group B streptococci

One-quarter of women have group B streptococcal vaginal colonization at some stage of their pregnancy. It is asymptomatic to the mother and generally only picked up incidentally on vaginal swabs taken for other reasons. It results in 1 in 65 of all neonatal deaths by causing overwhelming neonatal infection. If group B streptococcal infection is picked up on routine swabs, antibiotics should be given during labour to reduce neonatal infection. There is currently no national screening programme for group B streptococci in the United Kingdom.

5. B – Chickenpox

Chickenpox, caused by the varicella zoster virus (human herpesvirus 3), is spread via the airborne route. It has an incubation period of 3–21 days. Around 3 in 1000 pregnancies are affected. 90% of women are immune due to previous infection, which can be checked on booking bloods. If exposed to the virus, the non-immune pregnant woman should be offered varicella zoster virus immunoglobulin to reduce the chance of developing chicken pox.

If affected, a prodromal malaise and fever develops, followed by an itchy vesicular rash. Diagnosis is clinical and women should be advised to avoid other pregnant women. Acyclovir should be offered if the woman presents within 24 hours of developing the rash and she is at over 20 weeks' gestation; otherwise, treatment is supportive. The sequelae of maternal infection can be more serious compared to the general population, with a 10% risk of pneumonia and 1% mortality rate.

The fetus is at risk (1%–2%) of developing fetal varicella syndrome, particularly if infection occurs before 20 weeks, which involves dermatomal skin scarring, neurological defects, limb hypoplasia and eye defects.

Toxoplasmosis

Toxoplasma gondii is a protozoan parasite that comes from unwashed fruit and vegetables, raw/cured/poorly cooked meat, unpasteurized goats' milk, or contamination from soil or cat faeces. The incidence is 2 in 1000 pregnancies. 30% of women are immune due to previous infection. It is rare for mothers to display clinical features, although some develop flu-like symptoms. Treatment is with spiramycin. Fetal infection occurs in 40% of cases, with the majority occurring at higher gestations (severity is greatest at lower gestations). Fetal effects of *Toxoplasma* infection are miscarriage, stillbirth, hydrocephalus, deafness and blindness. Fetal infection can be diagnosed by amniocentesis or cordocentesis.

Cytomegalovirus

Cytomegalovirus affects 3 in 1000 live births. It is transmitted through urine, saliva and other bodily products. Maternal infection is typified by mild fever and malaise, after a 3- to 12-week incubation period. Diagnosis is confirmed by virology of bodily fluids. There is no treatment and therefore there is no benefit to screening. Fetal infection can be diagnosed using amniocentesis or cordocentesis. Around 10%–15% of infected fetuses are symptomatic at birth, showing chorioretinitis, microcephaly, skin rash, hepatosplenomegaly, jaundice and low birth weight. Consequences later in life include learning difficulties, visual impairment, progressive hearing loss or psychomotor impairment.

Parvovirus

Parvovirus B19 infection is spread by respiratory droplets, with an incubation period of 18 days. It is often seen in outbreaks at schools and manifests in children as erythema infectiosum – a 'slapped-cheek' appearance. Erythema infectiosum is also known as 'fifth's disease' – so called because it is the fifth of the six classic childhood skin rashes (the others being measles, chickenpox, rubella, scarlet fever and roseola infantum). In adults, parvovirus infection is often asymptomatic but can present with fever, malaise, arthralgia and a less marked rash. Among pregnant women with parvovirus infection, fetal death is seen in 9%. The second trimester holds the highest risk of fetal infection. The fetal sequelae are non-immune hydrops due to chronic haemolytic anaemia and myocarditis. *In utero* blood transfusion of hydropic fetuses may prevent demise. There are no long-term sequelae among survivors.

Parvovirus B19 is so called since it was first discovered in well B19 (row B, column 19) of a large series of Petri dishes.

THEME 2: FEMALE ANATOMY

1. H – Inferior vena cava
Venous drainage of the ovaries starts with the pampiniform plexus – a mass of veins in the broad ligament in close proximity to the ovary. The pampiniform plexus drains into a single ovarian vein, which leaves the pelvic cavity to journey upwards alongside the ovarian artery. The right ovarian vein drains directly into the vena cava. The left ovarian vein drains into the left renal vein and ultimately into the vena cava.

The ovarian arteries arise directly from the abdominal aorta, descend along the posterior abdominal wall, cross the external iliac arteries at the pelvic brim and enter the suspensory ligament of the ovary.

Pampiniform, from Latin *pampinus* = tendril (a thread-like structure of climbing plants used for support and attachment).

2. K – Pouch of Douglas
The relations of the vagina are as follows:

- Posteriorly (superior to inferior): pouch of Douglas, rectum, anal canal
- Laterally: levator ani, visceral pelvic fascia, ureters
- Anteriorly: base of the bladder, urethra

James Douglas, Scottish anatomist and physician (1675–1742).

3. D – Broad ligament
The broad ligament, rather than being a thin tube-like structure, is instead a double layer of peritoneum (continuous with the abdominal

peritoneum), which hangs suspended by the uterus, fallopian tube, ovary and other ligaments. The organs by which it is suspended divide the broad ligament up into its different sections:

- Uterus: mesometrium (the major part of the broad ligament)
- Uterine tube: mesosalpinx
- Ovary: mesovarium

The broad ligament also covers the ligament of the ovary, the suspensory ligament of the ovary and the round ligament of the uterus. It extends from the sides of the uterus to the lateral walls and floor of the pelvis, and assists in keeping the uterus in position.

4. A – Ampulla

Starting laterally, the parts of the fallopian tube are as follows: the infundibulum, ampulla, isthmus and uterine part. The infundibulum is the funnel-shaped distal end of the tube. It opens into the peritoneal cavity through a 2 mm gap at its base (the abdominal ostium). There are fimbriae (finger-like projections) at the end of the infundibulum, which aid the movement of the ovum into the fallopian tube. The ampulla is the longest and widest part and is where fertilization occurs. The isthmus enters the uterine horn and is thick walled. Finally, the uterine part of the fallopian tube passes through the uterine wall (intramural) and terminates in the uterine ostium to enter the uterine cavity.

> Infundibulum, from Latin *infundibulum* = funnel.
> Ampulla, from Latin *ampulla* = flask.
> Isthmus, from Greek *isthmus* = a connecting band (often used to describe a narrow strip of land that connects two larger land masses, like the Isthmus of Panama connecting the Americas).

5. J – Ligament of the ovary

The ligament of the ovary attaches to the medial aspect of the ovary and passes to the lateral edge of the uterus, posteroinferior to the uterotubular junction. It lies posterosuperiorly between the layers of the broad ligament to form the medial part of the mesovarium.

The round ligament of the uterus is a fibromuscular cord. This attaches anteroinferiorly to the uterotubular junction, lies anteroinferiorly between the layers of the broad ligament and travels to the lateral pelvic wall. It crosses the external iliac vessels and is transmitted, via the inguinal canal, to the subcutaneous tissue of the labium majus. The round ligament is the remnant of the fetal gubernaculum. The suspensory ligament of the ovary is part of the broad ligament (lateral part of the mesovarium). It connects the distal end of the ovary to the lateral wall of the pelvis and contains the ovarian vessels, lymphatics and nerves that run to and from the ovary.

1. D – Disseminated intravascular coagulation

This woman has presented with placental abruption, a complication that occurs in 1% of pregnancies. Placental abruption is when all or part of the placenta separates from the uterus before delivery. Abruption can be described as 'revealed' (visible *per vagina* blood loss) or 'concealed' (blood remains behind the placenta). Features include painful antepartum haemorrhage, a tender, 'woody-hard' uterus, maternal shock and fetal distress. Management includes ABC and urgent caesarean section if there is fetal distress. Complications of abruption include fetal death, postpartum haemorrhage (PPH) and disseminated intravascular coagulation (DIC).

DIC is a secondary event that involves pathological activation of coagulation pathways. The underlying condition leads to the local activation of coagulation mechanisms, which leads to widespread intravascular coagulation. This causes consumption of coagulation factors and platelets, leading to continued bleeding and additionally fibrin deposition, causing ischaemic organ damage. Obstetric conditions associated with DIC are antepartum haemorrhage/PPH, placental abruption, amniotic fluid embolism, preeclampsia/eclampsia and HELLP syndrome.

Clinical findings include generalized bleeding with end organ damage. A very abnormal coagulation screen is seen (increased prothrombin and activated partial thromboplastin times, reduced fibrinogen and low platelets) and a senior haematologist should be involved in the management. Management is two-fold: stop the bleeding and resuscitate with blood products. Replacement blood, fresh frozen plasma, cryoprecipitate and platelets may all be used. HDU- or ICU-level care may be required.

2. F – Uterine inversion

A fundal placenta lies at the most superior part of the uterus (i.e. at the top of the 'bump') and is a risk factor for uterine inversion, as is multiparity. Uterine inversion is a rare but serious complication often occurring as a result of mismanagement of the third stage of labour. It occurs when the uterine fundus has prolapsed into the uterine cavity (incomplete inversion) or even through the cervix/vulva (complete inversion), and often results from excessive cord traction or rapid decompression of the uterus. Patients suffer extreme abdominal pain with associated haemorrhage and circulatory collapse. Immediate replacement of the uterus to its anatomical position should be attempted by Johnson's manoeuvre: the fundus is cupped in the hand and pressure is applied in the direction of the posterior fornix to replace its position, and is held in place until a contraction occurs. Intravenous (IV) oxytocin can then help to maintain uterine contraction and allow the cervix to reform. Other methods to replace the uterus include hydrostatic measures or laparotomy. It is generally better to avoid the complication altogether by always using only gentle controlled cord traction with counter-traction on the uterus to deliver the placenta.

3. E – Shoulder dystocia

'Large for gestational age' (LGA) refers to babies above the 90th centile for weight at any gestational age. Macrosomia refers to fetuses with a weight of >4500 g. Factors predisposing to macrosomia include diabetes, obesity, multiparity, previous LGA baby, male fetus and large maternal stature. In diabetic mothers, high levels of glucose can cross the placenta and lead to macrosomia.

Delivery complications of macrosomic babies are failure to progress (with a higher requirement for caesarean section) and shoulder dystocia. This happens when the shoulders of the large baby become impacted on the symphysis pubis in the anteroposterior diameter. Even though the head of the baby has been delivered, the baby is unable to breathe due to compression of the thorax, so immediate action is required before the baby suffers from complications of asphyxia. A warning sign is when delivery of the chin is delayed or the head appears to recede following delivery. The woman is put into the McRobert's position (lying flat on her back with her knees pulled up to her shoulders) and suprapubic pressure is applied to push the fetal shoulder just above the symphysis pubis. These actions are usually successful, but if not, attempts can be made to deliver the posterior arm first in a diagonal diameter or to rotate the baby. More drastic alternatives are performed only when other methods have not been successful, including breaking the baby's clavicles or performing a symphysiotomy by incising the symphysis pubis under local anaesthetic. Trauma to the baby is common, including Erb's palsy and hypoxia.

4. B – Cord prolapse

Cord prolapse is when the umbilical cord passes through the cervix after the membranes rupture. It can occur with spontaneous or artificial rupture of membranes. It is more common in malpresentation such as breech or transverse lie, but can occur with a high head in cephalic presentation. The diagnosis is made when there are signs of fetal distress and the cord can be palpated in the vagina. Management is by immediate delivery, but while preparations for this are being made, the pressure must be taken off the umbilical cord. The mother assumes the 'all-fours' position (crawling position with her bottom up and her chest lowest) which uses gravity to stop the fetus from compressing the cord. Alternatively, the presenting part can be pushed upwards with two fingers of the examining hand, to relieve compression of the cord and to prevent cord spasm (both of which compromise fetal oxygen supply). If significant delay is expected (e.g. in the community), 500 mL of fluid via a catheter can be inserted into the bladder to aim for the same effect. Emergency caesarean section is performed unless the cervix is fully dilated and an instrumental or spontaneous delivery can be performed just as quickly.

5. G – Uterine rupture

Uterine rupture, along the previous uterine scar, in vaginal birth after caesarean section occurs in 22–74 per 10,000 cases, compared to virtually nil in those who do not labour and have a planned repeat section. The use of oxytocin to induce labour in a woman with a previous section increases the risk to 80 per 10,000, and prostaglandin administration increases the risk to 240 per 10,000. For more details on uterine rupture, see 'Complications of caesarean section', Theme 8, Paper 3.

THEME 4: CONTRACEPTION

1. E – Levonelle (levonorgestrel)

This is the most commonly used 'morning-after pill'. It is most effective when taken as soon as possible after unprotected sexual intercourse (UPSI), but can be used up to 72 hours later. It has no interactions with the progesterone-only pill (POP), unlike EllaOne. The patient must be told to return if she vomits within 2 hours of taking the tablet, that the next period may be early or late, that barrier protection should be used for 7 days and to seek medical attention if she experiences symptoms suggesting pregnancy (failure rates increase up to 72 hours after UPSI). The only contraindication is porphyria. Side effects are menstrual irregularities, nausea, lower abdominal pain, fatigue, headache, dizziness, breast tenderness and vomiting.

EllaOne

This is a new selective progesterone receptor modulator, licensed for emergency contraception up to 120 hours after unprotected intercourse or contraceptive failure. It inhibits or delays ovulation. It has been found to be at least as effective as progesterone-only emergency pills in some trials, but is of greater cost. Its side-effect profile is similar to Levonelle. Because it binds to progesterone receptors, it will reduce the efficacy of progesterone-containing contraceptives for the rest of the cycle. It should not be used in women taking medication to increase gastric pH (e.g. antacids or proton pump inhibitors).

2. C – Depo-Provera (medroxyprogesterone acetate)

Depo-Provera is a long-acting progesterone given by intramuscular injection, which lasts for 12 weeks, and is over 99% effective. It inhibits ovulation, thickens cervical mucus to prevent sperm reaching an egg and thins the lining of the womb to prevent implantation. It may protect against endometrial cancer and offers some protection from pelvic inflammatory disease. Depo-Provera is not affected by other medicines. Women must be counselled that there can be up to a 1 year delay in return to normal fertility. Up to 70% of women are amenorrhoeic at 1 year of use. Side effects include irregular periods, weight gain, headaches, acne, mood changes and breast tenderness. Breast cancer within the last

5 years is a contraindication, and caution must be used with significant cardiovascular disease, unexplained vaginal bleeding, molar pregnancy within the last 5 years, liver adenoma and diabetes with complications (nephropathy, retinopathy or neuropathy).

3. B – Cerazette (desogestrel)

Cerazette is a POP and is suitable for patients where combined pills are contraindicated, such as in this case (see 'Contraindications to contraception' – Paper 2 Answers, Theme 5). The progestogen in the pill thickens cervical mucus to prevent passage of sperm, thins the lining of the womb to prevent implantation and inhibits ovulation. It is up to 99% effective if taken correctly. The advantages are possible cessation of periods, although they can become irregular, and a quick return of fertility on stopping the POP. Disadvantages are the progesterone-related side effects and reduced efficacy with enzyme-inducing drugs. Cerazette is not effective if taken over 12 hours late (3 hours for other POPs) or after vomiting or severe diarrhoea. Contraindications are similar to those of Depo-Provera.

Nexplanon

Nexplanon is a small, flexible rod inserted below the skin of the upper arm that releases progestogen (similar mechanism of action as Depo-Provera). It is over 99% effective and works for 3 years. It can be removed at any time with a resumption of normal fertility. The advantage is that the patient does not have to remember to take contraception. The most frequent side effect is irregular vaginal bleeding; others include mood changes, breast tenderness and acne. Cautions and contraindications are the same as for oral progestogens.

Intrauterine device

The intrauterine device (IUD) is a small copper device which is inserted into the uterine cavity. The copper inhibits fertilization of the ovum and implantation into the endometrium. It is 98%–99% effective. Advantages are that it is long acting, contains no hormones and causes no delayed return to fertility. IUDs can remain *in situ* for 3–10 years depending on the type, but can be removed at any time. They are not affected by other medicines. The disadvantages are that periods may be heavier, longer and more painful, and there is an increased risk of ectopic pregnancy if the IUD fails. Infection risk is increased during the first 3 weeks postinsertion. Screening for existing infection is advised before an IUD insertion. Contraindications for IUDs are severe anaemia, recent sexually transmitted infection, unexplained uterine bleeding, a distorted or small uterine cavity, genital malignancy, active trophoblastic disease, pelvic inflammatory disease, immunosuppression and pregnancy. Contraindications that are specific to copper IUDs are copper allergy and Wilson's disease. IUDs can be used as emergency contraception up to 120 hours after unprotected intercourse.

4. J – Rifampicin

Hepatic enzyme inducers may considerably reduce the effectiveness of combined oral contraceptives and POPs, so additional contraception should be used. Examples of hepatic enzyme inducers include rifampicin, rifabutin, carbamazepine, griseofulvin, modafinil, nelfinavir, nevirapine, oxcarbazepine, phenytoin, phenobarbital, primidone, ritonavir and topiramate. This is an important list to know.

Doxycycline

The advice regarding such non-enzyme-inducing antibiotics and the oral contraceptive pill changed in 2011, and now no additional contraception needs to be advised, unless diarrhoea and vomiting occur.

Lisinopril

Oestrogens antagonize the hypotensive effect of angiotensin-converting enzyme inhibitors, so drugs such as lisinopril or ramipril may not be as effective in women taking the combined pill.

5. H – Mirena

The Mirena coil is a progesterone-only plastic intrauterine system. It is over 99% effective and works for 5 years. Mirena is licensed for contraception, treatment of primary menorrhagia and prevention of endometrial hyperplasia during oestrogen replacement. Advantages are that the patient does not have to remember to take contraception and, as the hormone is locally acting, progestogenic side effects and drug interactions are less frequent. Irregular bleeding is common in the first 3–6 months, but periods usually become lighter and shorter, are usually less painful and may stop completely. There is a minimal risk of infection during the first 3 weeks after insertion, and women are screened for sexually transmitted infections before fitting. Contraindications are the same as for other IUDs.

The progesterone-only pill (POP) or combined oral contraceptive pill (COCP) are not suitable for this patient as she is requesting long-acting reversible contraception (LARC). Mirena is first line for menorrhagia, so it is most suitable for this patient.

THEME 5: POSTPARTUM HAEMORRHAGE

PPH is defined as over 500 mL blood loss from the genital tract in a normal delivery, or less than 500 mL if associated with haemodynamic changes in the mother. Normal blood loss during delivery is 200–300 mL. Primary PPH occurs within 24 hours after birth, and secondary PPH ranges from 24 hours to 6 weeks postpartum. PPH is reported to occur in 5% of deliveries, although blood loss is often underestimated, so it is probably more common. Life-threatening PPH occurs in 1 in 1000 deliveries. Management includes anticipating risk so that preventative measures can be initiated. Resuscitation of the patient must be initiated while simultaneously identifying and treating the cause of the bleeding. Resuscitation includes ABC and aggressive fluid or blood replacement. If coagulopathy develops, a haematologist must be involved.

Causes of primary PPH include atonic uterus, perineal trauma, retained placenta or placental fragments, clotting disorders, uterine inversion, cervical tear, high vaginal tear and uterine rupture. Risk factors include antepartum haemorrhage, previous history of PPH, over-enlarged uterus due to multiple pregnancy, polyhydramnios, macrosomic fetus, fibroids, placenta praevia, prolonged labour, grand multiparity, uterine fibroids, chorioamnionitis and bleeding diathesis.

1. A – Atonic uterus

90% of PPH cases are caused by an atonic uterus. During the third stage of labour, the uterus compresses the intramyometrial blood vessels to stop bleeding. However, in some cases, this does not happen (hence the uterus is described as being atonic). It is more common if there was antenatal over-distention (twins/polyhydramnios), grand multiparity, antepartum haemorrhage, previous PPH, prolonged labour, full bladder or a retained placenta, as its physical presence prevents contraction of the uterus.

2. E – Infection

Infection is the most common cause of secondary PPH, and is often due to retained products of conception. Investigations include a high vaginal swab. All patients should be resuscitated if required and antibiotics administered. If there is significant bleeding, an examination under anaesthetic with evacuation of retained products of conception may be required.

3. A – Atonic uterus

Initial management of PPH (prior to surgical measures) includes emptying the bladder and rubbing up uterine contractions while medications are prepared and administered to contract the uterus. To 'rub up a contraction' means the uterus is massaged through the abdominal wall, or directly if the abdomen is open in theatre, and this will cause it to contract. In an otherwise-uncomplicated labour and pregnancy, the medications used are ergometrine and an infusion of oxytocin. For further persistent bleeding, carboprost (15-methylprostaglandin/Haemobate) can be given intramuscularly into the thigh or the myometrium, and misoprostol can be given *per rectum*.

4. A – Atonic uterus

Following exhaustion of the medical management options for atonic PPH, surgical options are attempted. A B-lynch suture is a uterine compression stitch that opposes the anterior and posterior walls to apply continuing compression. Other surgical approaches include insertion of a uterine balloon, over-sewing the placental bed, uterine artery or internal iliac artery ligation or hysterectomy.

5. F – Perineal Trauma

This can result from tears or from an episiotomy, which is a right mediolateral cut made at the posterior fourchette of the vagina. An episiotomy is usually performed during any instrumental delivery with the aim of avoiding uncontrolled perineal tears. If there is profuse bleeding, vessels can be clamped or packed while definitive repair is achieved. Genital tract injuries are more common after instrumental delivery. A high vaginal spiral tear is more likely to occur with a rotational instrumental delivery, such as with Kielland's forceps. A cervical tear is uncommon but can occur if the cervix was not fully dilated prior to delivery; they can bleed profusely and often need repair in theatre under anaesthetic.

Retained placenta: following delivery, the placenta should be examined for completeness. If retained products are suspected, and there is significant bleeding, manual removal of the placenta or its fragments is required. If this is suspected in a secondary PPH, an ultrasound scan can be used to confirm the diagnosis.

DIC is a possible consequence of a PPH and is the abnormal activation of the clotting cascade, leading to profuse bleeding and end organ damage (see Theme 3 in this paper for more details).

THEME 6: CERVICAL SCREENING

Cervical screening is a test looking for abnormal cells at the cervix. One in 20 women will have an abnormal test, but most will not lead to cancer, and they may return to normal on their own. Since the national screening programme began in the 1980s, the number of cervical cancer cases has reduced by 7% a year. Women are invited to screening every 3 years between 25 and 49 years of age, and every 5 years between 50 and 64 years of age in England, Wales and Northern Ireland. Scotland start screening earlier at 20 years of age and have 3-yearly tests until 60 years of age. Early detection of abnormalities, and treatment if necessary, can prevent up to 75% of cervical cancers.

Changes in the cervical cells are invariably caused by the sexually transmitted human papillomavirus (HPV). There are over 100 types; types 6 and 11 are associated with genital warts, but types 16 and 18 are high risk for cervical cancer and are present in 70% of all cervical cancers. There are 15 high-risk HPV (HR-HPV) serotypes and a HR-HPV triage test is performed on borderline and mildly dyskaryotic smears, and also as a test for cure following excisional treatment.

Samples are taken from the transformation zone of the cervix using a soft plastic brush and are tested using liquid-based cytology, which was implemented in 2008. At colposcopy, areas of cervical intraepithelial neoplasia (CIN) appear as white areas with well-defined edges on application of 5% acetic acid solution. There are also vascular changes typical of CIN seen at colposcopy.

There is vaccine for HPV (Gardasil). It is licensed for use in children of both sexes between 9 and 15 years, and females between 16 and 26 years, to assist in the prevention of cervical and vulval dysplasia and genital warts. These patients still require cervical screening to cover for infection prior to vaccination and the HR-HPV types not covered by the vaccine. Two injections are given, at 0 and 2 months in the <15 years of age cohort. Those >15 years of age at vaccination need another injection at 6 months. Current data suggest that immunity will be long term and it is unlikely that women will need any further boosters. Immunocompromised patients may still be re-infected despite a completed course.

1. F – Repeat in 3 years
If mild or borderline changes are found on a smear, it is then tested for HR-HPV. Because this patient is negative for HR-HPV, she can return for routine screening.

2. A – Colposcopy
A summary of the management of abnormal smears is as follows:

Smear result	HPV result	Action required
Negative – normal smear	Not required	Repeat smear in 3–5 years (routine recall)
Low grade (borderline changes or mild dyskaryosis)	Negative	Repeat smear in 3–5 years (routine recall)
	Positive	Colposcopy
High-grade (moderate or severe dyskaryosis)	Not required	Colposcopy
Glandular dysplasia	Not required	Urgent colposcopy
High-grade dyskaryosis ?invasion	Not required	Urgent colposcopy

If untreated, 20%–30% of women with CIN 3 will develop cervical cancer in the next 10 years. CIN 1 may rarely progress to CIN 2 or 3, but commonly regresses spontaneously or remains a persistent low-grade abnormality.

3. E – Repeat in 1 year
A new diagnosis of HIV should prompt initiation of yearly cervical smears with a colposcopic examination at the time of the first smear. If the patient is on highly active anti-retroviral treatment, this may have some effect on reducing the risk of HPV as well as HIV, but this is not proven, so higher surveillance is required presently.

4. C – Repeat in 6 months
At colposcopy, this woman was found to have abnormal cells, and went on to have a large loop excision of the transformation zone. This is the most common form of treatment, and involves removing the area of abnormal cells. Local anaesthetic is used, and a thin wire is used, heated with an electric current, to remove the area.

A cone biopsy is less frequently performed, which removes a larger area of abnormal cells, and is done under general anaesthetic.

A summary of the management of repeat smear tests after 6 months treatment is as follows:

Repeat smear test results posttreatment (test of cure)	HPV result	Action required
Negative or low grade (borderline changes or mild dyskaryosis)	Negative	Repeat smear in 3–5 years (routine recall)
	Positive	Colposcopy
High-grade (moderate or severe dyskaryosis)	Not required	Colposcopy
Glandular dysplasia	Not required	Urgent colposcopy
High-grade dyskaryosis ?invasion	Not required	Urgent colposcopy

5. H – Urgent colposcopy

This patient has persistent postcoital bleeding and an abnormal-looking cervix which requires investigation. A 'fast-track' 2-week wait referral can be initiated in view of the abnormal appearance of the cervix. She is in a new relationship which is a risk factor for sexually transmitted infections which may actually be the cause of her bleeding, but in view of the fact she has never had a smear, there is a risk of cervical cancer.

Invasive cervical cancer is the sixth most common malignancy in females. It is most common in the 45–55-year age group, and is rare before the age of 20. Cervical cancer occurs mainly in the squamous epithelium, with 75% being squamous cell carcinomas, 20%–25% adenocarcinoma and rarely adeno-squamous carcinoma. Less than 1% are due to melanoma, sarcoma or lymphoma. 80% of patients present with postcoital, intermenstrual or postmenopausal bleeding, and a minority with blood-stained vaginal discharge. Spread can occur to the vagina, pelvic side wall (involving the ureters, bladder or rectum) or via lymphatics to the pelvic nodes. Blood-borne metastases are rare. For more details on the staging and management of cervical tumours, see 'Management of endometrial and cervical cancer' (Paper 2 Answers, Theme 8).

THEME 7: MECHANISMS OF LABOUR

In order to answer these questions, it is important to understand the three stages of labour. A normal spontaneous labour should occur within 12 hours, which is to reduce the risk of complications related to its duration.

The latent first stage of labour is defined as the presence of painful contractions and some cervical change up to 4 cm. The established first stage of labour is when there are painful contractions and cervical dilatation of over 4 cm. The second stage is the time between full dilatation and delivery of the baby. This is initially passive, then active when the woman begins to push, as the fetal head descends towards the perineum. Finally, the third stage is from delivery of the baby to delivery of the placenta. During the second stage of labour, the relationship of the fetal head and body to the maternal pelvis changes to allow ease of passage. The ideal mechanism is with the presentation of a well-flexed fetal head, rotating into an occipitoanterior, vertex presentation for delivery. The vertex refers to the area of skull between the two fontanelles.

1. C – Engagement
This occurs when the largest part of the fetal head enters the brim of the pelvis, which is usually in the occipitotransverse diameter. Do not forget that the pelvic inlet is widest in the transverse diameter, and the outlet in the anterior–posterior diameter. Engagement often occurs before labour. On abdominal examination, engagement is measured as 'fifths' of the head palpable.

Descent is encouraged by uterine contractions, which accelerates when the membranes rupture.

2. F – Flexion
Flexion of the fetal head occurs passively throughout labour. With full flexion, the posterior fontanelle becomes palpable.

3. G – Internal rotation
The sloping inclination of the levator ani muscle encourages internal rotation of the head at the level of the ischial spines. This brings the sagittal suture of the head into the anterior–posterior plane of the pelvis, and the occiput rotates anteriorly towards the symphysis. If resistance occurs at this stage, the head may become engaged in the unfavourable occipitoposterior position. The head may later rotate 180° into a preferable occipitoanterior position. However, if the head remains occipitoposterior and there is extension of the neck, despite good contractions and maternal effort, an instrumental delivery may be required.

4. D – Extension
There is extension at the fetal neck as the occiput passes underneath the symphysis pubis and delivers. Tearing of the perineum can occur at this stage, which can be reduced by shorter, smaller, active pushes at this time and applying support to the perineum with a pad or swab.

5. E – External rotation (restitution)
Once the head is delivered, restitution is the reversal of the twist of internal rotation. This aligns the head with the shoulders, which descend in an oblique position. The shoulders are delivered in the anterior–posterior diameter, with the anterior shoulder delivered first under the symphysis pubis, sometimes with gentle downwards traction, followed by upwards traction for the other shoulder to be delivered.

THEME 8: COMPLICATIONS OF CAESAREAN SECTION

Caesarean sections account for 15%–20% of births in the UK. The lower-segment caesarean section (LSCS) has overtaken the classic midline uterine incision because of a lower complication rate. Indications for LSCS can be maternal (two previous LSCS, placenta praevia, maternal disease or maternal request) or fetal (breech, twin pregnancy if the first twin is not cephalic, fetal distress, cord prolapse or delayed first stage of labour). Complications include haemorrhage, gastric aspiration, infection and thromboembolic disease. LSCS can be performed under general or regional anaesthetic. The patient is positioned supine and tilted 15° to the left, to minimize aortocaval compression. Access to the uterus is via a transverse suprapubic (Pfannenstiel) incision.

Hermann Johannes Pfannenstiel, German gynaecologist (1862–1909).

1. F – Pulmonary embolism
This patient has a number of risk factors for thromboembolism and a pulmonary embolism (PE) is the most likely explanation for her hypoxia on air, low-grade pyrexia and lack of focal chest signs. Investigation is with a chest X-ray, compression duplex Doppler of the deep veins of the legs and, if these are normal, a ventilation-perfusion (V/Q) scan or CT pulmonary angiography (CTPA). A confirmed deep vein thrombosis or PE requires treatment initially with low molecular weight heparin (LMWH) moving onto warfarin when the risk of PPH is reduced. Risk factors for PE include any previous venous thromboembolism (VTE), thrombophilia, increased body mass index, prolonged hospital admission, medical comorbidities (heart or lung disease, systemic lupus erythematosus (SLE), cancer, inflammatory conditions, nephrotic syndrome or sickle cell disease), IV drug use, age >35 years, parity >3, smoker, any surgical procedure in the puerperium, gross varicose veins, systemic infection, immobility, preeclampsia, mid-cavity rotational operative delivery, prolonged labour and PPH.

Do not forget that thromboembolism is one of the leading causes of maternal mortality. The risk in pregnancy is six-times higher than in the general population. This is thought to be due to normal homeostatic changes that reduce the risk of haemorrhage at delivery, including increased clotting factor concentration and reduced fibrinolysis. Guidance to reduce the incidence of thromboembolic events includes the use of compression stockings and heparin prophylaxis for those with risk factors, with early mobilization where possible. All patients have a risk assessment done at booking and at subsequent hospital admissions, and receive advice which may just be early mobilization but can include thromboembolic deterrent stockings (TEDs) or antenatal or postnatal LMWH (incidence of thromboembolic disease 4–16:10,000).

2. J – Urinary tract injury
The close proximity of the urological tract to the uterus makes injury during caesarean section occasional but possible. Bladder injury must

be suspected in this scenario because of the low volume of blood-strained urine and the increasing lower abdominal pain in response to urine in the abdomen. Multidisciplinary care will be required with involvement of urologists (incidence: bladder injury 1:1000; ureteric injury 1:10,000).

3. C – Endometritis

Endometritis is the most likely answer as she is pyrexial and there is the risk factor of infection with prolonged rupture of membranes. Management should include a speculum for high vaginal and cervical swabs, blood cultures and blood tests for inflammatory markers. IV antibiotics should be administered until pyrexia settles for 24 hours as per local protocols. The baby should also be examined for signs of sepsis as it may have been affected by the same bacteria as the mother (incidence of any maternal infection 6:100).

4. K – Uterine rupture

Uterine rupture is an obstetric emergency that requires resuscitation of the mother and immediate delivery of the baby. The incidence of uterine rupture in vaginal birth after previous caesarean section is 35 in 10,000. Uterine rupture is usually associated with scar dehiscence from previous caesarean section (as in this scenario), but primary rupture can occur with obstructed labour, overzealous use of oxytocin, previous perforation during operative procedures and traumatic instrumental deliveries. The main symptoms are pain (abdominal or at the shoulder tip due to peritonism), fetal distress (seen on the cardiotocograph [CTG] as bradycardia), shock, vaginal bleeding or cessation of contractions. After delivery, the uterus is repaired or hysterectomy is performed, depending upon the site and extent of rupture, the woman's condition and parity.

5. B – Aspiration pneumonitis

Aspiration pneumonitis (Mendelson's syndrome) describes an acute lung injury that ensues after sterile gastric contents are inhaled into the lung. By contrast, aspiration pneumonia is an infectious process caused by the inhalation of pharyngeal secretions that are colonized by pathogenic bacteria (this will take longer to develop). Aspiration pneumonitis occurs in 1 in 3000 cases in which general anaesthetic is used and causes 10%–30% of anaesthetic deaths. Risk factors include absence of the gag reflex, difficult intubation, an inadequately emptied stomach, poor oesophageal sphincter tone, sedation and the pregnancy itself. Aspiration, as opposed to PE, is suggested by the findings at the right base and wheeze. To reduce the risk of aspiration pneumonitis, patients are offered drugs to reduce gastric volume (prokinetics; e.g. metoclopramide) and acidity (proton pump inhibitors; e.g. omeprazole) prior to caesarean section.

Curtis Lester Mendelson, American obstetrician and cardiologist (born 1913).

THEME 9: GYNAECOLOGICAL MALIGNANCIES

1. F – Vulva
Lichen sclerosus is a chronic autoimmune condition that is most common in postmenopausal women but can affect any age of both sexes. It causes a loss of collagen, leading to a thin epithelium, and affected lesions appear shiny, white and tight and are itchy or painful. Commonly affected areas are the labia, clitoris, perineum and perianal area. Treatment is with topical steroids. Suspicious areas of lichen sclerosus should be biopsied, as there is a 0%–9% risk of progression to vulval squamous cell carcinoma. Vulval intraepithelial neoplasia has less malignant potential than CIN, so lesions tend to undergo observation.

Vulval cancer accounts for 5% of gynaecological cancers, with a wide presenting age range. 90% are squamous carcinomas, with rarer forms including Bartholin's gland adenocarcinomas and Paget's disease of the vulva (a well-defined scaly, erythematous lesion caused by malignant change in the cells of the epidermal layer). Vulval carcinomas can present with pruritus, bleeding, pain/dyspareunia or a mass. Lesions spread slowly to local tissues, with lymphatic spread to inguinal nodes initially. Treatment varies from wide local excision to radical vulvectomy with bilateral node dissection. Local treatment with radiotherapy or systemic chemotherapy may also be effective.

2. D – Ovary
Ovarian cancer is the most common cause of gynaecological cancer death in westernized society. This is mainly due to its late and often advanced presentation and no current effective population screening. Endometrial cancer is the most common malignancy of the female genital tract.

3. A – Cervix
A very effective cervical screening programme is run to detect the presence of the HPV and changes in the cervix that may lead to cancer if left untreated. Screening is performed every 3 years from age 25 and every 5 years from ages 50–65. A further test called colposcopy is used if abnormalities are detected.

4. B – Endometrium
Endometrial tumours are invariably oestrogen dependent – hence many risk factors involve unopposed oestrogen exposure. Risk factors include exogenous oestrogen use (oestrogen-only hormone replacement therapy – no longer used in women with their uterus still *in situ*), obesity (androgens are converted to oestrogens in the peripheral fat), type 2 diabetes (independent of obesity), hypertension and pelvic irradiation for cervical cancer. Nulliparity and a late menopause are weak risk factors.

5. C – Fallopian tube

Fallopian tube cancer *per se* has been classified as rare, accounting for <0.3% of gynaecological cancers. However, it is now suspected that the majority of cancers that were initially thought to be ovarian are actually tubal in origin, therefore could actually be merged with ovarian cancers in 'tubo-ovarian' cancers. Therefore, these tumours are similar in presentation to ovarian cancers, with 70% being serous carcinomas. 'Hydrops tubae profluens' occurs in 10% of classified fallopian tube malignancies, where intermittent colicky pain settles with a sudden vaginal discharge of watery fluid. Spread is local, via the peritoneum and lymphatics, with metastases being present in around 50% of cases. The treatment options are much the same as for ovarian cancer.

THEME 10: THE INFERTILITY CLINIC

Reference ranges for females in the luteal phase:

Follicle-stimulating hormone	1.2–9 U/L
Luteinizing hormone	<14.7 U/L
Prolactin	53–360 U/L
Thyroid-stimulating hormone	0–5.7 mU/L
Sex hormone-binding globulin	26–110 nmol/L
Estradiol	101–905 pmol/L
Testosterone	0.2–2.9 nmol/L
Day-21 progesterone	>35 nmol/L suggests ovulation

A couple are said to be subfertile if conception has not occurred within 1 year of unprotected sex. Subfertility affects one in seven couples. Subfertility can be primary (where the woman has never conceived) or secondary (where she has previously conceived).

1. H – Premature ovarian failure

This woman has a low–normal estradiol despite a high luteinizing hormone (LH) and FSH. These results suggest premature ovarian failure (POF). Although the average age for the menopause in the UK is 51 years, a diagnosis of POF is only made in women less than 40 years (if the ovaries have never worked, it is termed primary ovarian failure). By the age of 40 years, the prevalence of POF is 1%. Most cases of POF are idiopathic, although a small proportion of patients have underlying disorders such as chromosome abnormalities (Down's syndrome, Turner's syndrome and fragile X syndrome), enzyme deficiencies or autoimmune conditions. Radiotherapy and chemotherapy can also cause premature menopause and of course a surgical menopause occurs if the ovaries are removed. POF occurs as a result of reduced follicle development or increased follicle atresia, and it causes amenorrhoea as well as other menopausal symptoms. *In vitro* fertilization can be performed, but donor eggs would be needed. The woman in this scenario may also need hormone replacement therapy for oestrogen deficiency to protect against osteoporosis.

2. G – Polycystic ovary syndrome

Polycystic ovary syndrome (PCOS; also known as Stein–Leventhal syndrome) is a common gynaecological disorder associated with menstrual disturbance and hyperandrogenism. PCOS can be diagnosed when two or more of the following criteria are present:

• Oligomenorrhoea or amenorrhoea (due to anovulation)
• Clinical or biochemical signs of androgen excess (hirsutism, acne, male pattern balding or high levels of testosterone)
• Ultrasound appearances of the ovaries: >12 follicles measuring 2–9 mm diameter or increased ovarian volume (>10 mL)

Remember that not all women with PCOS have polycystic ovaries on ultrasound scan, and not all women with the appearances of polycystic ovaries have the syndrome.

Diagnosis in this case is made from the oligomenorrhoea and high testosterone with low sex hormone-binding globulin. PCOS is associated with obesity, metabolic syndrome (type 2 diabetes, hypertension, dyslipidaemia, atherosclerosis and ischaemic heart disease) and dermatological conditions (hirsutism, acne and alopecia).

Because this patient is keen to conceive, weight loss is definitely the best initial management, as this may restart ovulation and, if she does become pregnant, a healthy weight means a lower-risk pregnancy. When she reaches a healthy weight, if she is still not ovulating, clomiphene can be considered. Clomiphene is an antioestrogen that occupies oestrogen receptors in the hypothalamus. This encourages ovulation by increasing FSH production. Ovulation is confirmed by a raised day-21 progesterone level. There is a risk of multiple pregnancy with clomiphene.

Michael Leo Leventhal, American gynaecologist (1901–1971).
Irving Freiler Stein, American gynaecologist (1887–1976).

3. B – Asherman's syndrome

Asherman's syndrome is the presence of intrauterine adhesions which can lead to reduction or absence of bleeding at the time of the periods, either because the endometrial lining is destroyed or because the blood is trapped inside as the outflow is blocked by the adhesions. It is caused by damage to the endometrial lining during suction evacuation of the uterus for miscarriage, termination or dilatation and curettage. Hysteroscopy and dissection of scar tissue may be helpful in Asherman's syndrome. Importantly, later in life, because the passage out of the uterus is blocked, postmenopausal bleeding would not be detected, so uterine cancer may be missed.

Joseph C. Asherman, Israeli gynaecologist (born 1889).

4. G – Polycystic ovary syndrome

This patient has more clinically evident symptoms of PCOS, with acne, hirsutism and oligomenorrhoea. Patients with PCOS are more susceptible to diabetes, endometrial cancer and dyslipidaemia (decreased high-density lipoproteins, increased triglycerides and increased low-density lipoproteins). Her ultrasound scan gives the characteristic appearance of polycystic ovaries.

5. D – Hypogonadotropic hypogonadism

Hypogonadotropic hypogonadism is caused by failure of the anterior pituitary to secrete the gonadotropins LH and FSH in order to stimulate ovulation. This is a form of secondary hypogonadism, as the fault is not from the gonads themselves, which may be functioning normally. Hypogonadotropic hypogonadism can be differentiated from POF, which has high gonadotropin levels. In this scenario, it is the excessive weight loss and exercise that has caused the reduction of gonadotrophin-releasing hormone (GnRH) secretion. The advice to this woman would be to normalize her weight and reduce her exercising. High stress levels can also cause a reduction in GnRH secretion.

Secondary amenorrhoea is defined as the absence of menses for 6 months in previously menstruating women. Causes can be divided into the following categories:

- Gonadal failure (POF)
- Pituitary dysfunction (pituitary tumour)
- Psychological causes (stress, travel and weight changes can reduce GnRH)
- Endocrine dysfunction (hypothyroidism)
- Oestrogen metabolism dysfunction (anorexia nervosa)

The most common pituitary tumours are benign adenomas, such as the prolactinoma. The excess prolactin secreted by these tumours inhibits gonadotropin release. Diagnosis of prolactinoma is by magnetic resonance imaging, and this tumour responds to dopamine agonists such as bromocriptine. Hypothyroidism should be screened for in all women with irregular menses and clinically suggestive symptoms. Low thyroxine (T_4) levels reduce negative feedback on the hypothalamic–pituitary axis, resulting in elevated prolactin and thyroid-stimulating hormone levels. In anorexia nervosa, there is less adipose tissue for androgens to be converted to oestrogens, resulting in lower circulating levels of the active metabolite estradiol.

Women can present with primary amenorrhoea as a cause of infertility. Turner's syndrome (45XO) is one of the more common genetic conditions, with an incidence of 1 in 2500 girls. The lack of one X chromosome gives rise to characteristic signs, including short stature and webbing of the neck. The ovaries in Turner's syndrome do not respond to gonadotropic hormones, and patients are almost universally infertile. Woman who present with primary amenorrhoea and infertility, and who have high levels of FSH, should be karyotyped to exclude Turner's syndrome.

Mayer–Rokitansky–Küster–Hauser syndrome (or müllerian agenesis) occurs in 1 in 4500 women and describes a failure of development of the embryonic müllerian ducts. It is characterized by a congenital absence of the uterus, cervix and the upper two-thirds of the vagina. Women have normal external genitalia, a 46XX karyotype and normal secondary sexual characteristics, as the ovaries are intact. These women need psychological support, and dilators or surgery can create a 'neovagina' to allow intercourse.

Practice Paper 4: Questions

THEME 1: METHODS OF DELIVERY

Options

A. Elective caesarean section
B. Emergency caesarean section
C. External cephalic version
D. Rotational forceps – Kielland's
E. Non-rotational forceps – Neville–Barnes
F. Normal delivery

For each of the following scenarios, select the most appropriate method of delivery. Each option may be used once, more than once or not at all.

1. A 30-year-old primigravida woman, with an epidural *in situ* and a delayed second stage, has been pushing for 2 hours and is now exhausted. On examination, the fetus is felt in the occipitoanterior position at 'station plus two'. The cardiotocogram is normal.
2. A 26-year-old woman in the antenatal clinic is at 39 weeks' gestation. She has had a previous classical caesarean section.
3. A 27-year-old woman who is in labour is fully dilated. On examination, a face presentation is felt, with the chin posteriorly.
4. A 32-year-old woman has been fully dilated for 1 hour and pushing for a further hour, but the baby has not yet delivered despite good maternal effort. On examination, the baby is in vertex presentation with an occipitoposterior position.
5. A 29-year-old woman is dilated at 10 cm. On examination, there is an occipitoanterior presentation with a flexed head. She has had one previous lower-segment caesarean section.

THEME 2: UROGYNAECOLOGY

Options

A. Abdominal colposuspension
B. Anterior repair
C. Botulinum toxin A
D. Hormone replacement therapy
E. Indwelling catheter
F. Intermittent self-catheterization

G. Mirabegron
H. Oxybutynin
 I. Periurethral injectables
J. Physiotherapy
K. Sacral nerve stimulation
L. Synthetic mid-urethral tape

For each of the following scenarios, select the next most appropriate management option. Each option may be used once, more than once or not at all.

1. A 56-year-old woman complains of urinary urgency and nocturia. She visits the toilet every hour, and sometimes 'doesn't make it'. She says she has tried 'those tablets that give you a dry mouth and some others that the doctor said worked differently', but has not had any success. She is asking about a day case procedure that will help with her symptoms. She previously had a cystocele repaired.

2. A 55-year-old woman suffers from urinary incontinence on coughing and laughing. She does not suffer from frequency or urgency. She passes urine once in the night. She has had three normal deliveries and a caesarean section, followed by a total abdominal hysterectomy 6 years ago. She smokes 15 cigarettes a day. On examination, she has a body mass index of 38 and has a caesarean section scar. Vaginal examination reveals no masses. She has incontinence on performing a Valsalva manoeuvre.

3. A 53-year-old complains of occasional incontinence. She has nocturia four times a night and passes urine 1–2 hourly. She has tried physiotherapy and bladder retraining without improvement. She has had two normal deliveries, and her menopause was 4 years ago. She has had a previous anterior repair. Apart from some scarring on the anterior vaginal wall, examination is unremarkable.

4. A 60-year-old woman has ongoing difficulties with overactive bladder symptoms. She has tried three different anti-cholinergic medications and has completed her conservative treatments with the urogynaecology nurse specialists. She does not want surgery.

5. A 45-year-old woman who has previously completed a full course of pelvic floor muscle training attends the gynaecology clinic with continuing complaints of leakage of urine when she coughs, laughs or sneezes. She has had urodynamic studies that show stress incontinence with no detrusor overactivity. She would like a minimally invasive effective treatment for stress urinary incontinence.

THEME 3: DRUGS IN PREGNANCY

Options
A. Carbimazole
B. Codeine phosphate
C. Ibuprofen
D. Doxycycline
E. Erythromycin
F. Gabapentin
G. Iodine-131
H. Ondansetron
 I. Promethazine
 J. Propylthiouracil
K. Thalidomide
L. Ursodeoxycholic acid

For each of the following scenarios, select the most appropriate drug. Each option may be used once, more than once or not at all.

1. A 32-year-old pregnant woman is diagnosed with Graves' disease. She expresses to her GP that she wishes to breastfeed and asks whether there is any medications that are safe for her to take.
2. A 24-year-old woman who is 12 weeks pregnant sees her GP complaining of persistent vomiting for several weeks and dizziness. She has 1+ of ketones in her urine and is requesting medication.
3. A 24-year-old woman, who has been complaining of a persistent itch, is diagnosed with obstetric cholestasis.
4. A 28-year-old pregnant woman is found to have pelvic inflammatory disease. The GP is wary that this commonly used antibiotic is contraindicated.
5. A 31-year-old breastfeeding woman requires analgesia following caesarean section. Paracetamol is not completely effective. Choose a suitable analgesic that is normally avoided during pregnancy.

THEME 4: PERIMENOPAUSAL HORMONES

Options

A. 17β-estradiol
B. Androstenedione
C. Follicle-stimulating hormone
D. Luteinizing hormone
E. Oestrone
F. Progesterone

For each of the following descriptions, select the most appropriate hormone. Each option may be used once, more than once or not at all.

1. There is reduced secretion of this hormone by the ovaries during the menopause.
2. This hormone is produced in peripheral adipose tissue.
3. The common precursor of oestrogens.
4. Measurement of this hormone supports the presence of ovulation.
5. A sustained high level of this is supportive of a diagnosis of menopause.

THEME 5: ACUTE PELVIC PAIN

Options

A. Acute appendicitis
B. Appendix abscess
C. Complete miscarriage
D. Corpus luteum cyst
E. Ectopic pregnancy
F. Incomplete miscarriage
G. Missed miscarriage
H. Mittelschmerz
 I. Pelvic inflammatory disease
 J. Threatened miscarriage
K. Torsion of ovarian cyst

For each of the following scenarios, select the most appropriate diagnosis. Each option may be used once, more than once or not at all.

1. A 35-year-old woman presents to the emergency department with sudden-onset severe colicky pain, focused around the left iliac fossa, and vomiting. She describes experiencing intermittent pain in this area over the last few months. Observations include heart rate 112 beats/minute and blood pressure 96/64 mmHg. Speculum examination reveals no *per vagina* bleeding, although there is left adnexal tenderness. A urinary pregnancy test is negative.

2. A 19-year-old student attends the emergency department with generalized abdominal pain and malaise. She complains of increased urinary frequency, a purulent vaginal discharge and pain on intercourse. On examination, her temperature is 38.2°C and there is cervical excitation. A urinary pregnancy test has been requested.

3. A 26-year-old woman presents to the emergency department with generalized cramping pains in her lower abdomen and amenorrhoea for 7 weeks. She feels faint and complains of heavy vaginal bleeding and describes large clots that she has passed. Examination reveals a tender lower abdomen. The cervical os is open and active bleeding is seen. Observations include pulse rate 110 beats/minute and blood pressure 110/64 mmHg. A urinary βhCG test is positive. An ultrasound scan demonstrates some tissue within the uterus.

4. A 25-year-old woman presents with right iliac fossa and shoulder-tip pain that has caused her to collapse. She is sexually active and is using the copper intrauterine device for contraception. On examination, she has a small abdominal mass in the right iliac fossa. There is guarding in this area with but no rebound tenderness. Cervical excitation is present. Observations include pulse rate 125 beats/minute and blood pressure 86/48 mmHg. A FAST scan in accident and emergency shows free fluid in the abdomen. A urinary pregnancy test result is awaited.

5. A 32-year-old woman complains of central abdominal tenderness which has moved to her right iliac fossa. She is sexually active and uses the Mirena coil for contraception. Abdominal examination reveals tenderness in the right iliac fossa with no masses. No abnormality is found on vaginal examination. Observations include pulse rate 110 beats/minute, blood pressure 132/84 mmHg and temperature 38.2°C. A urinary pregnancy test result is awaited.

THEME 6: GAMETOGENESIS

Options

A. Mature oocyte
B. Oogonia
C. Polar body
D. Primary oocyte
E. Primary spermatocyte
F. Primordial germ cell
G. Secondary oocyte
H. Secondary spermatocyte
 I. Spermatid
 J. Spermatogonia
K. Spermatozoa

For each of the following descriptions, select the correct term. Each option may be used once, more than once or not at all.

1. This cell is the starting point of both male and female gametogenesis.
2. This is the end product of spermatogenesis that is involved in fertilization.
3. A male cell that contains 23 single chromosomes prior to spermiogenesis.
4. A male cell that contains 46 double-structured chromosomes.
5. This is the by-product of female gametogenesis.

THEME 7: GENITAL INFECTIONS

Options

A. Bacterial vaginosis
B. Chancroid
C. Chlamydia
D. Genital candidiasis
E. Genital herpes
F. Genital warts
G. Gonorrhoea
H. Granuloma inguinale (Donovanosis)
I. Molluscum contagiosum
J. Scabies
K. Syphilis
L. Trichomoniasis

For each of the following scenarios, select the most appropriate diagnosis. Each option may be used once, more than once or not at all.

1. A 42-year-old man has developed multiple painful ulcers on his penis, with an associated phimosis. On examination, there is inguinal lymph node enlargement and a discharging sinus. A culture demonstrates *Haemophilus ducreyi*.
2. A 23-year-old female student presents with abdominal pain in the right upper quadrant. She has had multiple sexual partners with whom she used no barrier protection. When questioned further, she describes a vague history of dysuria and increased urinary frequency.
3. A 36-year-old woman attends the GP with a grey–white vaginal discharge that she says has a 'fishy' odour.
4. A 34-year-old woman attends the GP complaining of feeling generally unwell. She says that she is tired and mildly feverish, with headaches and an itchy diffuse skin rash. She also complains of pains in her joints. She noticed a painless ulcer on her labia that healed about 5 weeks previously. The last time she was sexually active was 2 months ago.
5. A couple in their 30s visit the GP. The woman works in a nursing home and is complaining of itching all over but particularly on her fingers and wrists, especially at night. Her partner says he developed a similar pattern of itching 3 weeks later, which has now spread to his penis.

THEME 8: TWINS

Options

A. Dizygotic dichorionic diamniotic
B. Dizygotic dichorionic monoamniotic
C. Dizygotic monochorionic monoamniotic
D. Monozygotic dichorionic diamniotic
E. Monozygotic monochorionic diamniotic
F. Monozygotic monochorionic monoamniotic

For each of the following descriptions, select the most appropriate terminology. Each option may be used once, more than once or not at all.

1. These are the most common types of twins.
2. These twins share the same amniotic sac.
3. These twins occur if division occurs at day 5 postfertilization.
4. If twins are of the opposite sex, they must be this type.
5. These are identical twins with a separate chorion, amnion and placenta.

THEME 9: ECTOPIC PREGNANCY

Options

A. Laparoscopy ± salpingectomy
B. Laparoscopy ± salpingotomy
C. Methotrexate injection
D. Repeat βhCG in 48 hours
E. Repeat βhCG in 72 hours
F. Repeat pelvic ultrasound in 48 hours
G. Urgent laparotomy

For each of the following scenarios, select the most appropriate management decision. Each option may be used once, more than once or not at all.

1. A 32-year-old woman, who had her last menstrual period (LMP) 8 weeks ago, returns for review. She presented 4 days ago with light vaginal bleeding, but denied pain. A pelvic ultrasound scan showed an empty uterus and a 2 cm × 1.6 cm echogenic mass adjacent to the left ovary with no free fluid. The hCG at that time was 625 IU/L. She had a repeat blood test at 48 hours (642 IU/L) and again today (630 IU/L). On examination, she is non-tender with blood pressure 116/68 mmHg and pulse 80 beats/min.

2. A 37-year-old woman presents with a 2-day history of sharp right iliac fossa pain and one episode of vaginal spotting. She is unsure of her LMP, but had a positive pregnancy test 1 month ago. Her past obstetric history is G5P3 + 1 (three children born by normal vaginal delivery and one left-sided ectopic 3 years ago). On examination, she has severe right adnexal tenderness, with blood pressure 95/55 mmHg and pulse 106 beats/min. An ultrasound scan shows an empty uterus, significant free fluid in the pouch of Douglas and a 4-cm dilated right fallopian tube. She has no desire to have more children and she was actually booked for sterilization.

3. A 29-year-old woman is referred from the emergency department with severe left iliac fossa pain and dizziness. Her LMP was 8 weeks ago and she has a positive pregnancy test. Past obstetric history is G2P1 (normal vaginal delivery). On examination, she appears unwell, with a blood pressure of 80/42 mmHg and pulse 130 beats/min. She has left iliac fossa tenderness and cervical tenderness on vaginal examination. Pelvic ultrasound done during stabilization shows a left adnexal mass, with a fetal heart beat and significant free fluid.

4. A 27-year-old primiparous woman who has been under investigation with the fertility team has attended with severe right iliac fossa pain and a positive pregnancy test. She is very happy until you inform her following the scan that she has an ectopic pregnancy. Her hCG is 2300 IU/L. She informs you that she had a hysterosalpingogram that showed a

blocked tube on the left side. She insists that she does not want to have to go through *in vitro* fertilization.

5. A 25-year-old woman presents to the emergency department with 3 days of heavy vaginal bleeding which is now settling, and lower abdominal discomfort. She says she has passed some large clots and says she thinks she has had a miscarriage. Her LMP was 6 weeks ago. Blood pressure is 124/80 mmHg and pulse 84 beats/min. She has no pain on examination. Pelvic ultrasound showed an endometrial thickness of 10 mm, with no gestational sac or fetal pole. There is no free fluid or adnexal masses. The βhCG is 841 IU/L.

Options

A. Abdominal circumference
B. Amniotic fluid volume
C. Biophysical profile
D. Head circumference
E. Crown–rump length
F. Femur length
G. Nuchal translucency

For each of the following scenarios, select the most appropriate measurement. Each option may be used once, more than once or not at all.

1. The most accurate parameter for assessment of gestational age in the first trimester.
2. From 14 weeks, this is the most reliable indicator of gestational age.
3. The most sensitive parameter to assess fetal growth and detect intrauterine growth restriction.
4. An abnormality on this test may suggest poorly functioning kidneys.
5. This can provide information regarding fetal neurological status and tone.

Practice Paper 4: Answers

THEME 1: METHODS OF DELIVERY

There is only limited information given in these scenarios. In real situations on the labour ward, many other factors are taken into consideration, including the views and skills of the obstetrician performing the delivery.

1. E – Non-rotational forceps – Neville–Barnes

Forceps are used to aid vaginal delivery, and are likely to be successful in this case as the baby is in a good position but the mother is tired. Forceps have two interlocking blades with a cephalic curve that fits around a baby's head. When correctly applied, they should lock together easily and not be forced. With all instrumental deliveries, a maximum of three contractions should be used to deliver the baby. If it requires more than this, then a caesarean section should be considered. The patient should have adequate analgesia (ideally a spinal or epidural), but if this is not possible, a pudendal nerve block can be used. Risks of all forceps deliveries include failure to deliver (requiring caesarean section), vaginal tears and fetal trauma, including facial bruising or abrasions.

Neville–Barnes forceps have both a cephalic curve to fit the baby's head, and a pelvic curve that follows the contours of the sacral hollow. These are used to aid delivery when rotation is not required, such as in this case where the baby is almost delivered at the occipitoanterior position but needs extra assistance.

Robert Barnes, English obstetrician (1817–1907).

2. A – Elective caesarean section

Elective caesarean sections are planned to occur before the onset of labour, but are generally not performed before 39 weeks. An elective section should be offered in certain conditions, including previous classical caesarean section, placenta praevia that is partially or completely obstructing the cervical os, multiple pregnancies if the first twin is not cephalic and in certain infectious diseases such as HIV with a high viral load or co-infection with hepatitis C. Maternal request is not an outright indication for caesarean section and the reasons for the request must be fully explored and a mental health team can be involved for women with anxiety about childbirth. A clinician may refuse a maternal request, but must instead refer her care to another healthcare provider for a second opinion.

A lower-segment caesarean section is the most common type of section, in which the incision is made in the lower uterine segment following reflection of the bladder. Classical caesarean sections, in which a vertical incision is made in the upper segment of the uterus, are uncommon, as there is a higher postoperative morbidity and risk of scar rupture in subsequent pregnancies.

3. B – Emergency caesarean section

Emergency caesarean sections are performed for either fetal or maternal emergencies. The urgency can be stated as category 1–4. A decision-to-delivery time of 30 minutes has been accepted as an audit standard for response to a category 1 caesarean section and 30–75 minutes for a category 2. Category 3 is a less urgent emergency and category 4 is an elective procedure. It is performed for failure to progress, fetal compromise or malposition (such as in this case) or maternal compromise. If the chin of the face was felt anteriorly, a normal delivery could have occurred, but a posterior chin will not deliver vaginally due to the large occiput.

4. D – Rotational forceps – Kielland's

Kielland's forceps are rotational forceps and do not have a pelvic curve, as this would damage maternal soft tissue during rotation. In this instance, rotation would be used to turn the baby to the occipitoanterior position followed by traction to deliver the baby. Such procedures are usually done in theatre so that a caesarean section could be undertaken if needed. Rotation of a baby can also be achieved manually or using a ventouse.

In ventouse deliveries, a suction cap is attached to the baby's head at a specific point before traction is commenced. A combination of traction and maternal effort can rotate the baby to an occipitoanterior position (if not in this position initially). There is an element of operator choice when determining whether forceps or ventouse is used.

Christian Kielland, Norwegian obstetrician (1871–1941).

5. F – Normal delivery

An occipitoanterior position with a flexed head is a favourable position, which should deliver with no complications or additional help being needed. Vaginal delivery is not contraindicated following one section, and is known as VBAC – vaginal birth after caesarean.

External cephalic version (ECV) is where a breech fetus is manually moved into a cephalic presentation through the maternal abdomen. 50% of ECVs are successful, and this is dependent on race, parity, uterine tone, liquor volume, engagement of the breech and whether or not the head is palpable. ECV should be offered to women with breech presentations from 36–37 weeks. Rarely, there are complications such as placental abruption, uterine rupture and foetomaternal haemorrhage, so ECV should be performed only where monitoring facilities and immediate delivery are available. Contraindications are antepartum haemorrhage in the previous 7 days, an abnormal cardiotocogram, major uterine abnormality, ruptured membranes and multiple pregnancy. Relative contraindications are small-for-gestational-age babies, proteinuric preeclampsia, oligohydramnios, major fetal anomalies, scarred uterus and unstable lie. Rhesus anti-D antibodies are given to all rhesus-negative women. Labours with a cephalic presentation following ECV are more likely to need obstetric intervention than cephalic ones without prior ECV.

Perineal tears can happen in normal deliveries, but can be more severe with operative delivery. Often an episiotomy (a mediolateral cut through the perineum) is performed if a tear is likely.

Tears are graded as follows:

- First-degree: injury to perineal skin only
- Second-degree: injury to perineum involving muscles but not the anal sphincter
- Third-degree: injury to perineum involving the anal sphincter complex
  - 3a: less than 50% external anal sphincter (EAS) thickness torn
  - 3b: more than 50% EAS thickness torn
  - 3c: both EAS and internal anal sphincter torn
- Fourth-degree: injury to perineum involving anal sphincter and anal epithelium

Third- and fourth-degree tears can lead to faecal incontinence. Obstetric anal injury is seen in 1% of vaginal deliveries. Risk factors include high birth weight (>4 kg), persistent occipitoposterior position, nulliparity, induction of labour, epidural, prolonged second stage (>1 hour), shoulder dystocia, midline episiotomy and forceps delivery.

THEME 2: UROGYNAECOLOGY

During the history you will often get an idea of the type of urinary incontinence (UI) the woman is suffering with – either stress, urgency or mixed. A bladder diary can also give valuable information about frequency and bladder capacity. Conservative treatment should be offered on the basis of the history alone, but if not successful, the patient should be offered urodynamic studies where further characterization of the incontinence can be undertaken.

1. C– Botulinum toxin A

At cystoscopy, the bladder wall is injected with botulinum toxin A. This reduces the unwanted muscle contractions seen in overactive bladders to reduce incontinence. Bladder overactivity must be confirmed on urodynamic studies first and the patient discussed by the MDT. The patient must be willing and able to self-catheterize as the botox can work too well, meaning the bladder does not empty.

James Marion Sims, American gynaecologist (1813–1883).

2. J – Physiotherapy

From the history, it sounds like this woman has stress incontinence, which is an involuntary loss of urine that occurs when the bladder pressure exceeds the urethral pressure in the absence of detrusor muscle contraction (e.g. when coughing and laughing). Conservative treatment can be started on clinical diagnosis after taking the history and examining the patient. Physiotherapy is the first-line treatment for stress incontinence and should be used for 3 months to assess full response. If this is not successful, then urodynamic studies are usually performed prior to proceeding to surgical treatments.

On examination, pelvic organ prolapse may also be noted, as childbirth is a causative factor for both these conditions. Stress incontinence becomes more common after the menopause as the supportive connective tissue around the pelvic floor begins to atrophy with the hypo-oestrogenic state.

It is important to discuss weight loss in this case (normal body mass index: 20–25) as this may improve symptoms and will also make surgery less risky. Other things to look out for are whether the patient has a chronic cough which could be treated and therefore would reduce the frequency of incontinence. Passing urine once at night is not considered abnormal so this woman would not be considered to have an overactive bladder.

Urodynamic studies are investigations used to measure detrusor pressures as the bladder is filled and 'provoked' with coughing. Transducers are placed in the rectum (to measure abdominal pressure) and the bladder (to measure intravesical pressure). Detrusor activity is calculated by subtracting the abdominal pressure from the bladder pressure. Normally, detrusor activity should not alter with filling or provocation. Involuntary detrusor contraction suggests detrusor overactivity. If leakage occurs with increases in abdominal pressure, in the absence of detrusor contraction, urodynamic stress incontinence is diagnosed.

3. H – Oxybutynin

An overactive bladder with or without incontinence occurs due to involuntary detrusor contractions. It accounts for 35% of female incontinence. Risk factors include previous surgery, multiple sclerosis and advancing age, although most cases are idiopathic. A urinary tract infection must be excluded. The diagnosis of detrusor overactivity is confirmed using urodynamic studies, which show detrusor contraction on filling or provocation. Conservative management is the first line which includes bladder retraining by either a physiotherapist or a urogynaecology specialist nurse to educate patients about urgency control and relaxation strategies. In those who do not find this effective, anticholinergic drugs may prove worthwhile (by causing relaxation of the bladder smooth muscle). Examples of anticholinergics include oxybutynin, tolterodine and darifenacin. Side effects of anticholinergics include headache and a dry mouth.

4. G – Mirabegron

This is a new treatment for overactive bladder symptoms. It is an alternative option when anticholinergic drugs are either not effective, contraindicated or the side effects mean they are not tolerated. It is a β-3-adrenoceptor agonist and works by activating β-3-adrenoceptors which relaxes the detrusor muscle, allowing the bladder to store more urine.

5. L – Synthetic mid-urethral tape

This is a tape that is inserted under the midsection of the urethra to provide extra support in this area and prevent stress leakage from the bladder. The vaginal wall behind the urethra is opened up, a tunnel is created on either side and the tape is threaded through both tunnels and exits the skin either behind the pubic bone or into the groin, to allow the urethra to be supported. It is usually performed under spinal or general anaesthetic and the patient returns home the same day as long as she can pass urine successfully.

Colposuspension is an abdominal procedure performed under general anaesthetic. Sutures are placed lateral to the bladder neck and are then sutured to the iliopectineal ligament, or the symphysis pubis. This acts to 'hitch up' the sagging bladder neck to improve continence.

Periurethral injectables are injected paraurethrally to bulk up the sphincter and prevent involuntary urinary loss from stress incontinence. They are done under local anaesthetic and require 'booster' injections. Efficacy is inferior to the tapes.

Hormone replacement therapy and anterior repair are not used in the treatment of UI.

THEME 3: DRUGS IN PREGNANCY

1. J – Propylthiouracil

The incidence of maternal hyperthyroidism is approximately 1 in 500 pregnancies. It usually predates pregnancy and 90% of cases are secondary to Graves' disease. Other causes include transient gestational hyperthyroidism, toxic multinodular goitre and a hydatidiform mole. Graves' disease is an autoimmune disorder due to circulating thyrotrophin receptor-stimulating antibodies (TRAb). The clinical diagnosis in pregnancy is difficult, as many symptoms frequently occur in normal pregnancy, such as tachycardia, heat intolerance and a cardiac flow murmur. High levels of TRAb can cross the placenta, causing fetal thyrotoxicosis; however, this is rare as IgG transfer is limited. Thyrotoxicosis in pregnancy can cause atrial fibrillation, abdominal pain, vomiting, diarrhoea and psychosis. There is a higher risk of preeclampsia, miscarriage, preterm labour and low birth weight.

The treatment of choice is either propylthiouracil or carbimazole. Of the two, propylthiouracil is preferred in early pregnancy (due to reduced placental transfer) and breast feeding (as it passes into breast milk less readily). Carbimazole is often used in the latter stages of pregnancy due to concerns of liver toxicity with propylthiouracil. The lowest dose of medication required is used to keep free thyroxine (T_4) levels at the upper limit of normal, and to reduce the risk of fetal hypothyroidism as a side effect. Thyroid function should be checked regularly, and serial ultrasound scans are performed to assess fetal growth. Radioactive iodine is contraindicated in pregnancy.

2. I – Promethazine

Around half of women experience nausea and vomiting during the early stages of pregnancy, but less than 2% of women go on to develop hyperemesis gravidarum. Hyperemesis gravidarum describes intractable vomiting that can lead to severe dehydration, metabolic disturbance and electrolyte imbalance, including hyponatraemia, hypokalaemia, ketonuria, raised transaminases and transient thyrotoxicosis.

Simple measures include avoiding triggers for nausea, and regular small amounts of food and fluids are recommended. Nine out of ten cases have settled by 16 weeks. If needed, an antiemetic such as promethazine (histamine H1 antagonist) is prescribed as first line. If this does not work, cyclizine (histamine H1 antagonist) or prochlorperazine (dopamine antagonist) can be used. Other antiemetics such as metoclopramide (dopamine antagonist) and occasionally ondansetron (a serotonin 5-HT$_3$ receptor antagonist) are used if vomiting is intractable.

If there is evidence of dehydration due to intolerance of oral fluids or significant ketonuria, hospital admission is required. Patients should remain nil-by-mouth until vomiting settles, while intravenous (IV) fluid resuscitation is given. Thiamine (vitamin B_1) supplements are sometimes indicated, to reduce the risk of Wernicke's encephalopathy. High-dose folic acid should be prescribed, as it is unlikely to have been well absorbed due to the vomiting.

Thalidomide was prescribed for morning sickness in the late 1950s and early 1960s, until it was found to be associated with severe birth anomalies. The most characteristic deformity associated with maternal thalidomide use is phocomelia, a shortening or absence of the long bones. In the most extreme cases, all four limbs are affected, so the hands and feet appear directly attached to the body (tetraphocomelia).

Phocomelia, from Greek *phoco* = seal + *melos* = limb.
Hyperemesis gravidarum, from Greek *hyper* = excessive + *emeticos* = vomit and Latin *gravida* = pregnant.
Carl Wernicke, German neurologist (1848–1905).

3. L – Ursodeoxycholic acid

Pruritus in pregnancy is common (around 20% of pregnancies), but the prevalence of itching due to abnormal liver function tests (LFTs) is less than 1%. In obstetric cholestasis, bile acids accumulate in the blood, causing jaundice and pruritus. There is a 40% recurrence rate in pregnancy, and it is common to have a positive family history. Itching typically involves the palms and soles, but can affect the whole body. It is important to rule out other causes of jaundice and pruritus, including hepatitis and gallstones. Screening blood tests include LFTs, γ-glutamyl transferase and bile acids. It may also be necessary to take a clotting screen, anti-smooth muscle antibody, anti-mitochondrial antibody and viral serology (hepatitis viruses, Epstein–Barr virus and cytomegalovirus). In obstetric cholestasis, transaminases, bile acids and bilirubin may all be raised. An ultrasound scan of the liver should also be performed.

Treatment includes chlorphenamine (an antihistamine) for pruritus and topical emollients. The lack of bile salts in the gut results in malabsorption of fat-soluble vitamins, including vitamin K, increasing the risk of postpartum haemorrhage and fetal intracranial bleeds. Oral vitamin K supplements may be required if prothrombin time is increased. Ursodeoxycholic acid, although not licensed for use in pregnancy, has been found to reduce the accumulation of bile acids and relieve pruritus. It is important to monitor and treat obstetric cholestasis, as there is a risk of premature birth, fetal distress and intrauterine death. Delivery is often offered early in view of the possible increased risk of intrauterine death.

4. D – Doxycycline

Doxycycline is not recommended in pregnancy. It is a tetracycline, which are known to cause fetal abnormalities and deposit in bones and teeth, delaying their growth. Breastfeeding mothers should also avoid doxycycline, as there is the additional side effect of staining the baby's teeth. Erythromycin, a macrolide, is a suitable alternative for pregnant or breastfeeding women. It is also the antibiotic of choice in premature rupture of membranes, as there is evidence that it may delay delivery and reduce maternal and neonatal infective morbidity.

5. C – Ibuprofen

Ibuprofen, a non-steroidal anti-inflammatory drug, is often effective for the pain experienced after a caesarean section. It should be avoided in late pregnancy, as it may cause premature closure of the ductus arteriosus. Ibuprofen is the second-line analgesic after paracetamol, which is safe to administer during pregnancy. Codeine is no longer recommended for use in breastfeeding women due to cases of neonatal respiratory depression.

THEME 4: PERIMENOPAUSAL HORMONES

The menopause is defined as the permanent cessation of menstruation due to failure of ovarian follicular development in the presence of adequate gonadotropin stimulation. The diagnosis is made retrospectively after 12 months of amenorrhoea. The average age of the menopause in the UK is 50.5 years. Premature menopause is diagnosed in those below 40 years, and can be due to autoimmune conditions, chromosomal abnormalities or as a result of radiotherapy or bilateral oophorectomy. The perimenopausal period, or climacteric, is of variable duration as the menstrual cycle lengthens and anovulation ensues.

The symptoms attributed to the menopause are largely due to oestrogen deficiency. Immediate effects of the menopause include vasomotor symptoms (hot flushes, night sweats, sleep disturbance, palpitations and dizziness) and psychological symptoms (low mood, irritability, poor memory and loss of libido). Intermediate effects, which can take a couple of years to develop, are atrophy of the vagina and vulva (→ atrophic vaginitis, manifesting in dryness, itching and dyspareunia), of pelvic tissues (→ prolapse) and of the urethral epithelium (→ dysuria, frequency and urgency). There is a 30% reduction in skin collagen. Long-term effects of the menopause include osteoporosis with subsequent pathological fracture (common sites include the distal radius, femoral neck and vertebrae), and an increase in the risk of atherosclerotic cardiovascular disease.

1. A – 17β-estradiol

Prior to the menopause, 17β-estradiol is the main oestrogen secreted by the ovaries. This is broken down into oestrone, and then oestriol. Gradually, the ovaries become resistant to gonadotropins, so gonadotropin levels become high, which can be measured to confirm the menopause.

2. E – Oestrone

After the menopause, the majority of the body's oestrogen is produced in peripheral fat.

3. B – Androstenedione

Oestrone is produced from the androgen androstenedione by the adrenal cortex (70%) and the ovary (30%). Obese women produce more oestrone in the peripheral adipose tissue, which is unopposed by progesterone, and they are therefore more at risk of endometrial hyperplasia and endometrial adenocarcinoma. Estradiol and oestriol are then produced from oestrone.

4. F – Progesterone

During the perimenopausal period, 60% of cycles remain ovulatory. This can be measured by luteal-phase progesterone (day 21 of the cycle, or 7 days before menstruation in longer cycles). In the 6 months prior to the menopause, progesterone levels indicative of ovulation occur in 5% of cycles. The estradiol produced by ovarian follicles at this time is insufficient to cause a mid-cycle surge of luteinizing hormone (LH), but is enough to cause some endometrial proliferation. Clinically, this is of more use during fertility investigations.

5. C – Follicle-stimulating hormone

Follicle-stimulating hormone (FSH) stimulates a follicle (sometimes two) to continue to increase in size and prepare for ovulation. The developing follicle secretes oestrogen into the circulation and this acts as negative feedback for FSH, and so FSH secretion would normally reduce. If no follicle is produced (due to menopause and the natural depletion of oocytes), the FSH will continue to rise in an attempt to stimulate development of a follicle. Menopause is generally a clinical diagnosis, but measuring FSH can be useful in premature ovarian failure.

THEME 5: ACUTE PELVIC PAIN

1. K – Torsion of ovarian cyst

Ovarian cysts are fluid-filled sacs that can grow to become as large as a grapefruit. The majority are benign and occur at child-bearing age. Women with ovarian cysts may complain of dull, intermittent, aching pains in the lower abdomen. The woman in this scenario, who has a negative pregnancy test, presents with sudden-onset severe, unilateral, colicky pain with shock. This history indicates torsion of an ovarian cyst. The pain may be intermittent if torsion is incomplete, and vomiting can occur. Her observations are concerning, showing tachycardia and hypotension. A delay in diagnosis can lead to irreversible ischaemia of the ovary. An urgent laparoscopy is needed and the pedicle untwisted. If possible, a cystectomy should be performed, although signs of ischaemia or necrosis may warrant oophorectomy.

2. I – Pelvic inflammatory disease

Pelvic inflammatory disease (PID) describes inflammation of the pelvic organs via ascending sexually transmitted infection (STI) from the genital tracts (although some cases occur following descending infections from local organs, such as the appendix). It is most common in 18–25-year-olds, with chlamydial infection causing 50% of cases and with gonorrhoea, mycoplasma, *Haemophilus influenzae*, cytomegalovirus, *Actinomyces* and herpes being decreasingly common causes. In 20% of cases, the causative organism is never found. Risk factors include unprotected sexual intercourse, multiple sexual partners, smoking and previous PID.

PID can be asymptomatic, being a retrospective diagnosis during investigation for infertility. However, patients may present with lower abdominal pain, deep dyspareunia, postcoital or irregular bleeding, menorrhagia or dysmenorrhoea, and a purulent discharge. Women with active infection are systemically unwell with fever, vomiting, anorexia and malaise. On examination, there is lower abdominal tenderness, cervical excitation, tenderness on pelvic examination and pyrexia. A urine sample and high vaginal and endocervical swabs must be taken. Treatment is with broad-spectrum antibiotics depending upon local guidelines (e.g. azithromycin, doxycycline and metronidazole) and analgesia. Contact tracing is recommended. Hospital admission may be needed to stabilize severe cases.

Complications include tubo-ovarian abscess, tubal infertility, ectopic pregnancy and chronic pelvic pain.

3. F – Incomplete miscarriage

Miscarriage is the most common complication of pregnancy. It is defined as the loss of pregnancy before 24 weeks. Underlying causes and risk factors of miscarriage include fetal abnormality (50%), infection (e.g. 'TORCH'), increasing maternal age, maternal illness (diabetes or renal disease), abnormal uterine cavity (intrauterine contraceptive device insertion or congenital septum) and medical intervention (amniocentesis or chorionic villus sampling). Note that exercise, intercourse and emotional trauma are not associated with miscarriage. Investigation into an underlying cause of miscarriage is performed if three miscarriages have occurred.

The woman in this scenario has had an incomplete miscarriage. This is where some fetal material has been passed, but some products of conception are retained in the uterus (these are visible on ultrasound scanning). The cervical os remains open until all the products have passed (whether that be spontaneous or with medical or surgical assistance).

Complete miscarriage is when the mother has experienced bleeding, all the fetal tissue has been passed, there are no products of conception on scanning and the cervical os is closed. In these cases, patients do not require further hospital follow-up.

A threatened miscarriage is when there is bleeding before 24 weeks, but the fetus is still viable and the cervical os is closed on examination. Only 25% of threatened miscarriages eventually miscarry.

A missed miscarriage (also known as a delayed or silent miscarriage) is when the fetus dies *in utero* and the cervix stays closed. There may or may not be bleeding in this case.

4. E – Ectopic pregnancy

An ectopic pregnancy is implantation of the embryo outside the uterine cavity, most commonly in the fallopian tube (but it can also happen in the cornua of the uterus, cervix, ovary or abdominal cavity). Ectopic pregnancies are becoming increasingly common in the UK, with an incidence of 11 in 1000 pregnancies. 50% occur in those with no predisposing risks, but risk factors include PID, previous tubal surgery, previous ectopic pregnancy, assisted reproductive techniques and endometriosis.

Presentation is variable and should be suspected in women of childbearing age with amenorrhoea, abnormal bleeding and abdominal pain, which can be associated with dizziness, fainting, shoulder pain or collapse. On examination, there is acute abdominal pain with cervical excitation or tender adnexae in a shocked patient. A transvaginal ultrasound is up to 93% accurate in detecting ectopic pregnancy, increasing with pregnancies over 5.5 weeks' gestation. Serial measurements of the human chorionic gonadotropin β-subunit (βhCG) are used to differentiate an ectopic from a viable uterine pregnancy and a spontaneous miscarriage. Presentation could be an incidental finding on an early pregnancy scan.

Management can be conservative, medical (methotrexate) or surgical, depending on clinical symptoms and future fertility desires. Risks and benefits should be considered and discussed with the patient. Rhesus D-negative women should be given anti-D.

Although this patient has a copper coil, she still has an ectopic pregnancy as they do not have 100% efficacy. This patient clearly needs urgent surgery which may be performed laparoscopically, but a laparotomy should be performed if she remains unstable despite resuscitation.

Mittelschmerz is a quick-onset, cramping pelvic pain (midline or unilateral) that occurs before or at the time of ovulation (day 14). It is more common in teenagers and older women. Persistent mittelschmerz may respond to the combined oral contraceptive pill, as this suppresses ovulation.

Corpus luteum cysts are normal findings as they are what is left in the ovary once the ova has been released. Enlarged or haemorrhagic corpus luteum cysts are the most common cause of pain in early pregnancy. These are found on ultrasound scan and are managed conservatively.

Mittelschmerz, from German *mittel* = middle + *schmerz* = pain ('pain that occurs mid-cycle').
Cornua, from Latin *cornu* = horn (as in a musical instrument).

5. A – Acute appendicitis
It is classic that appendicitis presents in this way with generalized pain localizing itself to the right iliac fossa. There is a pyrexia, tachycardia, localized tenderness and peritonism. Blood tests may show increased white blood cells and inflammatory markers. Urgent general surgical referral for appendectomy is required. Of course, the pregnancy test must be chased up as this woman could actually have an ectopic pregnancy, but this is less likely due to the use of the Mirena coil.

An appendix abscess is a collection of pus associated with appendicitis. An appendix mass may form when the omentum and bowel surround an inflamed appendix to wall it off. Patients with an appendix mass will have had several days of localized pain and pyrexia with a palpable mass in the right iliac fossa (confirmed with an ultrasound or computed tomography [CT] scan). Management is with fluids, analgesia and antibiotics. Drainage can be open or ultrasound/CT guided, with consideration of appendectomy.

THEME 6: GAMETOGENESIS

1. F – Primordial germ cell
2. K – Spermatozoa
3. I – Spermatid

4. E – Primary spermatocyte

5. C – Polar body

Spermatogenesis occurs when the adult male reaches puberty. It occurs under the influence of testosterone. The whole process of spermatogenesis takes 64 days. Primordial germ cells divide by mitosis and differentiate into spermatogonia, which lie immediately beneath the basement membrane of seminiferous tubules. As spermatogenesis progresses, the germ cells move from the basement membrane into the lumen of the seminiferous tubules. Spermatogonia divide by mitosis and differentiate into primary spermatocytes. Primary spermatocytes contain 46 double-structured chromosomes. These divide by meiosis. The primary spermatocytes initially complete the first meiotic division to give secondary spermatocytes. Secondary spermatocytes therefore contain 23 double-structured chromosomes, which complete the second meiotic division to give spermatids. Spermatids contain 23 single chromosomes. Spermatids undergo spermiogenesis (below) to give spermatozoa.

In summary, every primary spermatocyte eventually gives rise to four spermatid daughter cells, two with 22 + X chromosomes and two with 22 + Y chromosomes. Spermatozoa are the end products of spermatogenesis. They have undergone spermiogenesis, which is the process by which spermatids differentiate into the distinctly shaped spermatozoa. Spermatozoa are made up of a head (within which the nucleus lies) capped by the acrosome (containing hydrolytic enzymes), a middle piece that provides power for swimming (generated by large helical mitochondria) and a tail (the propulsion system made up of microtubules).

Oogenesis begins in females during intrauterine life and is a slow process, with many stages of division being arrested for long periods of time. It is more complicated than the male pathway, although the same principles are followed. Primordial germ cells are present in the wall of the yolk sac at the end of the third week of embryological development. They migrate by amoeboid movement to the developing gonads, where they arrive by the beginning of the fifth week. They then divide by mitosis and differentiate into oogonia. Oogonia differentiate into primary oocytes and become surrounded by follicular (epithelial) cells. These are collectively named primordial follicles. Primary oocytes contain 46 double-structured chromosomes and enter prophase of meiosis I. Division is arrested at the dictyotene phase of meiosis I, and the first meiotic division is completed only with the preovulatory LH/FSH surge to give a secondary oocyte and a polar body. The polar body is merely a useless by-product, which subsequently degenerates.

Secondary oocytes and polar bodies both contain 23 double-structured chromosomes. Meiosis I of the secondary oocyte is completed with the preovulatory LH/FSH surge, but further division of the secondary oocyte occurs only if fertilization occurs. With fertilization, the secondary oocyte divides by meiosis II to give a mature oocyte and a further polar body. The mature oocyte and its polar body both contain 23 single chromosomes. The initial polar body also undergoes meiosis II to give a further two polar bodies, both containing 23 single chromosomes.

Primary oocytes therefore eventually give rise to four daughter cells, all of which contain 22 + X chromosomes. However, only one of these is a mature oocyte, with the remaining three daughter cells being polar bodies.

THEME 7: GENITAL INFECTIONS

Remember, if anyone presents with a STI, they are at risk of carrying further infections so should have a full genito-urinary check-up.

1. B – Chancroid

Chancroid is caused by the Gram-negative bacterium *Haemophilus ducreyi*, and is found mostly in tropical countries. It is an ulcerative condition of the genitalia (single/multiple painful superficial ulcers) and develops within 1 week of exposure. Inflammation may lead to a phimosis. Enlargement and suppuration of inguinal lymph nodes may occur, leading to a unilocular abscess (buboes) that can rupture to form a sinus. Treatment is with appropriate antibiotics (e.g. erythromycin).

Lymphogranuloma venereum is an important differential, being a tropical STI caused by *Chlamydia trachomatis* serovars L1, L2 and L3. However, this gives a typically painless ulcer, followed by painful enlarged lymph nodes, with subsequent regional abscesses or fistulae. It may spontaneously remit, but can be treated with tetracyclines or erythromycin.

2. C – Chlamydia

This genital infection is caused by the Gram-negative organism *Chlamydia trachomatis* serovars D–K. Infection in women may be asymptomatic, although there can be abnormal vaginal discharge, dysuria and urinary frequency. Ascending infection can cause salpingitis and, if it enters the abdominal cavity, perihepatitis (Fitz-Hugh–Curtis syndrome) as in this patient, which leads to right upper-quadrant pain and tenderness. Chlamydial infection is a major cause of infertility and increases the possibility of ectopic pregnancy. In males, symptoms include mucopurulent discharge and dysuria (asymptomatic in 50%). Epididymo-orchitis is a complication. Diagnosis of chlamydia infection is by urine antigen detection or vaginal swab culture. Treatment is with antibiotics.

Chlamydia, from Greek *chlamys* = cloak (as chlamydia is often 'cloaked'; i.e. asymptomatic).
Thomas Fitz-Hugh Jr, American physician (1894–1963).
Arthur Curtis, American gynaecologist (1881–1955).

Gonorrhoea is the second most common STI, which is also frequently asymptomatic. Treatment is according to local guidance relating to antibiotic resistance. An intramuscular injection with ceftriaxone and a single dose of azithromycin is often recommended.

3. A – Bacterial vaginosis
Bacterial vaginosis (BV) is not an STI. It is an infection caused by mixed anaerobic flora (e.g. *Gardnerella* spp. and *Mycoplasma hominis*). It is often asymptomatic, but can cause a creamy-grey discharge with a fishy odour. There is no itching. The risk of preterm delivery and late miscarriage is higher if BV is present in early pregnancy; however, treatment with antibiotics (metronidazole) does not reduce the perinatal risks, and so should be used only in symptomatic women.

Genital candidiasis or 'thrush' is usually caused by *Candida* species and is a commensal of the vagina, but overgrowth of this is a common cause of vaginitis and vaginal discharge.

4. K – Syphilis (specifically secondary syphilis)
This woman has had a painless ulcer followed by systemic symptoms (fever, malaise, headache and skin rash). This history is indicative of secondary syphilis. For more information about syphilis, see 'Sexually transmitted infections' (Paper 1 Answers, Theme 4).

5. J – Scabies
Scabies is caused by the mite *Sarcoptes scabiei*, which burrows into the skin, where the female lays her eggs. Scabies is often a STI, but can be spread throughout households or institutions. Patients develop an intense itch, which is worse at night. This is caused by an allergic response to the eggs. The burrows made by the mite tend to be symmetrical and affect finger webs, sides of digits, flexor surfaces of wrists and the penis. Secondary infection of affected areas can occur. Immunocompromised patients can develop a more severe infestation, with thick hyperkeratotic crusting on affected areas. This is known as Norwegian scabies (first described in Norway in 1848 – it was originally thought to be a distant variant of leprosy).

Scabies, from Latin *scabere* = to scratch.

Genital herpes is caused by the DNA-containing herpes simplex virus (HSV) types 1 and 2. The infection remains prevalent due to asymptomatic shedding of the virus. Clinical features of primary infection include dysuria with painful, itchy lesions and occasionally urethral or vaginal discharge. Patients may also complain of constitutional symptoms (fever, headache, malaise and myalgia). Lesions are papular, vesicular or pustular; these crust and heal within 4 weeks. Examination may reveal inguinal lymphadenitis. HSV remains dormant in dorsal root ganglia, and reactivation occurs in 75% of cases. Recurrent attacks tend to be milder, shorter and not associated with systemic features. Diagnosis is by viral swabs. Severe infections can be managed with acyclovir.

Genital warts are most commonly caused by human papillomavirus types 6b and 11. Incubation is normally about 3 months, but warts may take up to 2 years to develop. When large warts coalesce, the appearance is known as condylomata acuminata. Genital warts increase in size during pregnancy, and wart-induced obstruction may be an indication for caesarean section. Management options include excision, cautery and immune modulator creams (podophyllin or imiquimod).

Condylomata acuminata, from Latin *condylomata* = knuckles + *acuminatum* = pointed.

Molluscum contagiosum is a viral skin disease causing multiple raised 'pearly papules'. It is a benign, self-limiting disease spread by skin-to-skin contact but is not sexually transmitted. It can be more marked in immunosuppressed patients, such as those with AIDS.

THEME 8: TWINS

Mono – single/one
Di – two
Zygote – initial cell when two gametes join
Chorion – outer membrane between fetus and mother
Amnion – inner membrane between fetus and mother

1. A – Dizygotic dichorionic diamniotic

Dizygotics are the most common type of twins (60%). They develop due to fertilization of two different ova, from the same or opposite ovaries, by two different sperm, and are therefore not identical. They can be of different sexes and are no more genetically similar than siblings would be. They are always dichorionic and diamniotic, which means that each fetus has its own chorion, amnion and placenta. Options B (dizygotic dichorionic monoamniotic) and C (dizygotic monochorionic monoamniotic) are nonsense.

2. F – Monozygotic monochorionic monoamniotic

Monozygotic twins result from the mitotic division of a single fertilized ovum (zygote) into identical twins. They may or may not share the same chorion and amnion, depending on when the mitotic division occurs. Monozygotic monochorionic monoamniotic twins are rare and occur when the mitotic division occurs after 9 days. If this occurs prior to the formation of the primitive streak, there will be a single amniotic cavity and chorion. If the division occurs after primitive streak formation, conjoined (Siamese) twins develop.

The term 'Siamese twins' comes from a famous pair of conjoined twins in the nineteenth century, Chang and Eng Bunker, who travelled the world with the circus. They were born in Siam (now Thailand).

3. E – Monozygotic monochorionic diamniotic

Monozygotic monochorionic diamniotic twins result if division occurs between 4 and 8 days (during formation of the inner cell mass). There is a single placenta but, if the amnion has not developed, each fetus will have its own amniotic membrane.

4. A – Dizygotic dichorionic diamniotic
5. D – Monozygotic dichorionic dizygotic

Monozygotic dichorionic dizygotic twins result if the division occurs at less than 3 days after fertilization (at the 'eight-cell' stage). The two embryos implant at separate sites and have a separate chorion, amnion and placenta. They will have the same structural appearance *in utero* as dizygotic twins do, but will be identical.

The incidence of twins is 1 in 100, and of triplets 1 in 1000. Predisposing factors are increasing maternal age and parity, personal or family history, race and assisted conception. Multiple pregnancies need greater monitoring, as fetal and maternal mortality and morbidity rates are higher. The mother has a greater risk of hyperemesis, miscarriage, hypertension and preeclampsia, gestational diabetes, polyhydramnios (especially with monozygotics), anaemia, antepartum and postpartum haemorrhages and placenta praevia. The fetal risks include increased peri-natal mortality, increased congenital abnormality, preterm labour, placental insufficiency or intrauterine growth restriction (especially in monozygotics), malpresentation, twin-to-twin transfusion and vanishing twin syndrome. Twin-to-twin transfusion is where, due to anastomosis of vessels in the single placental mass of a monochorionic twin pregnancy, one twin gains at the other's expense. One twin becomes anaemic, hypovolaemic, oligohydramniotic and growth restricted while the other one develops polycythaemia, hypervolaemia, polyuria and polyhydramnios. Laser ablation of placental vessels can be useful, although there are risks of fetal demise. Vanishing twin syndrome is where a fetus in a multiple-gestation pregnancy dies *in utero* and is subsequently reabsorbed by the mother (either partially or completely).

The delivery of twins requires special management. If the first twin is cephalic, a trial of labour is normally attempted regardless of the presentation of the second twin, but there is no definitive evidence comparing vaginal delivery with caesarean section. If the first twin is breech or transverse lie, a caesarean section is offered. Problems with delivery include cord prolapse, entanglement or knotting, locking, postpartum haemorrhage, thrombosis, fetal distress (especially in the second twin) and inefficient uterine activity after the first twin has been delivered.

THEME 9: ECTOPIC PREGNANCY

An ectopic pregnancy is where the fertilized ovum implants in any tissue other than the uterus. The 'other tissue' is most commonly the fallopian tube, but other sites include the ovary, cervix, caesarean section scar and abdomen. The incidence of ectopic pregnancy is around 11 per 1000 pregnancies. Patients may present with abdominal pain and vaginal bleeding. Initial investigations include a urinary pregnancy test, pelvic ultrasound and serum βhCG. Management depends on the clinical state of the patient and her future fertility requirements.

Ectopic, from Greek *ek* = away from + *topos* = place (i.e. in the wrong place).

All of the following options should be preceded by discussion with a senior doctor.

1. C – Methotrexate injection
This patient has been managed expectantly with 48-hour follow-up because she is clinically stable. The ultrasound scan suggests an ectopic pregnancy in the left adnexa, but there is no evidence of rupture, as she is haemodynamically stable and there is no free fluid in the pelvis (free fluid would suggest bleeding). Her serum βhCG has plateaued (i.e. has neither gone up by >63% [which would support a diagnosis of intrauterine pregnancy] nor down by >50% [which would suggest a miscarriage]). This therefore supports the diagnosis of an ectopic pregnancy that is not a failing pregnancy and therefore requires treatment but not surgical treatment as the patient is stable and has no pain.

Medical management with methotrexate is indicated when

- The patient is clinically stable with no evidence of active bleeding and no significant pain
- Serum hCG <1500 IU/L
- No intrauterine pregnancy
- Adnexal mass <35 mm, unruptured and no heartbeat

Methotrexate is an antimetabolite (a folic acid antagonist) that prevents fetal growth by interfering with DNA synthesis. It is often administered as a single intramuscular injection and the dose is calculated according to body surface area (50 mg/m^2). Serum βhCG is checked on days 4 and 7 postinjection and weekly until negative to ensure it continues to fall. Complete resolution can take many months and there is a 10% chance of tubal rupture following administration of methotrexate. Pregnancy should be avoided for 3 months after methotrexate.

2. A – Laparoscopy ± salpingectomy
There is a purposeful omission of the serum βhCG result in this scenario, as the clinical and radiological findings are sufficient to require a laparoscopy ± proceeding to salpingectomy/salpingotomy (salping-, from Greek *salpinx* = trumpet or tube – describing the shape of the fallopian tube). (This patient's βhCG level was in fact 5131 IU/L.) There is a 20-fold increased risk of ectopic pregnancy in patients who have had one previously. Patients require complete counselling regarding salpingotomy

(removal of the ectopic pregnancy with attempted preservation of the tube) and salpingectomy (removal of tube containing the ectopic pregnancy). This patient is likely to be a candidate for salpingectomy as she says she has completed her family.

Salpingectomy is found to have a lower postoperative risk of bleeding and fewer incidences of persistent trophoblastic tissue (i.e. unsuccessful removal of the pregnancy tissue). Salpingotomy is preferable in women who desire future fertility and who have a damaged or absent contralateral tube; however, they are at risk of a repeated ectopic pregnancy in future pregnancies.

Gabriele Fallopio, Italian anatomist (1523–1562).

3. G – Urgent laparotomy
This woman requires an emergency laparotomy due to haemodynamic instability and a live, bleeding ectopic pregnancy. Definitive management should, as always, be preceded by ABC. Assess the airway, give oxygen and assess breathing. Insert two large-bore cannulae and take bloods, including a group-and-save blood sample. Start IV fluids. Inform the senior doctor, the on-call anaesthetist and theatre. Experienced surgeons may attempt laparoscopy, but the aim is rapid cessation of bleeding.

4. B – Laparoscopy ± salpingotomy
This woman requires surgery as she has significant pain. However, unlike the patient in question 1, she is desperate to maintain her fertility. It is already known from the hysterosalpingogram (HSG) that the other tube is blocked, so if possible, this patient should be offered laparoscopic salpingotomy but must be informed that her risk of further ectopic pregnancy is very high and an early scan should be offered if she is pregnant in the future. Salpingotomy can be a more complicated operation and one in five woman may need further treatment. She should also be consented for a salpingectomy if bleeding or further tubal damage occurs during surgery. Women who undergo salpingectomy should be followed up with βhCG testing to ensure all functioning pregnancy tissue has been removed.

5. D – Repeat βhCG in 48 hours
This is a pregnancy of unknown location (PUL), which means she is, or has recently been, pregnant but it is not yet confirmed where the pregnancy is located. It is likely from the history that she has had a complete miscarriage, but unless products of conception are confirmed on scan or visualization at speculum, this cannot be guaranteed. As she has no symptoms, and the scan is not worrying, conservative management is appropriate and this includes measuring the hCG 48 hours later. If the hCG falls by greater than 50%, it is unlikely that the pregnancy is going to continue and a urine pregnancy test can be performed in 2 weeks' time. If positive at this point, she should return for assessment. All women with a PUL

should be advised regarding worsening symptoms, as an ectopic pregnancy cannot be excluded.

THEME 10: ULTRASOUND SCANNING IN PREGNANCY

Ultrasonography is an important investigative tool throughout pregnancy that is safe for mother and baby. Abdominal and transvaginal scans are used to assess the uterus and its contents, and the adnexae can be assessed if necessary to exclude pathology.

1. E – Crown–rump length

An ultrasound scan is the most widely used technique for the determination of gestational age. Women should be offered an early ultrasound scan between 10 and 13 + 6 weeks in order to accurately determine gestational age, fetal viability, fetal number and evidence of gross abnormality. This is often referred to as the 'dating scan'. This scan is important, as gestation becomes harder to define as the pregnancy progresses. Measurement of the crown–rump length (CRL) is the most accurate measurement of gestational age in the first trimester.

Nuchal translucency is used as part of the screening tool for Down's syndrome and is performed at 11 to 13 + 6 weeks. Nuchal translucency measures the lymphatic fluid that has accumulated under the skin at the back of the neck. An increased thickness of this fluid is an indicator of risk of chromosomal abnormality.

2. D – Head circumference

As the fetus grows, it becomes more flexed in shape, which makes the CRL unreliable. If the CRL measures more than 84 mm, which correlates to 14 weeks, the head circumference (HC) becomes a more reliable indicator of gestational age.

3. A – Abdominal circumference

Growth scans may be offered in a high-risk pregnancy, such as if there has been previous intrauterine growth restriction (IUGR). The abdominal circumference, HC, femur length and amniotic fluid volume are all measured and plotted on growth charts so not only absolute measurements can be noted, but also the trend of growth plotted against centiles. The most sensitive parameter for assessing growth with IUGR is the abdominal circumference. The growth velocity of the abdominal circumference will tend to slow if there is placental insufficiency as the fetus will redirect blood to the brain, meaning there is a lack of glycogen deposition in the liver. Pregnancies affected by IUGR have a higher risk of fetal distress during labour.

4. B – Amniotic fluid volume

Amniotic fluid is essentially fetal urine. It is produced by the kidneys and then swallowed in a constant cycle. Disruption to either of these mechanisms can alter amniotic fluid volume. Insufficient amniotic fluid (oligohydramnios) can be caused by fetal kidney abnormalities (polycystic kidneys or renal agenesis), placental insufficiency or ruptured membranes. Excess amniotic fluid (polyhydramnios) usually occurs in the third trimester, and is associated with diabetes, macrosomia, problems with fetal swallowing (oesophageal atresia) and multiple pregnancies. The volume is assessed at ultrasound scan by measuring the deepest pool of liquor that does not contain limbs or cord.

5. C – Biophysical profile

The biophysical profile is an assessment of fetal well-being. It is affected by factors suppressing the fetal central nervous system, such as hypoxia, infection and medication. The assessments look at fetal breathing movements, gross body fetal movement, fetal tone and amniotic fluid volume. A fetal cardiotocogram 'non-stress' test is also done. This gives reassurance that the fetus is not acidotic or neurologically depressed.

Doppler ultrasound is used to measure the velocity of blood flow during the cardiac cycle in the fetoplacental and uteroplacental circulation. The umbilical artery waveforms are used to predict fetal well-being. They give information about vascular resistance in downstream peripheral vessels, such as that which occurs within the placenta. The most useful observation is the absence or reversal of end-diastolic flow, suggesting progressive fetal deterioration.

The fetal normality scan (or '20-week scan') is a detailed structural scan performed to detect abnormality. If anomalies are detected, it allows time for parents to make difficult decisions. Biparietal diameter (BPD), HC and femur length are mandatory measurements. Abdominal circumference is optional, but is an accurate predictor of intrauterine growth restriction. 90% of congenital anomalies occur without risk factors, so screening is crucial. The fetal normality scan examines the following:

- Head shape and contents: hydrocephalus, anencephaly
- Spinal cord: spina bifida
- Abdominal shape and contents: exomphalos, gastroschisis
- Kidneys and renal pelvis: horseshoe kidney, hydronephrosis
- A four-chamber cardiac view: congenital heart defects
- Arms and legs: dwarfism, osteogenesis imperfecta, talipes
- Face and lips: cleft lip and palate

Practice Paper 5: Questions

THEME 1: ABDOMINAL PAIN

Options

A. Appendicitis
B. Constipation
C. Diabetic ketoacidosis
D. Gastroenteritis
E. Inflammatory bowel disease
F. Intussusception
G. Mesenteric adenitis
H. Mittelschmerz
I. Pancreatitis
J. Pneumonia
K. Urinary tract infection

For each of the following children presenting with abdominal pain, select the most likely diagnosis. Each option may be used once, more than once or not at all.

1. A 4-year-old girl presents to the emergency department with abdominal pain, located in the right loin and flank. She has vomited on two occasions in the last 24 hours, but her mother denies her vomiting up blood. Her temperature is 39.5°C.

2. A 2-year-old boy presents to the emergency department with abdominal pain. For the last 24 hours, he has been screaming and grabbing his abdomen. The episodes last for 15–30 minutes, during which he looks pale and is inconsolable. He then settles for a further 15–30 minutes before the pain starts again.

3. A 5-year-old boy presents to the emergency department with abdominal pain. He has been complaining of central abdominal pain for 24 hours. On examination, he is tender in the right iliac fossa and has a temperature of 37.6°C. On palpating the left iliac fossa there is pain on releasing your hand.

4. A 5-year-old boy presents with abdominal pain. He has had a slight fever and a sore throat for 24 hours and, since this morning, he has complained of central abdominal pain. Examination in the emergency department reveals tenderness throughout the abdomen and pharyngitis. He has a temperature of 39°C.

5. A 5-year-old boy presents with abdominal pain. He has had a slight fever for 24 hours and, since this morning, he has complained of central abdominal pain. His mother reports that he has been more lethargic than usual for the last few weeks. On examination, he has generalized tenderness throughout the abdomen, pharyngitis and laboured breathing.

THEME 2: APNOEA

THEME 2: APNOEA

Options
A. Gastro-oesophageal reflux
B. Hypoglycaemia
C. Intracranial haemorrhage
D. Obstructive sleep apnoea
E. Pertussis
F. Seizure
G. Sepsis

For each of the following scenarios, select the most likely cause of apnoea. Each option may be used once, more than once or not at all.

1. You are called urgently to the postnatal ward. A 24-hour-old infant stopped breathing for a number of minutes. The midwife gave resuscitation breaths, and the baby is now breathing again. The baby was born at term, although the mother's waters broke more than 24 hours prior to delivery. On examination, the baby is cool peripherally and tachycardic.
2. A 6-week-old infant presents to the GP. His mother reports that he is having frequent episodes in which he stops breathing for up to 30 seconds. He has occasionally turned blue. He often starts breathing again spontaneously, but sometimes needs a little stimulation. His mother noticed that these episodes occur in clusters after feeding.
3. You are called urgently to the postnatal ward to see the infant of a lady with gestational diabetes. The infant is now 24 hours old and had stopped breathing for a number of minutes. The midwife gave resuscitation breaths, and the baby is now breathing again. He was born at 36 weeks' gestation and weighs 2.4 kg. On examination he looks jittery, is cool peripherally and is tachycardic.
4. A 6-week-old infant presents to the emergency department. His mother reports that he has had a cough for a few days. The cough occurs in bouts, and a couple of times he has vomited towards the end of the paroxysm. Today, he had a bout of coughing and then stopped breathing and turned blue.
5. A 3-month-old infant presents to the emergency department. He was brought in by ambulance. The paramedic has been performing bag-and-mask ventilation since leaving the family home, as the infant was having a respiratory arrest. On intubating the child, you notice that his frenulum is torn. Once ventilated, examination reveals bruising around the chest wall.

THEME 3: IMMUNIZATION SCHEDULE

Options

A. Diphtheria
B. *Haemophilus influenzae* type b
C. Measles
D. Meningococcus C
E. Mumps
F. Pertussis
G. Pneumococcus
H. Polio
 I. Rubella
 J. Tuberculosis

For each of the following descriptions, select the most likely organism against which protection is given by vaccination. Each option may be used once, more than once or not at all.

1. A live vaccine given intradermally to at-risk babies.
2. An inactivated virus given intramuscularly to all babies at 2, 3 and 4 months, with a preschool booster and a further booster at 13–18 years.
3. An intramuscular killed vaccine protecting against a bacterial organism (Gram-negative diplococcus) given at 3, 4 and 12 months.
4. An intramuscular vaccine protecting against a bacterial organism given at 2, 3 and 4 months, with a preschool booster.
5. An intramuscular vaccine protecting against a Gram-positive anaerobic bacterial organism given at 2, 3 and 4 months, with a preschool booster followed by a booster at 13–18 years.

THEME 4: CHILD PROTECTION

Options

A. Accidental injury
B. Emotional abuse
C. Fabricated or induced illness
D. Neglect
E. Normal variant
F. Non-accidental poisoning
G. Non-accidental injury (physical abuse)
H. Pathological cause
I. Sexual abuse

For each of the following scenarios, select the most likely description from the above options. Each option may be used once, more than once or not at all.

1. A 2-year-old boy falls out of a first-floor window. His parents say that he was unattended at the time. He sustains a right-sided extradural haematoma resulting in a left hemiplegia.
2. A 3-month-old girl is found to have a fractured humerus. Her father says that she rolled off the changing mat onto a hard wooden floor.
3. A 3-week-old Asian child is referred by the health visitor, who has noticed bruising around the sacrum and buttocks. She suspects that the parents are smacking the baby for crying.
4. A 3-year-old boy is reported to have fallen from his tricycle and has not been using his right arm since. Examination is normal except for a diastolic murmur. X-ray reveals a fractured ulna and radius. The paediatric team perform a skeletal survey, which reveals Wormian bones of the skull vault.
5. A 12-month-old boy presents with a severe cough. On examination, the child is in respiratory distress, and suffers from paroxysms of coughing followed by a whoop. You also notice a widespread nappy rash, which improves rapidly while he is on the ward.

THEME 5: MANAGEMENT OF ASTHMA

Options

A. Two to ten puffs of inhaled short-acting β_2-agonist via spacer
B. Increase inhaled steroid to 400 µg/kg/day
C. Inhaled steroid 200–400 µg/kg/day
D. Intravenous (IV) aminophylline
E. IV infusion of magnesium sulphate
F. IV salbutamol
G. IV steroid
H. No further management required
 I. Nebulized short-acting β_2-agonist
 J. Oral leukotriene receptor antagonist
K. Oral steroids
L. Oxygen via facemask, two to ten puffs of inhaled short-acting β_2-agonist via spacer and oral steroid
M. Oxygen via facemask and two to ten puffs of inhaled short-acting β_2-agonist via spacer
N. Oxygen via facemask and nebulized short-acting β_2-agonist
O. Oxygen via facemask, nebulized short-acting β_2-agonist and oral or IV steroid
P. Regular inhaled short-acting β_2-agonist via a spacer

For each of the following children with asthma, select the next step in the management. Each case option may be used once, more than once or not at all.

1. A 4-year-old boy presents to his GP with a 6-month history of nocturnal cough and intermittent wheeze. On examination, he is small for his age and has mild eczema on his upper limbs.
2. A 3-year-old boy presents with poorly controlled chronic asthma. He is currently being managed with an inhaled short-acting β_2-agonist as required and 400 µg/kg/day of inhaled steroid. His mother wants to know whether there is anything else that you can do to help.
3. An 8-year-old girl presents with poorly controlled chronic asthma. She is currently being managed with an inhaled short-acting β_2-agonist as required, 800 µg/kg/day of inhaled steroid, a long-acting β_2-agonist and an oral leukotriene receptor antagonist. Inhaled theophylline was not previously successful. Her mother wants to know whether there is anything else that you can do to help.

4. A 3-year-old boy presents to his GP with an acute exacerbation of asthma. He has widespread wheeze, is too breathless to talk and has a heart rate of 140 beats/minute and a respiratory rate of 55 breaths/minute. The GP does not have the appropriate equipment to check the blood oxygen saturation.

5. A 4-year-old boy presents to the emergency department with an acute exacerbation of asthma. He is agitated, with oxygen saturations of 88% in air. He is demonstrating poor respiratory effort and has significantly reduced air entry.

THEME 6: INVESTIGATING THE FEBRILE CHILD

Options

A. Blood for culture and sensitivity
B. Blood for polymerase chain reaction
C. C-reactive protein
D. Chest X-ray
E. Cerebrospinal fluid for microscopy, culture and sensitivity
F. Cerebrospinal fluid for polymerase chain reaction
G. Full blood count
H. Limb X-ray
I. Urine for microscopy, culture and sensitivity

For each of the following children with a fever, select the investigation most likely to lead to a diagnosis. Each option may be used once, more than once or not at all.

1. A 2-year-old girl presents with a 4-day history of fever. The illness started with a cough. Her respiratory rate is 45 breaths/minute, saturations 94% in air, temperature 38.9°C and capillary refill time 1 second. There are crepitations at the left base on auscultation. Urine is negative on dipstick.

2. A 3-year-old girl presents with a fever for 2 days. She is drowsy and had a seizure causing twitching of the right side of the body for 4 minutes. Her respiratory rate is 30 breaths/minute, saturations 98% in air, temperature 38.3°C and capillary refill time 2 seconds. Urine is negative on dipstick.

3. A 6-month-old boy is admitted with persistent irritability. He is lethargic and is not feeding as well as usual. His respiratory rate is 30 breaths/minute, saturations 97% in air, temperature 38.0°C and capillary refill time 2 seconds. Urine is positive for leucocytes and nitrites on dipstick.

4. A 3-year-old boy presents with a 1-day history of being unwell. He appears shocked and has a 3-hour-old rash made up of urticaria and purpural spots. His respiratory rate is 30 breaths/minute, saturations 94% in air, temperature 39.0°C and capillary refill time 5 seconds. Urine is positive for leucocytes on dipstick.

5. A 2.5-year-old girl is admitted with a fever for 2 days. She has stopped walking and cries when changing her clothes. Her respiratory rate is 20 breaths/minute, saturations 99% in air, temperature 38.7°C and capillary refill time 1 second. Urine is clear on dipstick.

Options

A. Acquired hypothyroidism
B. Addison's disease
C. Bulimia nervosa
D. Congenital hypothyroidism
E. Cushing's disease
F. Cushing's syndrome
G. Hyperinsulinaemia secondary to diabetes
H. Lawrence–Moon–Biedl syndrome
 I. Obesity secondary to behavioural disorder
J. Polycystic ovarian syndrome
K. Prader–Willi syndrome
L. Primary obesity
M. Tricyclic antidepressant use

For each of the following patients who are clinically obese, select the most likely diagnosis. Each option may be used once, more than once or not at all.

1. An 8-year-old boy is clinically obese. As a baby, he was floppy and difficult to feed. He now has learning difficulties, and is constantly eating despite measures by his parents to hide food out of reach.

2. A 6-year-old boy is clinically obese. His body mass index is above the 95th centile. He has no other medical problems and examination is unremarkable. His mother says that she has tried everything to help him lose weight.

3. A 10-year-old boy is clinically obese and the shortest in his class. He had a renal transplant last year and his mother is worried that he is being bullied.

4. A 17-year-old girl is clinically obese. She has put a lot of weight on over the last year. She says that she is always tired and is becoming more constipated.

5. A 14-year-old girl is clinically obese. She has not started her periods yet and has severe acne. Among her investigations, a high insulin level is found.

THEME 8: HEART MURMURS

Options

A. Diastolic – second left intercostal space
B. Diastolic – second right intercostal space
C. Diastolic – fifth right intercostal space
D. Diastolic – apex
E. Ejection systolic – second left intercostal space
F. Ejection systolic – second right intercostal space
G. Pansystolic – fourth intercostal space, right adjacent to sternum
H. Pansystolic – fifth intercostal space, left adjacent to sternum
I. Pansystolic – apex
J. Systolic and diastolic – inferior to left clavicle

For each of the following conditions, select the most likely murmur that would be heard on auscultation of the heart (type of murmur – where heard best). Each option may be used once, more than once or not at all.

1. Ventricular septal defect
2. Mitral stenosis
3. Aortic stenosis
4. Patent ductus arteriosus
5. Pulmonary stenosis

THEME 9: DIARRHOEA

Options

A. Antibiotics
B. Cows' milk-free diet
C. Gluten-free diet
D. IV rehydration
E. Laxatives (e.g. Movicol)

F. No management required
G. Oral rehydration
H. Pancreatic enzyme supplements
I. Steroids

For each of the following children presenting with diarrhoea, select the most appropriate first step in the management. Each option may be used once, more than once or not at all.

1. A 5-year-old boy presents with diarrhoea. He has been passing approximately ten stools per day for the past 2 days. The stools are loose and have at times contained blood. He has had a fever and vomited three times yesterday. He attended a friend's party last weekend. On examination, he looks unwell. His blood pressure and pulse are normal and his eyes are not sunken. His peripheries are warm, but his lips are slightly dry.

2. An 18-month-old girl presents with diarrhoea. She has been passing five to ten stools per day for the past 6 months. Her mother reports that the stool is watery, smelly and that there are often food particles visible. The girl is thriving along her centile on the growth chart. On examination, she looks well, her blood pressure and pulse are normal, her eyes are not sunken, her peripheries are warm and her lips are moist.

3. A 16-month-old girl presents with diarrhoea. She has been passing 10–20 stools per day for the past 3 days. The stools are loose and smelly, but no blood is present. Her mother says that she had a fever, is irritable and vomited five times yesterday. She attends a nursery 3 days a week. On examination, she looks unwell, although her blood pressure and pulse are normal. Her eyes are sunken and she is cool around the edges, with a capillary refill time of 2 seconds. She was recently weighed for an immunization (12 kg), and today she weighs 11.5 kg.

4. A 19-month-old girl presents with diarrhoea. She has been passing five to ten stools per day for the past few months. Her mother reports that the stool is watery, although occasionally she will pass a large hard stool. The girl is thriving on her growth centiles. On examination, she looks well, her blood pressure and pulse are normal, her eyes are not sunken, her peripheries are warm and her lips are moist.

5. A 4-month-old, breastfed boy presents with diarrhoea. He has been passing five to ten loose stools per day for the past few months. The stool is watery and at times is flecked with blood. On examination, he looks well, he has widespread eczema, his blood pressure and pulse are normal, his eyes are not sunken, his peripheries are warm and his lips are moist.

THEME 10: HAEMATOLOGY AND HAEMATOLOGICAL MALIGNANCY

Options

A. Acute lymphoblastic leukaemia
B. Acute myeloid leukaemia
C. α-thalassaemia
D. β-thalassaemia
E. Glucose-6-phosphate dehydrogenase deficiency
F. Haemolytic–uraemic syndrome
G. Hodgkin's lymphoma
H. Non-Hodgkin's lymphoma
 I. *Plasmodium falciparum* infection
 J. Sickle cell disease
K. Spherocytosis
L. Splenic atrophy

For each of the following scenarios, select the most likely diagnosis. Each option may be used once, more than once or not at all.

1. A 2-year-old boy presents with chronic diarrhoea, abdominal distension and failure to thrive. His mother says that he has an itchy, vesicular rash on his upper limbs. A blood film reveals Howell–Jolly bodies and target cells.

2. A 3-year-old boy presents with multiple bruises all over his body. On examination, he has hepatosplenomegaly. A full blood count and blood film reveals anaemia, thrombocytopenia and blast cells.

3. A 4-year-old boy who has recently emigrated from Africa presents with fever. He is pale and acutely unwell. Blood film reveals signet-ring inclusions.

4. A 6-year-old boy who has recently emigrated from Africa presents with fever. He is pale and acutely unwell. Blood film reveals haemolytic fragments and Heinz bodies.

5. A 15-year-old boy who has recently emigrated from Africa presents with a prolonged history of fever. Examination reveals painless lymphadenopathy in the cervical region. Biopsy of the lymph nodes reveals Reed–Sternberg cells.

Practice Paper 5: Answers

THEME 1: ABDOMINAL PAIN

Abdominal pain is a common problem in children. It is also a highly non-specific symptom, so eliciting a diagnosis can be difficult. Symptoms associated with surgically correctable causes of acute abdominal pain include vomiting of bile, asymmetrical pain, local tenderness and peritonism.

1. K – Urinary tract infection

Urinary tract infections (UTIs) are relatively common in children, with 5% of girls having had a UTI by their second birthday. The most common causative organism is *Escherichia coli*. Other causative pathogens include *Proteus*, *Klebsiella*, *Enterobacter* and *Pseudomonas*. Infections located in the lower urinary tract (cystitis) will cause dysuria, urgency, wetting and generalized abdominal pain. This patient has an infection of the upper urinary tract (pyelonephritis), which causes more marked symptoms of high-grade fever and loin pain. The NICE guidelines* have attempted to standardize care of this common problem. Children with atypical or recurrent UTIs should have an ultrasound scan of the abdomen during the acute illness to rule out anatomical anomalies. Investigation for vesicoureteric reflux is no longer required routinely. If the UTI is recurrent or atypical in a child less than 3 years old, they should have renal function investigated with a dimercaptosuccinic acid (DMSA) scan (DMSA is a radiolabelled compound that becomes fixed in functioning proximal renal tubular cells. DMSA is not taken up by scarred, non-functioning areas of the kidney). The management of UTI is with oral or systemic antibiotics. Prophylactic antibiotics should not be prescribed routinely following a first UTI.

2. F – Intussusception

Intussusception is a surgical emergency. It affects children between the ages of 3 months and 3 years (most commonly between 6 and 18 months). Intussusception describes invagination of a proximal portion of bowel (the intussusceptum) into a distal segment (the intussuscipiens), most commonly at the ileocaecal junction. The blood supply to the telescoped

---

* Mori R, Lakhanpaul M, Verrier-Jones K. Diagnosis and management of urinary tract infection in children: Summary of NICE guidance. *BMJ* 2007; 335: 395–7.

bowel is compromised, resulting in tissue ischaemia and eventually necrosis. These children present with recurrent episodes of severe colicky abdominal pain, associated with pallor, screaming and drawing up of the legs. A sausage-shaped mass may be palpable in the right upper quadrant. The passage of blood and mucus *per rectum* (redcurrant jelly stools) is a late sign. Management is by resuscitation followed by reduction of the intussusception by a rectal air enema. If this is ineffective (25% of cases) then surgical reduction is required. Although intussusception can cause obstruction, these children would be vomiting and have abdominal distension, which is not found in this case.

3. A – Appendicitis

Acute appendicitis is the most common surgical emergency in childhood and adolescence. Inflammation of the appendix occurs secondary to obstruction of the appendiceal opening into the caecum. Obstruction can be by a faecolith (from Latin *faeco* = excrement + Greek *lith* = stone; 'piece of poo'), adhesions or lymphoid hyperplasia. Abdominal pain is initially central, but later shifts to the right iliac fossa due to localized peritonitis. Patients also have anorexia, nausea and vomiting, and a low-grade fever. (Only one-third of cases of appendicitis present with these characteristic findings.) Classically, there is pain over McBurney's point, which is found one-third of the way between the anterior superior iliac spine and the umbilicus. Rovsing's sign, in which palpation over the left iliac fossa causes right iliac fossa pain, may also be positive. If the inflamed appendix is adjacent to the bladder or rectum, then dysuria or diarrhoea can feature. Management is by appendicectomy.

Charles McBurney, American surgeon (1845–1913).
Niels Thorkild Rovsing, Danish surgeon (1862–1927).

4. G – Mesenteric adenitis

Non-specific abdominal pain is usually vague, central and colicky. Abdominal pain associated with a tachycardia and a flushed appearance often suggests an infective, extra-abdominal cause such as tonsillitis or otitis media. Mesenteric adenitis describes inflammation of the mesenteric lymph nodes that occurs following a viral upper respiratory tract infection. It presents with features similar to acute appendicitis, with the addition of high fever and evidence of viral infection (cervical lymphadenopathy and pharyngitis). Mesenteric adenitis is a self-limiting condition and, if it is suspected, management should initially be conservative to avoid unnecessary laparotomy.

5. C – Diabetic ketoacidosis

A large proportion of children with diabetes present initially with ketoacidosis. Diabetic ketoacidosis is a medical emergency with potentially severe complications. It must be managed carefully with rehydration and correction of the acidosis. Symptoms that suggest a diagnosis of diabetes include polydipsia (excessive thirst), polyuria, lethargy and weight loss. The symptoms of ketoacidosis include abdominal pain, nausea, vomiting and laboured breathing (the body's way of compensating for the acidosis by exhaling excess carbon dioxide). Ketoacidosis is often triggered by an acute infection, such as pharyngitis, which is found in this case.

THEME 2: APNOEA

Although there is no strict definition of apnoea, it can be roughly defined as the cessation of breathing for more than 20 seconds or for any period where the cessation of breathing is associated with pallor, cyanosis or a bradycardia. The causes of apnoea can be subdivided as follows:

1. Central: defect in neurological drive from respiratory centre
2. Obstructive: temporary blockage of the airway
3. Mixed: combination of central and obstructive

1. G – Sepsis

With this story, infection (sepsis, congenital pneumonia and/or meningitis) would be the most likely diagnosis. With a history of prolonged rupture of membranes of greater than 24 hours, sepsis is the most likely cause of apnoea, although it is also a risk factor for congenital pneumonia. You would need to perform a full septic screen that includes blood cultures, urine cultures, a lumbar puncture for cerebrospinal fluid (CSF) and a chest X-ray. The most common organisms causing sepsis in the neonatal period are group B streptococci and coliforms, which are acquired from the birth canal.

2. A – Gastro-oesophageal reflux

Gastro-oesophageal reflux (GOR) is a common problem in infants. Most cases in this age group are due to (transient) functional immaturity of the lower oesophageal sphincter (also known as physiological GOR) and do not require any medical management. Most cases resolve spontaneously by 12 months of age. Complications of reflux include apnoea in infants (this case), failure to thrive, aspiration, oesophagitis ($\rightarrow$ pain, bleeding and iron deficiency) and Sandifer's syndrome (dystonic movements of the head and neck that resemble seizures).

Most cases of GOR are diagnosed clinically, but it can be confirmed by measuring the lower oesophageal pH over a 24-hour period (pH study) or performing a barium swallow. In the pH study, a pH <4 for over 4 hours is indicative of reflux. Simple measures such as positioning the baby upright after feeding and thickening feeds are most likely to help. Medical treatments include drugs that increase gastric motility (erythromycin, metoclopramide or domperidone), antacids (Gaviscon), protein pump inhibitors (omeprazole) and H_2 receptor antagonists (ranitidine), though the evidence is not clear that these are actually beneficial. In severe, unresponsive cases, Nissen's fundoplication (where the fundus of the stomach is wrapped around the lower oesophagus to increase the effectiveness of the sphincter) is performed.

Rudolph Nissen, German surgeon (1896–1981).

3. B – Hypoglycaemia
In any emergency, your priority is to assess ABC. Remember always to check blood sugar (ABC-DEFG: Don't Ever Forget Glucose). In this case, one would list sepsis as a differential, but a blood sugar would confirm the diagnosis rapidly. Hypoglycaemia is defined as blood glucose <2.6 mmol/L. Neonates are commonly asymptomatic when hypoglycaemic, but may present with jitteriness, convulsions, hypotonia, lethargy and apnoea. Infants at risk of hypoglycaemia are babies at <37 weeks' gestation, babies <2.5 kg, intrauterine growth restriction and babies born of mothers with diabetes or who were on β-blockers for preeclampsia. Prolonged, symptomatic hypoglycaemia can cause permanent neurological disability. Management of hypoglycaemia is by feeding (or intravenous [IV] glucose if the infant cannot be fed).

4. E – Pertussis
Respiratory infections associated with apnoea include respiratory syncytial virus (RSV), bronchiolitis and pertussis (whooping cough). Localized airway infections such as tonsillitis, retropharyngeal abscess and epiglottitis can cause obstructive apnoea.

5. C – Intracranial haemorrhage
Physical abuse (non-accidental injury [NAI]) can present in many ways. This case has many of the classic signs of physical abuse (bruising around the chest wall and torn frenulum). Vigorously shaking babies causes subdural haemorrhage by rupturing the small subdural vessels.

Frenulum, from Latin *frenulum* = little bridle (a bridle being the straps that fit over a horse's head to help control it).

THEME 3: IMMUNIZATION SCHEDULE
The following information is summarized from the National Health Service website, www.nhs.uk/vaccinations.

1. J – Tuberculosis
The bacille Calmette–Guérin (BCG) vaccine protects against tuberculosis (TB). The aim of the UK BCG immunization programme is to immunize those at increased risk of developing severe disease and/or of exposure to TB infection. The largest population who are immunized are infants (aged 0–12 months) with a parent or grandparent who was born in a country where the annual incidence of TB is 40/100,000 or greater. The vaccination is usually offered shortly after birth.

2. H – Polio

The live oral polio vaccine has been replaced by inactivated polio vaccine (IPV). This is to remove the risk of vaccine-associated paralytic polio.

3. D – Meningococcus C

Meningococcus (*Neisseria meningitidis*) is a Gram-negative diplococcus that is currently the leading cause of pyogenic meningitis in the UK. There are at least 13 subtypes of meningococcus, which can cause both meningitis and sepsis. This vaccine only protects against meningococcus type C.

4. F – Pertussis

The pertussis vaccine is a suspension of killed organisms. Immunization does not give total protection, and protection is not lifelong. Immunized infants will have a milder illness if they are infected. By having a high level of herd immunity (i.e. immunizing as many children as possible), the most vulnerable group (infants in the first few months of life) are protected.

5. A – Diphtheria

Diphtheria is now rare in developed countries thanks to the protection given by the combined diphtheria, tetanus and pertussis (DTaP) vaccine. This has now been combined with IPV and the *Haemophilus influenzae* type b vaccine (Hib) to make up a pentavalent vaccine. Tetanus is also a Gram-positive anaerobic organism and is also now rare in developed countries due to immunization programmes.

The current immunization programme (March 2015) up to the age of 18 years is as follows:

- 2 months: DTaP/IPV/Hib, pneumococcal, rotavirus
- 3 months: DTaP/IPV/Hib, meningitis C (Men C), rotavirus
- 4 months: DTaP/IPV/Hib, pneumococcal (PCV), Men C
- 12–13 months: Hib/Men C, measles, mumps and rubella (MMR), PCV
- 2, 3 and 4 years: influenza vaccine
- Preschool: DTaP/IPV, MMR
- Girls 12–13 years: human papillomavirus
- 13–18 years: tetanus, diphtheria, IPV, Men C

THEME 4: CHILD PROTECTION

Safeguarding the wellbeing of children is important. This subject is complex and continuously evolving. Any healthcare professional working with children needs to be aware of the signs of presentation and the points of referral. If you have concerns about the safety of a child you must discuss this with someone. Never keep these concerns to yourself.

1. D – Neglect

This child has most likely suffered an accidental injury (option A). However, he was not appropriately supervised and the consequences for him are significant, therefore this is neglect (option D). It is important to consider that the account given may not be true and that this injury may have been inflicted, making NAI (option G) a less likely but important differential.

Physical injury can be inflicted deliberately, but can also be caused by a failure to provide a safe environment. The following should initiate a higher level of suspicion of inflicted injury (NAI):

- Discrepancy between injury/presentation and history given
- Change in history over time or between different people
- Delay in presentation
- Unusual reaction to the injury
- Repeated injuries
- History of NAI or suspicious injury in a sibling
- Other signs of neglect or failure to thrive

2. G – Non-accidental injury (physical abuse)

Any fractures in non-mobile children are suspicious. Most fractures in mobile children are accidental. A fall onto a hard surface would not be completely unreasonable, but this question is testing your knowledge of normal childhood development. Children are able to roll from their front onto their back at 24 weeks and from their back to their front at 28 weeks. It is therefore very unlikely that a 3-month-old could roll off their change mat. The story does not fit with the injury, and therefore you must suspect NAI. Remember that developmental milestones are not set in stone and therefore a child protection assessment would include a full assessment of development.

3. E – Normal variant

Although you would need to examine this baby to confirm your diagnosis, this sounds like a Mongolian blue spot. These are normal birthmarks and therefore 'normal variants'. They are found more commonly in Asian and Afro-Caribbean children. They usually fade by 1 year of life, but some persist.

4. H – Pathological cause

This child has sustained a serious injury considering the mode of trauma. Child protection should be considered seriously; however, pathological causes should be ruled out. This is a case of osteogenesis imperfecta type I, an autosomal dominant condition. This results in bony fragility, which causes recurrent fractures and deformity. Wormian bones may be seen on skull X-ray (these are irregular, isolated bones found within skull sutures – they are not fractures). The sclerae are blue, and the condition is associated with conductive hearing deafness (50% of cases) and aortic valve regurgitation – hence the diastolic murmur in this case. The 'named doctor' is a consultant (usually paediatric) responsible for giving advice on child protection matters within a hospital.

5. D – Neglect

Neglect can present in many ways: failure to thrive, poor development of emotional attachment and delayed development, speech and language. In this case, the child has contracted pertussis (whooping cough) because of a failure to be taken for immunization. Neglect may also present with inadequate hygiene such as a severe nappy rash, which improves rapidly with adequate care. It is important to note that parents have the right to choose not to have their children immunized; however, in combination with other signs of neglect, this should alert your suspicions to a child who is not being adequately cared for.

THEME 5: MANAGEMENT OF ASTHMA

Asthma is the most common chronic respiratory disorder affecting children. The British Thoracic Society guidelines for the management of asthma are the gold standard in the UK (they can be found at www.brit-thoracic.org.uk). All children seen in hospital with an acute exacerbation of asthma should have their long-term management reviewed, their inhaler technique assessed and a clear discharge plan provided along with a follow-up appointment with their GP.

1. P – Regular inhaled short-acting β_2-agonist via a spacer

This boy has a new diagnosis of asthma and should be started on step 1 of the management ladder. He should be reassessed later and, if this has not been effective, then an inhaled steroid should be added. At this age (under 5 years), all inhalers should be given through a spacer device to maximize their effect. The diagnosis of asthma is supported in this case by the atopic picture (eczema).

For reference, the management of asthma follows a stepwise approach, summarized as follows:

- Step 1: short-acting β_2-agonist (salbutamol or terbutaline)
- Step 2: step 1 + low-dose inhaled steroid (budesonide or fluticasone)
- Step 3: step 2 +
  - <5 years of age: leukotriene inhibitor (monteleukast)
  - ≥5 years of age: high-dose inhaled steroid and long-acting β_2-agonist
- Step 4: step 3 + fourth drug (e.g. theophylline or an anticholinergic)
- Step 5: step 4 + oral steroid (prednisolone)

2. J – Oral leukotriene receptor antagonist

This child is under 5 years of age and is receiving a good dose of inhaled steroid. Check that compliance and technique are good. The mother has asked whether there is anything else that can be given: an oral leukotriene receptor antagonist (e.g. monteleukast) is the next available treatment. Oral leukotrienes are very useful at this age, as they can be sprinkled onto foods such as yoghurt or cereal. Children over 5 years of age could have the inhaled steroid increased and a trial of a long-acting β_2-agonist (e.g. salmeterol or formoterol).

3. K – Oral steroids

This girl is on a significant regimen of medications. It would be very important to check compliance and technique. It is often possible to check compliance by finding out whether repeat prescriptions are being collected appropriately. If on theophylline, compliance can be monitored using a theophylline blood level. It is important to check compliance in this case, as the next step would be oral steroids. If this child has not already been referred, they should be referred to a respiratory paediatrician.

4. L – Oxygen via facemask, two to ten puffs of inhaled short-acting β_2-agonist via spacer and oral steroid

This is a severe exacerbation of asthma. Features of severe asthma are

- Patient is too breathless to talk or feed
- Respiration rate ≥50 breaths/minute
- Pulse ≥140 beats/minute
- Peak flow ≤50% predicted or best

Considering that the patient is at the GP surgery, he should be managed with the above step (oxygen/inhaled β_2-agonist/steroid). Oxygen should be employed if available. The child will need to be safely transferred to a paediatric assessment unit for further monitoring and treatment.

5. O – Oxygen via facemask, nebulized short-acting β_2-agonist and oral or IV steroid

This is a life-threatening exacerbation of asthma. Features of life-threatening asthma are

- Fatigue or exhaustion
- Decreasing consciousness
- Silent chest or poor respiratory effort
- Peak flow ≤33% predicted or best

The above measures should be performed (oxygen/nebulized β_2-agonist/steroid). Frequent use of nebulized short-acting β_2-agonists (salbutamol) is described as 'back-to-back nebs', in which each nebulizer is immediately followed by another. This child is very sick, and will probably need admission to a paediatric intensive care unit. He is likely to need IV salbutamol and/or IV aminophylline; however, one should reassess response to the initial management prior to commencing these agents. In a child over 5 years of age, IV magnesium sulphate can also be used.

THEME 6: INVESTIGATING THE FEBRILE CHILD

Infectious diseases remain a major cause of childhood mortality and morbidity in the UK. A fever in a child usually indicates an underlying infection. A full blood count and C-reactive protein (CRP) are very useful in febrile children who do not have a confirmed focus for infection. However, they will not provide a diagnosis. Neutrophilia suggests a bacterial infection and lymphophilia suggests a viral infection, but these are not hard-and-fast rules. CRP is an acute-phase protein produced by the liver. Raised levels are a sign of inflammation, not just infection.

1. D – Chest X-ray

This girl has community-acquired pneumonia. The diagnosis can be made clinically, although radiology can confirm pulmonary consolidation. Tachypnoea is one of the most sensitive signs of pneumonia in children of this age. Attention must be paid to oxygenation, nutrition and hydration. In this case, the patient is not compromised and so can be treated at home with oral antibiotics.

2. F – Cerebrospinal fluid for polymerase chain reaction

This girl with fever and seizures has viral encephalitis. Warning signs of encephalitis are focal neurological signs, focal seizures (as in this case) and a decreased level of consciousness. The investigation most likely to yield a diagnosis would be CSF for polymerase chain reaction (PCR) of herpesviruses. She should be treated with IV broad-spectrum antibiotics and aciclovir until the results from the CSF are obtained.

3. I – Urine for microscopy, culture and sensitivity

This boy, with fever and a dipstick positive for nitrites and leucocytes, is likely to have a UTI. Although empirical antibiotics can be commenced, a sample of urine is still required for microscopy, culture and sensitivity, as the child is below 3 years of age. Getting a good-quality urine sample at this age is difficult. The gold standard is a clean-catch urine which involves sitting the child on a sterile pot. Other methods, such as bag and or pad collections, risk contamination and incorrect diagnosis and so should not be used. In some sick children, catheter insertion or suprapubic aspiration can be used to obtain urine prior to starting antibiotics.

4. A – Blood for culture and sensitivity

This boy, who presents with high fever and a purpuric rash, has sepsis caused by the Gram-negative diplococcus *Neisseria meningitidis*. Blood for culture and sensitivity would be the first-line investigation, although PCR can also be employed. Meningococcal disease can present as meningitis, sepsis or both. Evidence shows that children presenting with meningitis alone have a better prognosis.

5. A – Blood for culture and sensitivity

This girl is febrile and is refusing to walk. It is likely, therefore, that she has osteomyelitis or septic arthritis. Radiology will not show any abnormality until later in the disease course. An ultrasound scan of the joints would be more useful. This girl should initially be treated with empirical IV antibiotics, but before this, blood cultures and joint aspiration should be sent for in order to look for the offending organism.

THEME 7: OBESITY

Body mass index (BMI) is a standardized measurement used in adults, and can also be used in adolescents and children. A BMI >95th centile in children and >30 kg/m^2 in adolescents is the definition of obesity. Management options include treating the cause, lifestyle changes, behavioural therapy, physical activity and dietary advice.

1. K – Prader–Willi syndrome

Prader–Willi syndrome can present in the neonatal period with hypotonia and poor feeding. Later in life, children gain excessive weight due to hyperphagia (excessive appetite). Other features include hypogonadism, strabismus, low IQ and characteristic facial features (narrow forehead, olive-shaped eyes, anti-mongoloid slant and carp-shaped mouth).

Laurence–Moon–Biedl syndrome is associated with learning difficulties, but is also characterized by progressive visual impairment (due to retinal changes), digital anomalies (polydactyly and syndactyly), hypogenitalism and nephropathy.

2. L – Primary obesity

Obesity among children is increasing. Primary obesity is the most common cause, and other disorders associated with obesity are rare. Pathological causes account for less than 1% of cases. In most cases, obesity is the result of a positive energy balance that is stored as adipose tissue.

3. F – Cushing's syndrome

Cushing's syndrome describes the clinical features caused by adrenal steroid excess. The most common cause is iatrogenic steroid administration – in this case, steroids used as an immunosuppressant postrenal transplant. Patients with Cushing's present with moon-like faces, plethora, acne, buffalo hump (interscapular fat pad), truncal obesity, growth arrest (i.e. poor height), easy bruising, hypertension, hypogonadism, cataracts and/or glucose intolerance. Cushing's disease is excess corticosteroid secretion secondary to a pituitary tumour.

Addison's disease is primary autoimmune-mediated adrenocortical failure. The adrenal cortex secretes three things: glucocorticoids, mineralocorticoids and adrenal androgens. These usually feed back to the anterior pituitary to reduce adrenocorticotropic hormone (ACTH) secretion. Therefore, if the adrenal cortex fails, there are many consequences: reduced glucocorticoids (hypoglycaemia and weight loss), reduced mineralocorticoids (hyperkalaemia, hyponatraemia and hypotension), reduced adrenal androgens (decreased body hair and libido) and ACTH excess (increased pigmentation in sun-exposed areas, pressure areas, palmar creases, buccal mucosa and recent scars). The diagnosis of Addison's disease is by the short synacthen test. In this investigation, plasma cortisol levels are measured before and after the administration of a single intramuscular or IV dose of ACTH. Normally, the administration of ACTH will result in a rise in cortisol. If there is an inadequate rise in cortisol on the second reading, adrenal insufficiency is indicated. Management of Addison's disease is with the replacement of glucocorticoids and mineralocorticoids (with hydrocortisone and fludrocortisone).

Thomas Addison, English physician (1795–1860).
Harvey Cushing, American neurosurgeon and endocrinologist (1869–1939).

4. A – Acquired hypothyroidism

Congenital hypothyroidism presents early in life with coarse facial features, large tongue, hoarse cry, hypotonia, lethargy, umbilical hernia, constipation and prolonged jaundice. This is now rarely made as a clinical diagnosis due to screening using the Guthrie card.

Acquired hypothyroidism, which develops later in life, is more common. Iodine deficiency is the most common cause of acquired hypothyroidism worldwide. In iodine adequacy, autoimmune disease (Hashimoto's thyroiditis) is the most common cause in childhood and adolescence. Patients present with short stature (due to poor height growth and delayed skeletal growth), intolerance to cold, constipation, lethargy and weight gain. Signs may include goitre, bradycardia and slow relaxation of tendon reflexes. Autoantibodies to thyroid peroxidase (an enzyme required to make thyroxine) may be found. Treatment is with thyroid replacement (thyroxine).

Hashimoto Hakaru, Japanese physician (1881–1934).

5. J – Polycystic ovarian syndrome

The cause of polycystic ovarian syndrome (PCOS) is unknown. Girls with PCOS are classically tall, obese and hirsute. They suffer from amenorrhoea, dysfunctional menstrual bleeding and infertility. Biochemical features include raised testosterone and raised luteinizing hormone. Metabolically, these girls have raised cholesterol levels and insulin resistance, which predisposes them to diabetes. In this case, the raised insulin level is not due to diabetes but to the PCOS. For more information on PCOS, see 'The infertility clinic' (Paper 3 Answers, Theme 10).

THEME 8: HEART MURMURS

Heart murmurs are a relatively common finding in children, and many pathological lesions have distinct patterns of murmurs. Murmurs are caused by turbulent blood flow, usually through valves but also through vessels and heart chambers. Most murmurs are innocent (non-pathological), such as vibratory murmurs and venous hums. The following features suggest an innocent murmur: quiet, asymptomatic, louder during fever/exercise, varying during respiration/posture and systolic.

Heart murmurs are graded according to their intensity:

- Grade I: faint murmur (usually only cardiologists can hear)
- Grade II: quiet murmur
- Grade III: moderate/loud intensity, no thrill
- Grade IV: loud murmur, with a thrill
- Grade V: very loud murmur with a thrill (still requires stethoscope to hear)
- Grade VI: very loud murmur with a thrill (can be heard close to chest wall without a stethoscope)

1. H – Pansystolic – fifth intercostal space, left adjacent to sternum

A ventricular septal defect is the most common congenital cardiac lesion in children. The murmur is pansystolic, which means that it is heard throughout systole. This murmur is caused by shunting of blood from the high-pressure left ventricle to the low-pressure right ventricle.

2. D – Diastolic – apex

Mitral stenosis is almost always caused by rheumatic fever, which in itself is now rare in the UK. The murmur is found at the end of diastole and is heard best in the mitral region (fifth intercostal space, left side, midclavicular line – the apex).

3. F – Ejection systolic – second right intercostal space

In mild cases, aortic stenosis will usually cause no symptoms in early life. As the child gets older, the stenosis may become more severe due to calcification of the valve. In critical aortic stenosis, heart failure will ensue rapidly after birth. The murmur is systolic and is heard loudest at the second right intercostal space parasternally (the aortic area). The murmur is associated with an ejection click and the murmur may be conducted to the neck (carotids).

4. J – Systolic and diastolic – inferior to left clavicle

Patent ductus arteriosus is a common problem in preterm newborns. The fetal circulation remains patent, causing heart failure due to blood shunting from the systemic to the pulmonary circulation. The murmur is described as a 'machinery murmur' that is often both systolic and diastolic. It is heard best inferior to the left clavicle.

5. E – Ejection systolic – second left intercostal space

The murmur of pulmonary stenosis is systolic and heard best in the second left intercostal space parasternally (pulmonary area). The degree of pulmonary stenosis varies greatly between patients. Most cases are mild and will not affect the child's health. Critical stenosis will often present rapidly when the ductus arteriosus closes, and will cause early death unless diagnosed early. Management is with dilatation of the stenosis using a balloon or surgical correction.

THEME 9: DIARRHOEA

Diarrhoea is defined as stools of increased frequency, volume and fluidity. Acute diarrhoea has a short onset and duration; chronic diarrhoea is present for over 2–3 weeks. Most cases of diarrhoea in children are due to viral infections, and the key is assessing and treating any dehydration.

1. G – Oral rehydration

Using natural routes of hydration/rehydration is always optimal, as there is less risk of electrolyte imbalance. This child has gastroenteritis, which is likely to be bacterial in origin. Although he is unwell, he has not yet become dehydrated. At this point, no treatment would be required except advice to his parents about good hydration and hand-washing. Antibiotics and adsorbent or stool-bulking drugs (e.g. loperamide) should be avoided in gastroenteritis. Organisms that cause bacterial gastroenteritis include *Campylobacter*, *Salmonella* and *Shigella* spp., as well as *Escherichia coli*. The most serious complication of bacterial gastroenteritis (other than profound dehydration and shock) is haemolytic–uraemic syndrome, which can cause acute-onset renal failure and anaemia.

2. F – No management required

This is a case of 'toddler's diarrhoea'. Most cases of toddler's diarrhoea can be diagnosed clinically, often with the description of food in the diarrhoea ('carrots and peas' diarrhoea) in the otherwise-well child. However, it is important not to miss more sinister diagnoses. Many centres will send stool for blood, ova and parasites, pH, bacterial cultures and reducing substances (sugars suggestive of carbohydrate malabsorption). No management is required except reassurance that the child is normal. Most cases resolve with age.

3. G – Oral rehydration

This girl has gastroenteritis, most likely caused by a virus. Many children receive IV rehydration too early. With patience and perseverance, most cases of gastroenteritis can be managed with oral rehydration/hydration. If the child is under 2 years of age and refusing oral fluids, then a nasogastric tube can be sited, thus allowing the gastrointestinal tract to be used for fluid intake. This girl is dehydrated, as she has sunken eyes and dry mucous membranes. Weights are very useful in children, and in this case we can see that she is less than 5% dehydrated (mild dehydration). The most common cause of viral gastroenteritis is rotavirus, which, along with RSV bronchiolitis, keeps paediatric wards and GP surgeries busy during the winter months. Rotavirus vaccination was introduced into the UK immunization programme in 2013, and is given in two doses (at 2 and 3 months).

4. E – Laxatives (e.g. Movicol)

This is a case of overflow diarrhoea secondary to constipation. Constipation is a vicious cycle in this age group: children learn that it is painful to pass large hard stools, and so retain the stool, which gradually becomes harder, thus making the child more constipated. Eventually, these children lose sphincter tone, and proximal soft stools bypass the impacted stool. This is known as overflow diarrhoea. Treatment is complex and reassurance is important. Laxatives such as Movicol (a macrogel) and lactulose work by holding water in the stool (osmotic laxatives). These agents require a good fluid intake to work. It is important to inform the parents that the overflow diarrhoea may become a little worse before the constipation improves. Treatment can take months to years to complete.

5. B – Cows' milk-free diet

Proteins found in cows' milk, and occasionally soy-based milk, can cause an enterocolitis in infancy. Management is with a trial of hydrolyzed formula (e.g. Nutramigen®), or by eliminating cows' milk from the diet of a breastfeeding mother. There are other, more sinister causes of rectal bleeding in infants that should be considered. These include haemorrhagic disease of the newborn, anal fissures, volvulus, intussusception, polyps, Meckel's diverticulum and infection.

THEME 10: HAEMATOLOGY AND HAEMATOLOGICAL MALIGNANCY

1. L – Splenic atrophy

Howell–Jolly bodies are basophilic nuclear remnants in the cytoplasm and are a sign of asplenism (as the spleen normally removes such fragments). Causes of splenic atrophy and asplenism include surgical removal of the spleen, sickle cell disease and coeliac disease (this case). The rash on the upper limb is dermatitis herpetiformis (which confusingly has nothing to do with herpes) and is associated with coeliac disease. Target cells are red blood cells, which demonstrate increased staining in the middle of an area of pallor. They are found in obstructive liver disease, sickle cell disease, asplenism, thalassaemia and iron-deficiency anaemia.

William Henry Howell, American physiologist (1860–1945).
Justin Marie Jolly, French haematologist (1870–1953).

2. A – Acute lymphoblastic leukaemia

Leukaemia is caused by the proliferation of a single bone marrow stem cell following malignant transformation.

Acute lymphoblastic leukaemia (ALL) is the most common leukaemia in children, and is caused by the clonal proliferation of lymphoid precursor (blast) cells that have been arrested at an early stage of development. The blast cells infiltrate the marrow and lymphoid tissue, causing pancytopenia and lymphadenopathy, respectively. The central nervous system (CNS) can also be affected, causing headache, vomiting, meningism, cranial nerve palsy and seizures. Treatment is with supportive measures such as transfusion and antibiotics, as well as with chemotherapy. Chemotherapy is traditionally delivered in three main stages: remission induction, consolidation and maintenance, which can be for a number of years. Since patients with ALL are at high risk of developing neurological disease, they are often given CNS prophylaxis in the form of intrathecal methotrexate and radiotherapy. The prognosis of ALL is good with appropriate treatment.

Acute myeloid leukaemia

Acute myeloid leukaemia (AML) is caused by the proliferation of myeloid precursor cells. The presentation of AML is variable. Many sufferers are completely asymptomatic and are diagnosed incidentally, whereas others become very unwell very quickly. Marrow failure caused by blast infiltration results in anaemia, thrombocytopenia and neutropenia (resulting in the clinical features of easy bleeding, bruising and multiple infections). Investigation usually shows a significantly raised white blood cell count. Cellular inclusions called Auer rods that are seen on microscopy are pathognomonic of AML. The management of AML involves blood and platelet transfusion, treatment of secondary infections and chemotherapy. Stem cell transplantation may be considered. The prognosis of AML is worse than that of ALL. This condition is generally seen in adulthood and is rapidly fatal if untreated. Patients with Down's syndrome are at increased risk of both ALL and AML, with the risk of AML being highest in the first 3 years of life.

3. I – *Plasmodium falciparum* infection

This boy has malaria. Malaria is caused by *Plasmodium* parasites, which are transmitted through the bite of the female *Anopheles* mosquito. The incubation period is 3 weeks. Patients present with abrupt-onset fever and rigors. The fever peaks every 3 or 4 days. Other features are abdominal pain, diarrhoea, headache and flu-like symptoms. Malaria is diagnosed on thick and thin blood films. Thick films allow detection of parasites; thin films reveal the species responsible and the determination of parasitaemia (measured as the percentage of erythrocytes infected). Complications of malaria include haemoglobinuria ('black water fever' – from severe haemolysis), acute renal failure and cerebral malaria (fits and coma). Cerebral malaria is the main cause of death.

4. E – Glucose-6-phosphate dehydrogenase deficiency

Glucose-6-phosphate dehydrogenase (G6PD) is an enzyme that reduces oxidative stress by reducing glutathione levels within red cells. G6PD deficiency is an X-linked disorder common in West Africa, southern Europe, the Middle East and Southeast Asia. Patients are usually asymptomatic until oxidative stress causes haemolytic anaemia. Common triggers include fava broad beans (broad bean-induced haemolysis is termed favism), drugs (including antimalarials and sulphonamide antibiotics) and infections. Treatment is supportive, although transfusions may be required for acute haemolytic crises. Heinz bodies are denatured haemoglobin aggregates that are found in the cytoplasm of red blood cells. They result from oxidant stress (e.g. G6PD deficiency) or haemolysis. Recessive carriers of the G6PD mutation are protected against malaria.

5. G – Hodgkin's lymphoma

Lymphomas are diseases caused by malignant proliferation of the lymphoid system. Hodgkin's lymphoma classically presents with asymmetrical painless lymphadenopathy, usually in the form of a single rubbery lymph node in the cervical, axillary or inguinal region, which may become painful after alcohol ingestion. Disease spread to the mediastinal nodes may occur and cause dyspnoea and superior vena cava obstruction. Approximately 20% of patients suffer systemic symptoms such as weight loss, sweating, fever, pruritis and general lethargy (these are known as 'B' symptoms). Diagnosis is usually based on lymph node biopsy showing pathognomonic Reed–Sternberg cells. Computed tomography scanning can help confirm the diagnosis, and is often used for staging. Early-stage disease is managed with radiotherapy alone. In advanced and bulky disease, the combination of radiotherapy and chemotherapy is often employed. The prognosis of Hodgkin's lymphoma is good, with a 70% chance of cure even in later stages of disease. Increasing age and the presence of systemic symptoms indicate a poorer prognosis.

Thomas Hodgkin, British physician (1798–1866).
Dorothy Reed Mendenhall, American paediatrician (1874–1964).
Carl Sternberg, Austrian pathologist (1872–1935).

Other haematological terms

- Anisocytosis: red cells are of varying sizes (haemoglobinopathies and anaemias)
- Basophilic stippling: RNA inclusion bodies in the cytoplasm
- Burr cells (echinocytes): cell membrane with a serrated appearance
- Helmet cells: red cell fragments indicating microangiopathic haemolysis haemolytic uraemic syndrome (HUS)
- Poikilocytosis: red cells are of varying shapes
- Schistocytes: another term for helmet cells (above)
- Spherocytes: small, spherical, densely stained cells

Poikilocyte, from Greek *poikilos* = irregular.
Aniocytosis, from Greek *anisos* = unequal.
Schistocyte, from Greek *schistos* = split.

Practice Paper 6: Questions

THEME 1: VOMITING

Options

A. Appendicitis
B. Duodenal atresia
C. Exomphalos
D. Gastroenteritis
E. Gastro-oesophageal reflux
F. Gastroschisis
G. Incarcerated inguinal hernia
H. Intussusception
I. Malrotation with volvulus
J. Meckel's diverticulum
K. Overfeeding
L. Pyloric stenosis
M. Sepsis
N. Testicular torsion
O. Urinary tract infection

For each of the following infants presenting with vomiting, select the most likely diagnosis. Each option may be used once, more than once or not at all.

1. A 2-month-old, bottle-fed infant presents with vomiting. He has been vomiting milk up to five times a day for the last 2 days. The vomiting is associated with loose stools and he has been having up to ten bowel motions a day for 3 days. His temperature is 37.1°C. On examination, his blood pressure and pulse are normal, his eyes and fontanelle are not sunken, his peripheries are warm and his lips are moist.

2. A 2-month-old, bottle-fed infant presents with vomiting. He has had bilious vomiting for the past 24 hours. On examination, he looks very unwell, he is tachycardic, his eyes and fontanelle are sunken and his capillary refill time is 5 seconds. His blood pressure is normal. He has a firm mass in his groin.

3. A 2-month-old, bottle-fed infant presents with vomiting. He vomits small amounts of milk into his mouth, which he then swallows. This has been a problem since the first few weeks of life. He is often very irritable after feeds and arches his back. On examination, his blood pressure and

pulse are normal, his eyes and fontanelle are not sunken, his peripheries are warm and his lips are moist.

4. A 2-month-old, bottle-fed infant presents with vomiting. He is described as a 'greedy baby'. He vomits large amounts of milk after feeds. This has been a problem since the first few weeks of life. On examination, his blood pressure and pulse are normal, his eyes and fontanelle are not sunken, his peripheries are warm and his lips are moist.

5. A 2-month-old, bottle-fed infant presents with vomiting. This has steadily been getting worse over the last 5 days. He is now eager for feeds, and shortly after taking milk will forcefully vomit. On examination, his blood pressure is normal, he is tachycardic, but his eyes and fontanelle are not sunken, his peripheries are warm and his lips are moist. However, he has lost weight since he was last weighed at 6 weeks of age.

THEME 2: THE CHILD WITH A LIMP

Options

A. Developmental dysplasia of the hip
B. Fracture
C. Genu varus
D. Ligamental strain
E. Osgood–Schlatter disease
F. Osteomyelitis
G. Perthes' disease
H. Septic arthritis
 I. Slipped capital femoral epiphysis
 J. Spontaneous haemarthrosis
K. Talipes equinovarus
L. Transient synovitis

For each of the following children presenting with a limp, select the most likely diagnosis. Each option may be used once, more than once or not at all.

1. A 14-year-old boy presents with a limp and left knee pain of 24 hours' duration. He is systemically well and is afebrile. On examination, he appears overweight. His left leg is externally rotated and shorter than the right.

2. A 6-year-old boy presents with groin pain and a limp. The groin pain is exacerbated by exercise. On examination, you notice a leg-length discrepancy. He is systemically well and afebrile. There is no history of medical problems.

3. A 7-year-old boy presents with hip pain and a limp of acute onset. He denies pain at rest. He has been unwell for the few days prior to admission with a low-grade fever and a coryzal illness. He is reluctant for you to move the affected leg, which has a decreased range of movement.

4. A 24-month-old boy presents with a limp. Since waking this morning, he has not been using his left leg and is unable to weight-bear. He has a temperature of 39.5°C and looks systemically unwell. You attempt to examine the range of movement of the affected limb, but this elicits severe pain. The left knee is red, hot and swollen.

5. A 16-month-old boy presents with a limp. His mother has noticed that, since he started walking 2 months ago, he has had a limp, although it does not appear to cause him any discomfort. He is systemically well and is afebrile.

THEME 3: COUGH

Options

A. Aspiration of vomit
B. Asthma
C. Bronchiolitis
D. Croup
E. Cystic fibrosis
F. Foreign-body inhalation
G. Pertussis
H. Pneumonia

For each of the following children presenting with a cough, select the most likely diagnosis. Each option may be used once, more than once or not at all.

1. An 18-month-old girl presents with a recurrent cough, which is occasionally productive. She is small for her age. Her mother reports episodes of wheeze.

2. A 2-year-old boy presents with a cough. The cough has been present for the last 3 days. He was previously well. On examination, he has a temperature of 38.9°C and a respiratory rate of 55 breaths/minute. There is no wheeze.

3. A 4-year-old boy presents with a recurrent cough, which is worse at night. He is small for his age. The cough has been present for the last 12 months and interrupts his sleep.

4. A 6-month-old boy presents with a cough. The illness began 4 days ago with a runny nose and a mild fever. Over the last 24 hours, he has developed a high-pitched cough associated with a wheeze. On examination, fine crepitations are heard throughout both lung fields.

5. A 2-year-old boy presents with a cough, which started suddenly this afternoon at a children's party. He is otherwise well and has a temperature of 36.5°C. On examination, there are reduced breath sounds on the right side.

THEME 4: CHROMOSOMAL DISORDERS

Options
A. 45XO
B. 47XXX
C. 47XXY
D. 47XY (13)
E. 47XY (18)
F. 47XY (21)
G. 69XXY
H. Fragile X syndrome

For each of the following scenarios, select the most likely karyotype. Each option may be used once, more than once or not at all.

1. You are performing the postnatal check on a 3-day-old girl. She has swollen hands and feet, and you find it difficult to palpate her femoral pulses.
2. You are asked to see a 1-hour-old baby. He is dysmorphic, with a small chin and low-set ears. He also has a small head and rocker-bottom feet.
3. A 15-year-old boy presents to the general paediatrics clinic. He and his family are concerned as he has not entered puberty yet. He is tall for his age and has small, firm testes. He is a shy boy and has had some behavioural problems at school.
4. You are asked to see a 1-hour-old baby. He is dysmorphic with a round face. On examination, you notice that he is very floppy.
5. A 5-year-old boy presents to the outpatient clinic. He has learning difficulties, a large head and large testicles. He has quite a characteristic facial appearance, with a prominent forehead and large ears.

THEME 5: ARTHRITIS

Options
A. Acute rheumatic fever
B. Enteropathic arthritis
C. Haemarthrosis
D. Hand–foot syndrome
E. Leukaemia
F. Monoarticular juvenile idiopathic arthritis
G. Pauciarticular juvenile idiopathic arthritis
H. Polyarticular juvenile idiopathic arthritis
I. Psoriatic arthropathy
J. Reactive arthritis
K. Septic arthritis
L. Still's disease
M. Systemic lupus erythematosus
N. Transient synovitis

For each of the following children presenting with painful joints, select the most likely diagnosis. Each option may be used once, more than once or not at all.

1. A 12-year-old boy presents with painful joints. He recently had a bout of gastroenteritis, which he blames on a 'dodgy doner kebab'. His stools were loose and contained blood. He was previously well. On examination, both his knee joints are tender and hot.

2. A 12-year-old boy presents with painful joints. He is known to have sickle cell disease and was out sledging today in the freshly fallen snow. The joints of his fingers on both hands are now red, hot and swollen.

3. A 12-year-old boy presents with painful joints. For 2 months, he has complained of having painful wrist joints. Both wrists are affected, and on examination they appear red, hot and swollen. He is otherwise systemically well and has had no recent illness.

4. A 12-year-old boy presents with painful joints. He recently had a sore throat, which was confirmed as a streptococcal infection on throat swab. He has an unusual rash over his trunk and upper limbs associated with a fever. The rash is made up of pink rings and is not itchy.

5. A 12-year-old boy presents with painful joints. He recently had a bout of gastroenteritis, which he blames on a 'dodgy doner kebab'. His stools were loose and contained blood. He says that his stools had contained blood for at least a month prior to the bout of gastroenteritis. On examination, both knee joints are tender and hot.

THEME 6: JAUNDICE IN THE NEWBORN

Options

A. Abdominal X-ray
B. Abdominal ultrasound
C. Blood cultures
D. C-reactive protein
E. Conjugated bilirubin level
F. Full blood count
G. Group and Coombs' testing
H. Metabolic screen
 I. No further investigation required
 J. Sweat test
K. Thyroid-stimulating hormone
L. TORCH screen
M. Unconjugated bilirubin level
N. Urea and electrolytes

For each of the following neonates/infants presenting with jaundice, select the most likely investigation that will reveal the underlying cause. Each option may be used once, more than once or not at all.

1. You are asked to see a 12-hour-old baby urgently on the delivery suite. He stopped breathing for a few seconds and needed stimulation to terminate the apnoea. He is jaundiced, irritable and not feeding well. His mother's waters broke over 24 hours before he was born.

2. You perform a baby check on a 12-hour-old baby. He is clinically well but significantly jaundiced. His mother is from India and had two children before moving to the UK.

3. A GP refers a 5-week-old infant who is jaundiced. His mother reports that his stools are white like chalk. On examination, the infant is clinically well but markedly jaundiced.

4. A health visitor refers a 10-day-old infant who is clinically well but jaundiced. The jaundice was first noticeable after 3 days when a bilirubin level was sent for and found to be below the treatment level for phototherapy. He was initially breastfed, but his mother has just given up and started bottle feeding, as he was not gaining weight.

5. You are asked to see a 24-hour-old newborn baby. He is small for his dates and was born at 37 weeks' gestation. On examination, you notice that he has a small head and is jaundiced. Palpation reveals a large liver. While you are present, the baby has a seizure.

THEME 7: SEIZURES

A. Anaesthesia and intubation
B. Buccal midazolam
C. Buccal diazepam
D. Intravenous (IV) dextrose
E. IV lorazepam
F. IV phenytoin
G. No treatment required
H. Oral antiepileptic medication (e.g. sodium valproate)
 I. Oral antipyretics
 J. Oral antibiotics
K. Oral diazepam
 L. Rectal diazepam
M. Rectal paraldehyde

For each of the following children, select the most appropriate next step in management once airway, breathing and circulation have been assessed and facial oxygen has been applied. Each option may be used once, more than once or not at all.

1. A 3-year-old boy presents with fitting. There is no history of epilepsy and he is on no medication. The seizure started 5 minutes ago and has now stopped. He has a fever of 38.9°C and on examination you notice an inflamed left ear drum. His mother says that he has been pulling at his ear all day. His blood sugar is 5.0 mmol/L.

2. A 3-year-old boy presents with fitting. There is no history of epilepsy and he is on no medication. He started fitting 40 minutes ago. The seizure is continuing despite attempts at medical termination. His blood sugar is 4.7 mmol/L.

3. A 3-year-old boy presents with fitting. There is no history of epilepsy and he is on no medication. He started fitting 15 minutes ago. The ambulance crew has given a single dose of rectal diazepam en route. On your arrival, the emergency department registrar has had two attempts at inserting a cannula, but has been unsuccessful. His blood sugar is 5.6 mmol/L.

4. A 3-year-old boy presents with fitting. There is no history of epilepsy and he is on no medication. He started fitting 20 minutes ago. He had an IV cannula sited on arrival and his blood sugar is 4.5 mmol/L. He has had two doses of IV lorazepam, but continues to fit.

5. A 3-year-old boy presents with fitting. There is no history of epilepsy and he is on no medication. His mother says that he has been having these fits for a few months. They always occur when he has hurt himself. Today, he bumped his head and started crying. He then stopped breathing and turned blue. On falling to the floor, there was a brief period where he was twitching his legs. He has now fully recovered. His blood sugar is 3.5 mmol/L.

THEME 8: FEVER AND A RASH

Options

A. Erythrovirus (fifth disease)
B. Hand, foot and mouth disease
C. Henoch–Schönlein purpura
D. Kawasaki's disease
E. Measles
F. Meningococcal meningitis
G. Meningococcal sepsis
H. Mumps
I. Roseola
J. Rubella
K. Scarlet fever
L. Varicella zoster

For each of the following descriptions, select the most likely diagnosis. Each option may be used once, more than once or not at all.

1. A 2.5-year-old boy presents with a fever and a rash. The rash is found mostly on his trunk, and is made up of papules, vesicles and pustules. There are lots of scratch marks over his torso. The onset of fever coincided with the rash.

2. A 2.5-year-old boy presents with a fever and a rash. Five days ago, he was in contact with a girl at nursery who has chickenpox. His mother says that, after this contact, he became miserable and had a runny nose; a few days later, he developed a pink rash moving from his face down to his trunk. On examination, he has some white spots in his mouth.

3. A 2.5-year-old boy presents with a fever and a rash. On the day prior to his admission, he had been a little irritable and had a high fever. He had vomited once. On the following morning, he was not rousable and had a red rash over his lower limbs. On examination, he is cold and tachycardic and has a capillary refill time of 5 seconds.

4. A 2.5-year-old boy presents with a fever and a rash. He had been a little hot this morning, but his mother sent him to nursery after giving him some paracetamol. She has now brought him to the emergency department because she is concerned that he has been slapped around the face at nursery.

5. A 2.5-year-old boy presents with a fever and a rash. His mother is concerned that he is having an allergic reaction, as he has been hot all day, has a red rash that feels like goose-pimples and now his tongue is red and swollen. You examine his throat, which reveals an inflamed pharynx.

THEME 9: FAILURE TO THRIVE

Options

A. Antiretrovirals
B. Cardiac catheter laboratory plugging
C. Open cardiothoracic surgery
D. Change in milk formula
E. Creon with feeds
F. Fundoplication
G. Gluten-free diet
H. No treatment required
 I. Oral domperidone
 J. Oral metronidazole
K. Oral nystatin
L. Oral omeprazole
M. Oral rifampicin, isoniazid and pyrazinamide
N. Psychological intervention
O. Total parenteral nutrition

For each of the following children presenting with failure to thrive, select the next step in management. Each option may be used once, more than once or not at all.

1. A 4-month-old boy is failing to thrive. He has gastro-oesophageal reflux, shown on pH studies, and is being treated with feed thickeners, positioning, antacids, a proton pump inhibitor and a hypermotility drug. He continues to cry and arch his back after feeds. He has also occasionally stopped breathing and becomes cyanosed after feeds.

2. A 6-month-old girl is failing to thrive. On examination, she is small and breathless. Examination of the chest reveals a murmur heard throughout systole and diastole. The murmur is loudest below the left clavicle.

3. A premature infant develops necrotizing enterocolitis. A laparotomy is performed and the majority of the small and large bowel is resected.

4. A 2-year-old girl is failing to thrive. She has chronic diarrhoea and bloating. She is originally from India and arrived in the UK 12 months ago. An upper gastrointestinal endoscopy is performed and a duodenal biopsy is taken, which reveals partial villous atrophy with motile trophozoites.

5. A 2-year-old girl is failing to thrive. She has chronic diarrhoea and bloating. She is originally from Libya and arrived in the UK 12 months ago. An upper gastrointestinal endoscopy is performed and a duodenal biopsy is taken, which reveals total villous atrophy and no organisms.

THEME 10: HAEMATURIA

Options

A. Benign familial haematuria
B. Drug ingestion
C. Food ingestion
D. Glomerulonephritis
E. Haemolysis
 F. Haemorrhagic cystitis
G. Henoch–Schönlein purpura
H. Hypercalciuria
 I. Nephrotic syndrome
 J. Polycystic kidney disease
K. Porphyria
L. Renal/bladder tumour
M. Rhabdomyolysis
N. Stress haematuria

For each of the following scenarios, select the most appropriate diagnosis. Each option may be used once, more than once or not at all.

1. A 12-year-old boy presents to the clinic having recently started treatment for tuberculosis. He has developed painful purple lesions on his lower limbs and reports that he has started 'weeing blood'. The urine dipstick is negative for blood, protein, leucocytes and nitrites.

2. A 15-year-old boy reports that his urine has turned red. He has not changed his diet and is otherwise clinically well. He is a regular cross-country runner and took part in a road race the day before presentation. A urine dipstick is positive for blood and negative for protein, leucocytes and nitrites. He is followed up, and two repeat urine samples have no blood in them.

3. A 16-year-old girl has recently been started on the oral contraceptive pill. She presents shortly after with abdominal pain and vomiting. She reports that her urine has turned red. A dipstick is negative for blood, protein, leucocytes and nitrites.

4. A 3-year-old boy presents with red urine. He is clinically well, although he did have a perioral rash with yellow crusting 2 weeks prior to admission. He is systemically well and has no other symptoms. On examination, you find no signs other than a raised blood pressure. Urine is positive for blood and protein, but negative for leucocytes and nitrites. A full blood count is normal, with a normal blood film.

5. A 4-year-old boy returns to the ward after surgery to remove a brain tumour. The nursing staff notice that his urine is red. A urine sample is taken, and is positive for blood but negative for protein, leucocytes and nitrites.

Practice Paper 6: Answers

THEME 1: VOMITING

1. D – Gastroenteritis

This history (vomiting and diarrhoea) is suggestive of gastroenteritis. A malrotation of the gut would usually present with bilious vomiting. Infective causes such as meningitis and a urinary tract infection should be in your differential diagnosis, but the lack of pyrexia in this case makes these less likely. Gastroenteritis is unusual in this age group, although it is more common in bottle-fed infants. The most important step is assessing and treating any degree of dehydration and ruling out more sinister infective causes. Educating parents on how to sterilize bottles is important in preventing gastroenteritis.

2. G – Incarcerated inguinal hernia

This child is unwell. Bilious vomiting in this age group is a sign of bowel obstruction and should be taken seriously. In this case, the infant has an incarcerated inguinal hernia, as revealed by the firm mass in the groin. (Testicular torsion can present with a firm mass in the scrotum with vomiting, but this is unlikely to be bilious.) As the bowel becomes obstructed, fluid shifts into the bowel, which becomes oedematous and inflamed. The first step in managing this child is treating the severe dehydration, followed by reduction of the hernia and possible resection of necrotic bowel. There has been more than one cardiorespiratory arrest due to incarcerated inguinal hernias, so take them seriously.

3. E – Gastro-oesophageal reflux

True vomiting is the forceful ejection of stomach contents. Gastro-oesophageal reflux (GOR) is technically not vomiting but rather regurgitation, where stomach contents are ejected effortlessly. In infants, the lower oesophageal sphincter is not competent, so the passive reflux of acidic gastric contents into the oesophagus and oral cavity can cause significant symptoms. Aspiration can occur with GOR, causing chronic cough, wheeze and recurrent pneumonia in childhood. The first steps in management are conservative (e.g. positioning) and adding feed thickeners. Later steps include antacids (Gaviscon), prokinetics (erythromycin), H_2 receptor antagonists (ranitidine) and proton pump inhibitors (omeprazole). The evidence is still not clear as to whether these medical strategies are effective.

4. K – Overfeeding

Overfeeding with milk is rare in breast-fed babies. In bottle-fed babies, taking excessive volumes of milk causes distension of the stomach, which then ejects (vomits) the milk. A good feeding history is essential in any baby presenting with vomiting. Infants should take 150–180 mL/kg/day of milk.

5. L – Pyloric stenosis

The presentation of non-bile-stained projectile vomiting soon after feeds in a hungry baby is suggestive of pyloric stenosis. Pyloric stenosis is hypertrophy of the circular muscle of the pylorus. This causes gastric out-flow obstruction. It characteristically presents at between 2 and 7 weeks of age and it most commonly affects firstborn males (4 males:1 female). Apart from projectile vomiting, affected babies may be 'constipated' and lose weight. Often, these children are not clinically dehydrated, as the body compensates for the chronic fluid loss. A characteristic hypo-chloraemic, hypokalaemic, metabolic alkalosis results from vomiting stomach acid and renal replacement of H^+ for K^+. A pyloric stenosis mass can sometimes be palpated by giving the baby a 'test feed': when the baby is given milk, visible gastric peristalsis may be seen over the epigastrium, and the pylorus is felt as an olive-shaped mass in the upper abdomen. If the diagnosis is in doubt, an ultrasound scan can be performed. After initial rehydration, management is by Ramstedt's pyloromyotomy, during which the muscle of the pylorus is cut longitudinally down to the mucosa. The baby can tolerate milk feeds a few hours after the operation.

Conrad Ramstedt, German surgeon (1867–1963).

Duodenal atresia is the congenital absence or closure of a portion of the duodenum. Around one-third of babies with duodenal atresia have trisomy 21 (Down's syndrome). Affected babies present at birth with bile-stained vomiting and abdominal distension. Diagnosis is confirmed by the presence of a double-bubble sign on the abdominal X-ray. This rep-resents the presence of air in the stomach and proximal duodenum only, and not in the distal intestines. Treatment is by duodeno-duodenostomy.

Gastroschisis (Greek *gastro* = belly + *schisis* = cleft; 'split belly') is a defect in the anterior abdominal wall adjacent to the umbilicus. Abdominal contents, such as the liver and intestines, can herniate through this defect, but there is no sac covering the contents. Management of gastroschisis is by immediately covering the exposed viscera with cling film, followed by surgical repair. Gastroschisis is rarely associated with other congenital malformations.

Exomphalos is the herniation of abdominal contents through the umbilicus. The herniated viscera are surrounded by a sac (as out-pouching of the peritoneum), and this structure is known as an omphalocele. Surgical closure of the defect is required. 50% of cases of exomphalos are associated with other congenital malformations, such as trisomies and cardiac defects.

Meckel's diverticulum is a congenital diverticulum that contains gastric-type mucosa. It is an example of a true diverticulum (Latin *diverticulum* = by-road). A true diverticulum incorporates all the layers of the wall from which it arises. Conversely, a false diverticulum is made up of only the inner layer of the normal bowel wall, an example being colonic diverticula. There is a rule of twos surrounding Meckel's diverticulum: it is found 2 feet proximal to the ileocaecal junction, it is 2 inches in length and it occurs in 2% of the population. Most Meckel's diverticula are incidental findings, but the most common presentation is painless rectal bleeding. Some may present with acute inflammation, similar to acute appendicitis. Because Meckel's diverticula contain gastric mucosa, they are susceptible to peptic ulceration. Diagnosis is confirmed by a technetium-99m scan. The radiolabelled technetium is taken up only by gastric-type mucosa, so the scan will highlight the stomach as well as a diverticulum in the right iliac fossa. Treatment is by resection if required.

Johann Friedrich Meckel, German anatomist (1781–1833).

THEME 2: THE CHILD WITH A LIMP

1. I – Slipped capital femoral epiphysis
Slipped capital femoral epiphysis (SCPE) describes posterolateral displacement of the femoral head. Slippage occurs though the femoral head growth plate. It occurs most commonly in boys aged 10–15 years during their adolescent growth spurt, and is associated with obesity, micro-genitalia, hypothyroidism and a tall stature. 20% of cases are bilateral. SCPE presents with a limp and hip pain referred to the knee. It may follow minor trauma. There may be restriction in abduction and internal rotation of the hip. The diagnosis is confirmed on X-ray of the affected hip. Management is by surgical pinning of the epiphysis. Complications of SCPE include premature epiphyseal fusion and avascular necrosis.

2. G – Perthes' disease
Perthes' disease (or Legg–Calvé–Perthes' disease) is a degenerative disease of the hip. There is ischaemia of the femoral head involving the epiphysis and adjacent metaphysis (resulting in avascular necrosis). This is followed by revascularization and reossification over 2–3 years. Perthes' disease is five-times more common in boys and usually occurs at between 2 and 10 years of age. It presents with insidious-onset hip pain (which may be referred to the knee) and a limp. It is bilateral in 10% of cases. Diagnosis is by lateral X-ray of the affected hip, which shows an increased density and reduced size of the femoral head. The femoral head later becomes fragmented and irregular.

Management in mild disease is by bed rest and traction. In more severe cases, the femoral head needs to be 'covered' by the acetabulum so that it can act as a mould for the reossifying epiphysis. This is achieved by maintaining the hip in abduction or by surgical femoral osteotomy. The prognosis of Perthes' disease is usually good. However, if the child is under 6 years of age, or if more than half of the epiphysis is involved, there is an increased risk of deformity of the femoral head, with subsequent degenerative osteoarthritis in adult life.

Georg Clemens Perthes, German surgeon (1869–1927).

3. L – Transient synovitis
Transient synovitis (irritable hip) is the most common cause of acute hip pain in prepubescent children (between 3 and 8 years), and often follows a viral infection. It is often a diagnosis of exclusion. Features include sudden-onset hip pain that radiates to the knee, mild fever, a slight limp and a reduced range of movement, especially external rotation. There is no pain at rest and minimal systemic symptoms. Investigations, such as full blood count, acute-phase reactants (e.g. C-reactive protein), blood cultures and joint X-rays are negative. Ultrasound investigation may demonstrate an effusion. Management is with analgesia and rest. Irritable hip usually resolves in 7–10 days.

4. H – Septic arthritis
Septic arthritis is a medical emergency. It often affects a single joint and should always be considered with the presentation of a hot, swollen, tender joint with a restricted range of movement in an unwell patient. Septic arthritis is an infection within the synovial joint, most often caused by *Staphylococcus aureus* infection. It is most common in the hip and knee. Risk factors for developing septic arthritis include being very old or very young, intravenous (IV) drug use, diabetes and having preexisting joint complaints. X-ray is normal in the early stages, but an ultrasound scan should be performed and joint aspiration done to culture organisms. Management of septic arthritis is with surgical washout of the joint and IV antibiotics (e.g. flucloxacillin and benzylpenicillin) until the patient is clinically well, followed by a several weeks of oral antibiotics. Complications of septic arthritis include joint destruction (leading to arthritis), spread of infection to the bone (osteomyelitis) and ankylosis (bony fusion across the joint).

5. A – Developmental dysplasia of the hip
Developmental dysplasia of the hip (DDH; or congenital dislocation of the hip) is a spectrum of disorders ranging from partial subluxation to frank dislocation of the hip. DDH is found in 1 in 1000 births, and it is six-times more common in females. The left hip is more likely to be dislocated than the right. Risk factors for DDH include a positive family history, breech delivery, spinal/neuromuscular abnormalities (e.g. spina bifida and talipes equinovarus) and oligohydramnios.

Neonatal screening for DDH is by two methods: Barlow's test (the hip can easily be displaced posteriorly out of the acetabulum on adduction of the leg with posterior pressure) and Ortolani's manoeuvre (the femoral head can be reduced back into the acetabulum on abduction of the leg with anterior pressure). These tests are routinely done at birth and 6 weeks of age. These manoeuvres have a good positive predictive value (i.e. if the examination is positive, the patient has DDH) but a very poor negative predictive value (i.e. many patients with a normal examination are later found to have DDH). DDH may present with asymmetrical skinfolds, limited abduction, shortening of the affected limb and limp. If spotted early, DDH responds to conservative treatment. The hips can be placed in a restraining device (Pavlik harness) for several months. Progress should be monitored by ultrasound or X-ray. If conservative measures fail, open reduction and femoral osteotomy may be required. Necrosis of the femoral head is a potential complication of DDH.

Sir Thomas Barlow, English physician and paediatrician (1845–1945).
Marino Ortolani, Italian paediatrician (1904–1983).

In talipes equinovarus ('clubfoot'), the foot is inverted and plantar flexed. Talipes is the most common congenital abnormality, occurring in around 1 in 500 births. Half of cases are bilateral. Clubfoot may be secondary to intrauterine compression (from oligohydramnios) or a neuromuscular disorder (such as spina bifida). This condition must be managed, otherwise the deformity will persist. Options include passive stretching and strapping. If deformity is severe, then corrective surgery is required.

Osgood–Schlatter disease is a condition characterized by transient inflammation of the growth plate (i.e. osteochondritis) of the tibial tuberosity where the patellar tendon attaches. It is most common in active boys in their early teens. Features include pain and swelling around the tuberosity that is worse on activity, especially leg extension. Treatment is with rest and analgesia.

Spontaneous haemarthrosis describes recurrent acute swellings in joints of children due to underlying haemophilia. Trivial trauma may result in bleeding into the joint, most commonly the knee, and this is known as haemarthrosis. Haemophilia is an X-linked recessive deficiency of factors VIII or IX. Recurrent haemarthroses result in pain, stiffness and early osteoarthritis.

Genu varus (or bowlegs) is a deformity characterized by medial angulation of the lower leg at the knee (the term 'valgus' describes the opposite deformity). Most cases of genu varus in children under 2 years of age are non-pathological (i.e. a normal variant). The most common pathological cause of genu varus is rickets, which is a deficiency of vitamin D resulting in a lack of calcium absorption with subsequent skeletal and dental deformities. Another cause of genu varus in children is Blount's disease, in which asymmetrical growth of the tibial physis results in a progressive varus deformity at the knee (i.e. the lateral part of the tibia grows quicker than the medial side). Blount's disease is more common in Scandinavian and Afro-Caribbean children.

The original Latin words *varus* and *valgus* had the opposite meanings to their modern uses in medicine. *Varus* meant 'knock-kneed' and *valgus* meant 'bowlegged', because the Latin words actually described the position of the leg at the hip joint rather than at the knee joint. (Latin *genu* = knee.)

Talipes equinovarus, from Latin *talus* = ankle + *pes* = foot + *equinus* = horse-like + *varus* = inward (inward turning of the ankle and foot, like a horse).

Walter Putnam Blount, American orthopaedic surgeon (1900–1992).
Robert Bayley Osgood, American orthopaedic surgeon (1873–1956).
Carl Schlatter, Swiss physician (1864–1934).

THEME 3: COUGH

1. E – Cystic fibrosis

Cystic fibrosis (CF) is the most common autosomal recessive condition in Caucasian populations in the UK, affecting 1 in 2500 live births. CF is caused by an abnormal gene coding for the CF transmembrane regulator protein, located on chromosome 7. The most common mutation in CF is the ΔF508 mutation. The poor transport of chloride ions and water across epithelial cells of the respiratory system and pancreas exocrine glands in CF results in an increased viscosity of secretions. The range of presentations is varied, including recurrent chest infections, failure to thrive from malabsorption and liver disease. In the neonatal period, infants may present with prolonged neonatal jaundice, bowel obstruction (meconium ileus) or rectal prolapse.

The gold standard investigation for CF is the sweat test. The abnormal function of sweat glands results in an excess concentration of sodium chloride (NaCl) in sweat. Sweat is stimulated by pilocarpine iontophoresis, collected on filter paper and analysed.

Normal sweat NaCl concentration: 10–14 mmol/L
Sweat NaCl concentration in CF: 80–125 mmol/L

At least two sweat tests should be performed, as diagnostic errors and false positives are common.

Management options in CF include physiotherapy (for respiratory secretions), antibiotics (for prophylaxis and treatment of lung infections) and pancreatic enzyme supplements (to prevent malabsorption). Complications include diabetes mellitus, hepatic cirrhosis, infertility in males, severe pulmonary hypertension and cor pulmonale, as well as chronic lung infections (*Pseudomonas* spp. and *Burkholderia cepacia*). Many cases of CF are now being picked up early since the introduction of a national screening programme assessing immunoreactive trypsin (IRT) levels on the Guthrie card at day 8 of life. IRT is a pancreatic enzyme with levels that are raised in CF.

2. H – Pneumonia

Fever and a respiratory rate >50 breaths/minute in a child under 3 years of age are strongly suggestive of pneumonia. Lower respiratory tract infections (pneumonias, 'chest infections') can be caused by both viruses and bacteria. Although aspiration can cause similar findings, there are no risk factors in this case that suggest aspiration (e.g. neurological pathology). Chest signs such as crepitations are less reliable in children, and often will not be heard at all. It is paramount that you check the respiratory rate, as most children with pneumonia will be tachypnoeic. Upper respiratory tract infections can cause very similar findings, but the child is less likely to be tachypnoeic. Evidence of lower respiratory tract infections may be seen on chest X-ray. Treatment of bacterial infections is with appropriate antibiotics (and oxygen if required).

3. B – Asthma

This boy has asthma. Asthma can present in a number of ways, including cough (often worse at night), wheeze, shortness of breath and failure to thrive. Sleep is interrupted, which can affect school performance. Note that GOR can also cause a night cough and should be considered as a differential.

Asthma is the most common chronic illness in childhood, affecting up to 15% of all children. The underlying pathophysiology is chronic inflammation of the bronchial mucosa, with airway hyper-reactivity. Trigger factors (e.g. exercise, viral infections, allergens, cold air and severe emotions) cause bronchoconstriction, mucosal oedema and excess mucus production. This leads to airway narrowing and the typical features of asthma. Asthma is associated with atopy, a condition in which individuals produce substantial amounts of immunoglobulin E antibodies following trivial exposures to everyday antigens. It tends to run in families. Other atopic conditions include allergic rhinitis (obstruction of nostrils causing sniffing, sneezing and a runny nose), eczema, allergic conjunctivitis, urticaria/angioedema and food/drug allergies. When allergic rhinitis occurs only in summer due to high pollen counts, it is known as 'hay fever'. If it occurs throughout the year, it is called 'perennial rhinitis'.

A diagnosis of asthma can be confirmed by demonstrating reversible airflow obstruction using a peak flow meter (this can only be done above the age of 5 years). If peak flow significantly improves following administration of a bronchodilator, then asthma is suggested. The management of asthma follows a stepwise approach, summarized as follows:

- Step 1: short-acting β_2-agonist (salbutamol or terbutaline)
- Step 2: step 1 + low-dose inhaled steroid (budesonide or fluticasone)
- Step 3: step 2 +
  - <5 years of age: leukotriene inhibitor (monteleukast)
  - ≥5 years of age: high-dose inhaled steroid and long-acting β_2-agonist
- Step 4: step 3 + fourth drug (e.g. theophylline or an anticholinergic)
- Step 5: step 4 + oral steroid (prednisolone)

Acute exacerbations of asthma may require admission to hospital. Immediate treatment of acute asthma is with high-flow oxygen (via a facemask), bronchodilating nebulizers (β_2-agonists and anticholinergics) and steroids. Features of severe asthma are being too breathless to talk or feed, respiration rate ≥50 breaths/minute, pulse ≥140 beats/minute and peak flow ≤50% predicted or best. Features of life-threatening asthma are fatigue/exhaustion, decreasing consciousness, a silent chest, poor respiratory effort and a peak flow ≤33% predicted or best.

4. C – Bronchiolitis
Bronchiolitis is very common. It keeps paediatric wards busy during the winter months and can be life threatening, especially to at-risk groups (premature babies, heart disease, etc.). Bronchiolitis is caused by viruses, most commonly respiratory syncytial virus. Respiratory distress (intercostal recession, head bobbing and nasal flaring) and wheezing are caused by obstruction of the small airways. Auscultation may reveal fine inspiratory crepitations. Bronchiolitis can be confirmed by taking swabs of nasopharyngeal secretions (nasopharyngeal aspirate). Most infants do not require admission, although some may need support for hydration and oxygenation. Antibiotics, steroids and bronchodilators are not effective.

5. F – Foreign-body inhalation
Foreign-body inhalation is most common in toddlers, as they are prone to putting objects in their mouths. The most common offenders are small foodstuffs. Most foreign bodies present immediately. However, some may be delayed by weeks to months before symptoms develop. At the time of swallowing, the child has sudden-onset cough, wheeze or breathlessness. If the object is stuck in the larynx, it causes a croupy cough and stridor. If the object becomes stuck in the bronchus, there may initially be no symptoms until an infection develops several days later. Inhaled foreign bodies may be diagnosed by radiography, but rigid bronchoscopy will confirm the diagnosis and remove the offending object.

For information on the diagnosis and investigation of respiratory problems in children and adults, put your textbooks away and use the excellent British Thoracic Society Guidelines.*

THEME 4: CHROMOSOMAL DISORDERS

1. A – 45XO (Turner's syndrome)

Most cases of Turner's syndrome result in early miscarriage (approximately 95%). Despite this, the incidence remains approximately 1 in 2500 live-born females. The features of Turner's syndrome are lymphoedema of the hands and feet in the neonatal period, webbed neck (*in utero* oedema causes the webbing), short stature, wide carrying angle, widely spaced nipples, coarctation of the aorta and infertility. Girls with Turner's syndrome will have normal to low-normal intelligence.

Henry Turner, American endocrinologist (1892–1970).

2. E – 47XX (18) (Edwards' syndrome)

Most children with Edwards' syndrome die early in infancy, with fewer than 10% surviving beyond 1 year of age. The clinical features of Edwards' syndrome are low-set ears, small chin, microcephaly, overlapping fingers, rocker-bottom feet, cardiac defects (especially ventricular septal defects), renal anomalies and learning disability.

Patau's syndrome, or 47XX (13), is characterized by structural defects of the brain, small eyes, polydactyly and cardiac/renal malformations. Most babies with Patau's syndrome do not survive beyond 1 year of age.

John Hilton Edwards, British geneticist (1928–2007).
Klaus Patau, German geneticist (1908–1975).

3. C – 47XXY (Klinefelter's syndrome)

Klinefelter's syndrome is the most common cause of male hypogonadism, occurring in 1–2 per 1000 male births. These patients have small, firm testes, are tall and have behavioural problems, delayed speech and gynaecomastia. Testosterone therapy is sometimes used to improve the development of secondary sexual characteristics.

47XXX (triple X syndrome) is the presence of an extra X chromosome in females. Although some patients have mild learning disabilities, most do not have any unusual dysmorphic or medical problems, and are usually able to conceive. As such, triple X syndrome is rarely diagnosed.

The triploidies 69XXY, 69XXX and 69XYY result from fertilization of an egg by two sperm. They are estimated to occur in about 2% of conceptuses. Most affected babies are miscarried, although some live to be a few months of age.

Harry Fitch Klinefelter, American endocrinologist (born 1912).

---

* British Thoracic Society guidelines (www.brit-thoracic.org.uk)

4. F – 47XY (21) (Down's syndrome)

This is the most common trisomy, with an incidence of 1 in 600 births. Dysmorphic features include a round face, large tongue, small ears, flat occiput, a single palmar (simian) crease and spots on the iris (Brushfield's spots). Other problems are severe learning difficulties, congenital heart defects (especially atrioventricular septal defects), duodenal atresia, visual/hearing impairment and early-onset Alzheimer's disease. Babies with Down's syndrome are strikingly hypotonic.

John Down, in his '*Observations of an Ethnic Classification of Idiots*' (1866), thought that 'mentally challenged' children of different races had different characteristics. His description of the Mongolian 'idiot' (as having a flat, broad face, oblique eyes, large tongue, single palmar crease and coarse speech) was later recognized as a (race-independent) chromosomal abnormality, and was named Down's syndrome.

John Langdon Down, British physician (1828–1896).

5. H – Fragile X syndrome

Strictly speaking, fragile X syndrome is an X-linked recessive rather than a chromosomal disorder. There are multiple (>200) CGG trinucleotide repeats on the X chromosome. Many female carriers of fragile X syndrome have mild learning difficulties. Affected boys will have moderate learning difficulties (average IQ is 50), macrocephaly, macro-orchidism, large ears, a long face and a prominent mandible and forehead. Down's and fragile X syndromes are the most common genetic causes of severe learning difficulties in children.

THEME 5: ARTHRITIS

1. J – Reactive arthritis

Reactive arthritis is the most common cause of an acute arthritis in children. It is defined as a sterile synovitis occurring after an infection outside the joint. The infections are usually gastrointestinal or genitourinary in origin. Common organisms include *Shigella*, *Salmonella*, *Campylobacter*, *Yersinia* and *Chlamydia* spp. Transient synovitis tends to affect children at between 3 and 10 years of age. It tends to follow viral rather than bacterial infections.

2. D – Hand–foot syndrome

Preschool children with sickle cell disease can present with 'hand–foot syndrome'. They have tender swelling of the hand and wrists or feet. Such episodes can be precipitated by stress or cold. The incidence of septic arthritis and osteomyelitis, especially by *Streptococcus* and *Salmonella* spp., is increased in sickle cell anaemia.

3. G – Pauciarticular juvenile idiopathic arthritis

Juvenile idiopathic arthritis (JIA) was previously referred to as juvenile chronic arthritis or juvenile rheumatoid arthritis. JIA is defined as joint inflammation persisting for 6 weeks or more, with initial onset in a person under 16 years of age, in the absence of another specific cause. Diagnosis is clinical, and relies on ruling out other causes of arthritis. JIA is classified according to the number of joints affected:

- Monoarticular: single joint
- Pauciarticular: ≤4 joints (also known as oligoarticular)
- Polyarticular: >4 joints

Pauciarticular JIA usually occurs in younger children, affecting the knees, ankles and wrists most commonly. Polyarticular JIA is more common in girls of all ages, usually symmetrically involving the hands and wrists. Complications of JIA include chronic anterior uveitis, flexion contraction of the joints and amyloidosis. Management options include physiotherapy, simple analgesia (non-steroidal anti-inflammatory drugs [NSAIDs]), intra-articular steroid injections and disease-modifying anti-rheumatic drugs (e.g. methotrexate and ciclosporin).

Still's disease is a systemic form of juvenile arthritis that is thought to be an autoimmune disorder. It usually begins at the age of 3–4 years and is more common in girls. Features of Still's disease include intermittent high pyrexia and a salmon-pink rash with aches and pains of the joints and muscles. Other features are hepatosplenomegaly, lymphadenopathy and pericarditis. Inflammatory markers such as C-reactive protein will be raised; however, antinuclear antibody and rheumatoid factor are usually negative. Management options include physiotherapy, resting splints, NSAIDs, disease-modifying drugs (e.g. methotrexate and ciclosporin) and steroids. The younger the age of onset of Still's disease, the worse the prognosis.

Sir George Freidrich Still, English physician (1861–1941).

4. A – Acute rheumatic fever

Rheumatic fever is predominantly a disease of the developing world, and is usually seen in children between 5 and 15 years of age. The condition develops 2–4 weeks after a group A β-haemolytic streptococcal pharyngitis. In susceptible individuals, the antibodies formed against the bacterial carbohydrate cell wall cross-react with antigens in the heart, joints and skin in a process known as molecular mimicry. The immune response in the heart causes myocarditis, pericarditis and endocarditis, resulting in valve destruction, conduction defects, arrhythmia and congestive cardiac failure.

The diagnosis of rheumatic fever is made using the modified Duckett Jones criteria, requiring either two major criteria or one major and two minor criteria plus evidence of streptococcal infection (e.g. serial anti-streptolysin O [ASO] titres).

Modified Duckett Jones criteria
Major:

- Pancarditis
- Polyarthritis

- Sydenham's chorea (St Vitus' dance)
- Erythema marginatum
- Subcutaneous nodules

Minor:

- Fever
- Arthralgia
- High erythrocyte sedimentation rate or white cell count
- Heart block

In this case, the boy has erythema marginatum, arthralgia and a fever. Serial ASO titres were found to be rising, revealing a recent streptococcal infection.

Pancarditis can present with murmurs, including mitral regurgitation, aortic regurgitation (in 50%) and the Carey Coombs murmur (a soft mid-diastolic murmur that occurs due to nodule development on mitral valve leaflets). Sydenham's chorea includes choreiform movements, emotional lability and explosive speech. The polyarthritis is often fleeting, affects the large joints and is characteristically responsive to aspirin. Subcutaneous nodules are small, firm and painless, and are best felt over the tendons or bones.

The treatment of rheumatic fever requires antibiotics (usually penicillin), analgesia, NSAIDs and bed rest. Steroids are sometimes indicated in severe cases. Following the acute phase, patients require prophylactic antibiotics prior to invasive procedures such as tooth extraction in order to protect against bacteraemia and subsequent bacterial endocarditis.

> Chorea, from Latin *chorea* = dance.
> Saint Vitus' dance (*chorea sancti viti* in Latin) was a festival of the Middle Ages celebrating Vitus, the patron saint of dancers, actors and comedians.
> Carey Franklin Coombs, English cardiologist (1879–1932).
> T. Duckett Jones, American physician (1899–1954).
> Thomas Sydenham, English physician (1624–1689).

5. B – Enteropathic arthritis

Enteropathic arthritis is an asymmetrical pauciarticular arthritis (oligoarthritis) predominantly affecting the larger joints of the lower limb. It occurs with underlying inflammatory bowel disease. It is difficult to distinguish between ulcerative colitis (UC) and Crohn's disease from the history, although UC is more commonly associated with bloody stools. Other extraintestinal features of inflammatory bowel disease include clubbing, erythema nodosum (painful lesions on the lower legs), anterior uveitis (inflammation of the anterior eye causing acute pain, photophobia and blurring), ankylosing spondylitis, hepatobiliary disease (primary biliary cirrhosis), pyoderma gangrenosum (deep, necrotic ulcers with a dark-red border usually occurring on the leg) and perianal disease (skin tags, fissures and fistulae).

THEME 6: JAUNDICE IN THE NEWBORN

As many as 50% of newborn babies will be clinically jaundiced in the first week of life. Bilirubin is produced by the breakdown of fetal haemoglobin, which is replaced with adult haemoglobin. Most infants will not need any intervention or any investigation as long as they do not break any of the following rules:

- Jaundice is not apparent in the first 24 hours of life
- The infant is clinically well, and remains clinically well
- The serum bilirubin is below treatment level
- The jaundice has resolved by 14 days (21 days in preterm infants)

High levels of unconjugated bilirubin can cross the blood–brain barrier and cause permanent neuronal damage (kernicterus). Jaundice can be treated with phototherapy, which converts unconjugated bilirubin into non-toxic isomers that are excreted. In reality, one would rarely perform a single blood test in an infant with jaundice, instead ordering a series of investigations together as a 'jaundice screen'. In this question, the examiner is looking to see whether you can assess the diagnosis and the investigation that comes with it. In day-to-day clinical life, always remember to take a serum bilirubin level, as this will determine whether phototherapy is required.

1. C – Blood cultures

This infant is likely to have a bacterial sepsis associated with prolonged rupture of membranes. Common organisms include group B streptococci, *Escherichia coli*, *Listeria* spp., *Staphylococcus aureus* and other streptococci. A full blood count and C-reactive protein may be helpful, but will not provide a diagnosis. A blood culture is needed. IV empirical antibiotics should be started immediately.

2. G – Group and Coombs' testing

This is likely to be a case of rhesus haemolytic disease of the newborn. The mother's blood group should be taken, along with a group and Coombs' test performed on the baby's blood. The blood group will tell you whether they have the same blood group and rhesus status; the Coombs' test will tell you whether there is a haemolysis occurring. Rhesus disease is now uncommon in the UK due to the use of anti-D immunoglobulins in rhesus D-negative mothers to prevent the production of antibodies. All pregnant women have their blood group taken early in pregnancy, and then infants of rhesus-negative mothers will have their blood taken from the umbilical cord immediately after birth, though some 'slip through the net' and still develop haemolytic disease in future pregnancies.

3. B – Abdominal ultrasound

This child has prolonged jaundice with white stools. The most important diagnosis to rule out is biliary atresia. Any baby jaundiced beyond 14 days of life should have conjugated bilirubin levels measured. If there is a high conjugated fraction (>25 μmol/L), then biliary atresia is likely. This, however, does not confirm the diagnosis, as there are other causes of a prolonged conjugated jaundice. Biliary atresia can be seen on liver ultrasound or on a non-excreting hydroxyiminodiacetic acid scan. If biliary atresia is diagnosed early enough (before 6–8 weeks), surgery can be performed and will result in a relatively good outcome. Later diagnosis has a higher risk of the child requiring a liver transplant. It is for this reason that parents should never be reassured that jaundice >14 days is 'breast milk'/physiological jaundice unless a blood conjugated fraction has been performed.

4. I – No further investigation required

This is most likely to be a case of 'breastfeeding'/physiological jaundice. There are many hypotheses regarding why breastfeeding can cause jaundice, but all are still yet to be proven. The key here is that the infant is well, that the jaundice was not present in the first 24 hours after birth and that it is below treatment level. If the jaundice is still present after 14 days, he will need to have conjugated bilirubin levels.

5. L – TORCH screen

All of the congenital infections in the TORCH mnemonic cause jaundice.

T	Toxoplasmosis
O	Other (e.g. syphilis)
R	Rubella
C	Cytomegalovirus (CMV)
H	Herpes simplex

The most common of these is CMV, which may be associated with hepatomegaly. Features common to all TORCH infections are low birth weight, prematurity, jaundice, microcephaly, seizures, anaemia, failure to thrive and encephalitis. There are other causes of seizures and this child will need to be admitted to the special care baby unit for investigation and treatment.

THEME 7: SEIZURES

In any seizure, the priority is first to assess and rule out any compromise of airway, breathing and circulation. Check for and treat any hypoglycaemia (ABC-DEFG: Don't Ever Forget Glucose). The Advanced Life Support Group has drawn up algorithms for managing both paediatric and adult seizures. Make sure that you are familiar with these.

1. I – Oral antipyretics

This boy has most likely had a febrile convulsion. For a seizure to be defined as a 'febrile convulsion', it must meet the following criteria:

- Seizure associated with a temperature >38°C
- Developmentally normal child
- Age less than 6 years (some would also say age older than 6 months)
- No evidence of an intracranial infection/inflammation
- No previous afebrile seizure
- No acute metabolic disturbance which could cause a seizure

There is often a family history of febrile seizures. Evidence suggests that antipyretics such as paracetamol and ibuprofen do not reduce the risk of febrile convulsions (so if you marked 'no treatment required', you would be given a correct response in your exam). However, if a child is in pain (earache in this case) or has a fever, then symptomatic relief is appropriate. Acute otitis media does not routinely need antibiotic management.

2. A – Anaesthesia and intubation

This boy is in status epilepticus. Status epilepticus is defined as generalized convulsions lasting 30 minutes or longer, or successive convulsions lasting over 30 minutes without recovery between seizures. When a child has been fitting for a period of longer than 20 minutes, an anaesthetist should be contacted, as there is a good chance that the child will need rapid anaesthesia (by rapid sequence induction) for intubation and ventilation.

3. B – Buccal midazolam OR L – Rectal diazepam

Benzodiazepines are the mainstay of early seizure treatment. They can be given intravenously (lorazepam), rectally (diazepam) or buccally (midazolam). Getting intravenous access is important, but if this is not possible, then there are other routes of administering antiepileptic medications. Buccal midazolam is probably more effective than rectal diazepam for terminating seizures. However, rectal diazepam would also be an appropriate answer to this question. One must be aware that benzodiazepines – by any route – can cause respiratory depression. When a child is fitting, you should continually reassess ABC and keep an appropriately sized bag and mask to hand.

4. F – IV phenytoin

This child is not yet in status epilepticus, but is still having a significant seizure that requires terminating. He has had two doses of benzodiazepine, and so the next step is a phenytoin infusion. Failing this, the next step is intubation and ventilation.

5. G – No treatment required

This child is having breath-holding attacks. These usually commence in the first few years of life. They are often preceded by physical or emotional trauma. After a brief period of crying, the child will hold their breath and will become cyanotic. They will then become hypotonic and potentially lose consciousness. Some children subsequently display seizure-like activity (tonus or clonus). No investigation or treatment is required. Behavioural steps may help, and some families find that blowing on the face or splashing the face with water may terminate the event.

THEME 8: FEVER AND A RASH

1. L – Varicella zoster

Chickenpox is caused by the varicella zoster virus, which is spread via the respiratory route with an incubation period of 14–21 days. Clinical features include fever and an itchy rash found predominantly on the trunk and scalp. The rash is made up of pustules and vesicles, which eventually crust over. The onset of fever coincides with the pustular phase of the rash. Complications of chickenpox include secondary bacterial infection (staphylococcal or streptococcal), pneumonitis and conjunctival lesions. Postinfective ataxia (cerebellitis) is a rare complication that presents with ataxia several weeks after infection. Purpura fulminans (widespread vasculitis of the skin and subcutaneous tissues) and stroke are very rare complications.

In immunocompromised patients, primary varicella infection can result in disseminated haemorrhagic infection with a 20% mortality rate. If a pregnant woman develops chickenpox in the first trimester, there is a 2% risk that the baby will develop fetal varicella syndrome (characterized by limb hypoplasia, microcephaly, cataracts, growth retardation and skin scarring). Treatment of chickenpox is generally supportive, although the antiviral aciclovir should be given to adolescents and immunocompromised individuals. Human varicella zoster immunoglobulins are administered prophylactically to immunocompromised patients who are at high risk of infection.

2. E – Measles

Measles is caused by an RNA virus that is transmitted by droplet infection. There is an incubation period of 10–12 days. The incidence has decreased since the introduction of the vaccine has led to herd immunity. Children with measles tend to be miserable, with fever, coryza, cough, conjunctivitis and a maculopapular rash that starts at the face and spreads downwards onto the trunk. The fever and coryza precede the rash by around 4 days. Koplik's spots (white pinhead spots on the buccal mucosa) are pathognomonic for measles. Complications of measles include otitis media, pneumonitis, myocarditis and encephalitis. Encephalitis, which occurs in 1 in 5000 cases a few weeks after initial infection, is characterized by headache, lethargy, convulsions and coma. Long-term sequelae of measles encephalitis include epilepsy, deafness, hemiplegia and learning difficulties. Subacute sclerosing panencephalitis is a very rare complication that begins 7 years after initial infection. Features include gradual loss in neurological function, progressing to dementia and death.

Management of measles is symptomatic and children should be isolated. Measles is a notifiable disease.

Henry Koplik, American physician (1858–1927).

3. G – Meningococcal sepsis

Meningococcal disease is caused by the Gram-negative diplococcus *Neisseria meningitidis*. Meningococcal disease can present with meningitis alone (15%), septicaemia alone (25%) or both meningitis and septicaemia (60%). The incubation period is 2–10 days. Affected children often present with non-specific symptoms: headache, poor feeding, lethargy and photophobia. This is followed by shock, fever and a non-blanching purpuric rash. In this case, the signs suggest septicaemia as the likely disease rather than meningitis. In meningitis, examination may reveal Kernig's sign (when the hip is flexed with the knee bent, pain is felt on attempting to straighten the leg) and Brudzinski's sign (flexion of the neck causes the leg to be drawn up due to meningeal irritation). A bulging fontanelle, neck stiffness and opisthotonus (lying with an arched back) are late signs of meningitis. The offending organism can be cultured (from pharyngeal swabs, blood cultures, aspirates of skin lesions or cerebrospinal fluid), although diagnosis is increasingly relying on polymerase chain reaction. Treatment is with resuscitation and immediate IV antibiotics (e.g. cefotaxime).

Josef Brudzinski, Polish paediatrician (1874–1917).
Vladimir Mikhailovich Kernig, German neurologist (1840–1917).

4. A – Erythrovirus (fifth disease)

Fifth disease (also known as erythema infectiosum or slapped-cheek syndrome) is caused by droplet-borne parvovirus B19 infection (now called erythrovirus). It has an incubation period of 6–14 days. Affected children present with an appearance of slapped cheeks followed by a maculopapular rash on the limbs, malaise and fever. Complications include arthralgia and aplastic anaemia. All children with fifth disease should have a full blood count to exclude pancytopenia from aplastic anaemia.

Fifth disease is so called because it is the fifth of the six classic childhood skin rashes (the others being measles, chickenpox, rubella, scarlet fever and roseola infantum).

5. K – Scarlet fever

Scarlet fever is caused by the group A β-haemolytic streptococcus (*Streptococcus pyogenes*), which has an incubation period of 7 days. Children present with tonsillitis, an erythematous rash predominantly on the trunk and a sore coated tongue (strawberry tongue). Desquamation (peeling) of the skin of the palms and soles may occur towards the end of the illness. Diagnosis is made by culturing group A streptococci from throat swabs. A retrospective diagnosis can be found by finding a rising

ASO titre on serial testing (2 weeks apart). Complications include otitis media, acute nephritis and rheumatic fever.

Roseola infantum (exanthema subitum) is caused by human herpesviruses 6 and 7, and presents with high fever and malaise followed by a generalized macular rash. Diagnosis is confirmed by finding evidence of the virus in serum.

Hand, foot and mouth disease is caused by enteroviruses (e.g. coxsackievirus). It results in a painful papulovesicular eruption on the palms, soles, mucous membranes and occasionally the buttocks.

THEME 9: FAILURE TO THRIVE

1. F – Fundoplication
This child has severe GOR disease, which is being managed medically. Feed thickeners make milk more viscid and reduce reflux into the oesophagus. Antacids and proton pump inhibitors (e.g. omeprazole) do not prevent reflux, but rather reduce the acidity of the stomach contents and therefore reduce irritation within the gullet. Hypermotility drugs (e.g. domperidone) reduce the tone in the pylorus and aid emptying of the stomach to reduce reflux. All of these steps have failed in this child, and he is symptomatic with failure to thrive and apnoea after feeds. The next step in management is surgical correction – fundoplication – which involves wrapping the fundus of the stomach around the lower part of the oesophagus.

2. B – Cardiac catheter laboratory plugging
This child has a patent ductus arteriosus, causing heart failure. Heart failure commonly causes failure to thrive for two reasons: first, the workload of the heart is raised due to increased right atrial filling pressures; and second, these children are often too breathless to feed effectively. The heart failure should initially be treated with diuretics, such as furosemide and spironolactone. The patent ductus should then be plugged via a catheter inserted into the femoral artery. Only if this fails should open cardiothoracic surgery be performed.

3. O – Total parenteral nutrition
Necrotizing enterocolitis is a life-threatening condition occurring in the neonatal period. It occurs primarily in premature infants who are milk-fed. The exact cause is not yet known. There is ischaemia of the bowel and infection by bowel organisms. Babies present with bile-stained vomiting, bloody diarrhoea and abdominal distension. This is rapidly followed by shock. Abdominal X-ray shows dilated bowel loops and thickening of the bowel wall with intramural air. Management is initially medical with broad-spectrum antibiotics to cover both aerobes and anaerobes, but often the affected bowel needs to be resected. If only small lengths of bowel remain, then nutrition is not possible through the gut. Nutrition

therefore needs to be provided parenterally (intravenously) – usually through a central line. Calories, fat, protein, vitamins and minerals all need to be administered. These children often have a stormy course, as they get frequent central line infections.

4. J – Oral metronidazole

This girl has giardiasis (also known as beaver fever, because of the occurrence of campers getting the disease from drinking contaminated water that was inhabited by beavers, although the reality is that *Giardia* can live in the gastrointestinal tract of many animals). The motile trophozoites and the villous atrophy are diagnostic. *Giardia lamblia* is a flagellate protozoal parasite, passed via the faeco–oral route, which attaches itself to the intestinal wall but does not invade it. Chronic infection causes malabsorption, particularly of carbohydrates and fat. The malabsorption of fat can result in deficiency of fat-soluble vitamins (vitamins A, D, E and K). A duodenal biopsy identifying trophozoites suggests giardiasis. Stool cultures can be taken to look for cysts. Treatment is with oral metronidazole.

5. G – Gluten-free diet

Causes of villous atrophy include coeliac disease, temporary gluten intolerance secondary to gastroenteritis, cows'/soy milk intolerance, giardiasis, severe combined immunodeficiency, postchemotherapy, kwashiorkor and tropical sprue. The most common cause would be coeliac disease, especially with a history of chronic diarrhoea, abdominal distension and failure to thrive.

Coeliac disease ('coeliac', from Greek *koiliakos* = abdominal), which affects 1 in 1000 in the UK, is caused by an adverse immunological response to the gliadin fraction of gluten. Children normally present with failure to thrive following the introduction of the gluten cereals barley, wheat and rye. Symptoms include general irritability, diarrhoea, abdominal distension, buttock wasting, iron-deficiency anaemia and growth failure. Diagnosis is by jejunal biopsy, which demonstrates villous atrophy and crypt hyperplasia, although screening for autoantibodies is often performed in the first instance (anti-gliadin and anti-endomyseal antibodies). Treatment is with a lifelong gluten-free diet, which results in rapid resolution of symptoms. Conditions that are associated with coeliac disease include small-bowel lymphoma, dermatitis herpetiformis (an intensely itchy vesicular rash found on the extensor surfaces) and other autoimmune diseases (e.g. thyroid disease, pernicious anaemia and vitiligo).

THEME 10: HAEMATURIA

Haematuria can be described as either microscopic (>5 red cells per high-power field) or macroscopic (visible to the naked eye). Remember that red urine is not always blood; other causes include drug ingestion (below), porphyrinuria, methaemoglobinaemia and food ingestion (beetroots and blackberries). All patients with significant haematuria should have the following investigations performed: blood pressure, full blood count, serum creatinine and complement C3/C4 levels, urine for culture, 24-hour urine collection for creatinine, protein and calcium and an ultrasound scan of the urinary tract.

1. B – Drug ingestion

This boy is being treated for tuberculosis. The anti-tuberculous drug rifampicin commonly causes red urine and purple tears as side effects. Other anti-tuberculous drugs (and their side effects) are isoniazid (hepatitis and peripheral neuropathy), pyrazinamide (hepatitis, photosensitivity and gout), streptomycin (nephrotoxicity and ototoxicity) and ethambutol (optic neuritis). The painful purple lesions on the legs are erythema nodosum (Henoch–Schönlein purpura could be a differential, but the dipstick is negative for blood). Causes of erythema nodosum include sarcoidosis, leprosy, inflammatory bowel disease, streptococcal throat infections, tuberculosis and certain drugs (sulphonamide antibiotics and the oral contraceptive pill [OCP]).

2. N – Stress haematuria

Stress haematuria (also known as 'march haematuria' or 'exercise-induced haematuria') occurs after vigorous forms of exercise. It is painless (i.e. no dysuria, loin pain, etc.) and is of short duration. Important differentials here would be isolated asymptomatic haematuria and benign familial haematuria. The former is ruled out by the history of vigorous exercise, and the latter by the repeated samples being clear, plus the lack of affected family members. One should also consider glomerulonephritis, but again this is less likely, as the dipstick is negative for protein.

3. K – Porphyria

This girl has recently started on the OCP. This is used to control periods, for certain skin conditions and for birth control. If she is sexually active, she is at risk of urinary tract infections (also known as haemorrhagic cystitis if there is haematuria). However, the dipstick is completely negative, even for blood. Pyelonephritis can cause haematuria with a dipstick negative for leucocytes and nitrites; however, the dipstick would be positive for blood.

This girl has acute intermittent porphyria (AIP) with an acute attack induced by the OCP (attacks can also be induced by alcohol). The porphyrias are a group of disorders caused by a defect in the production of the enzymes necessary for haemoglobin synthesis. AIP is autosomal dominant. The clinical features are caused by the accumulation of the porphyrins (haemoglobin precursors) and include acute abdominal pain, vomiting and constipation, neuropathy, seizures and psychoses. The urine can turn reddish-brown on standing. Diagnosis is made on sending stool, urine and blood for porphyrin measurement.

Porphyria, from Greek *porphura* = purple pigment. This may be a reference to the 'purple' discoloration of the bodily fluids of affected patients.

4. D – Glomerulonephritis

This boy has asymptomatic, macroscopic haematuria associated with proteinuria and a raised blood pressure (nephritic syndrome) from glomerulonephritis. Underlying causes of glomerulonephritis include postinfectious glomerulonephritis, immunoglobulin A (IgA) nephropathy, Alport's syndrome, haemolytic–uraemic syndrome (HUS) and nephritis. This boy has postinfectious glomerulonephritis following impetigo from group A streptococcal infection (although impetigo is more commonly caused by staphylococci). IgA nephropathy causes haematuria 2 days after an upper respiratory tract infection and is associated with Henoch–Schönlein purpura.

HUS is characterized by a triad of acute renal failure, microangiopathic haemolytic anaemia and thrombocytopenia. It is the most common cause of acute renal failure in childhood. Most cases are associated with prodromal infectious diarrhoea, most often the verocytotoxin-producing *Escherichia coli* strain 0157:H7.

Alport's syndrome is characterized by a triad of glomerular basement membrane degeneration, sensorineural deafness and ocular abnormalities. It is the second most common inherited cause of chronic renal failure (after polycystic disease). An X-linked mutation causes degeneration of type IV collagen, found in the basement membrane, cochlea and eye.

Cecil Alport, English physician (1880–1959).

5. M – Rhabdomyolysis

Cranial surgery can be extensive and take prolonged periods of time. This predisposes to the development of rhabdomyolysis. Rhabdomyolysis is the breakdown of muscle fibres with release into the blood of myoglobin, which is excreted into the urine. The result is acute renal failure. Although the red urine is caused by myoglobin rather than blood, it still causes a positive dipstick to blood. Treatment is with IV rehydration to aid excretion of myoglobin and prevent renal failure. Rhabdomyolysis is classically caused by crush injuries, but can also be caused by prolonged periods of inertia with pressure on the muscles.

Practice Paper 7: Questions

THEME 1: CONSTIPATION

Options

A. Anal dilatation
B. Behavioural therapy
C. Bowel resection
D. Ethylenediamine tetraacetic acid chelation
E. Gastrograffin enema
F. Laxatives
G. Manual evacuation
H. Oral enzyme supplements
I. Thyroid-stimulating hormone
J. Thyroxine

For each of the following children with constipation, select the next most appropriate step in management. Each option may be used once, more than once or not at all.

1. A 12-year-old boy is constipated. He opens his bowels on average once each week. He describes this as being incredibly painful, 'like a tearing pain'. On wiping, he has noticed blood on the toilet paper. Examination is very painful, and a skin tag is present at the anal verge.

2. A 6-year-old boy is constipated. He is a challenging child who has some behavioural problems and has recently started eating dirt from the garden. He presents to the emergency department with acute-onset abdominal pain, vomiting and headache. On examination, he is unable to walk properly. You perform a full blood count, which reveals a haemoglobin of 8.4 g/dL with a mean cell volume of 72 fL. A blood film reveals basophilic stippling.

3. A newborn presents having failed to open his bowels by 48 hours of life. On performing a rectal examination, you note a normal-sized rectum. When you withdraw the examining finger, there is an explosion of meconium from the rectum.

4. A 6-month-old boy presents with constipation. He recently moved from China. He has coarse facial features and a large tongue. He is behind on his developmental milestones. Examination is unremarkable except for an umbilical hernia.

5. A newborn presents having failed to open his bowels by 48 hours of life. Apart from this, he is clinically well. He has an older sibling with cystic fibrosis.

THEME 2: ANAEMIA

Options

A. Blood film
B. Haemoglobin electrophoresis
C. No investigation at this point
D. Plasma viscosity
E. Schilling test
F. Serum ferritin levels
G. Serum folate levels
H. Serum iron levels
I. Serum lead levels
J. Serum urea and creatinine

For each of the following cases presenting with anaemia, select the investigation most likely to give a diagnosis at this point. Each option may be used once, more than once or not at all.

1. A 4-year-old girl presents with acute-onset pain in the fingers of her left hand. She had been playing in the snow with her brothers earlier that day. She is normally fit and well, but was feeling under the weather a week ago, with a high temperature and flushed cheeks. A full blood count reveals a haemoglobin of 5 g/dL.

2. A 4-year-old girl presents with a fever and productive cough, and is found to have a lower respiratory tract infection. A routine full blood count reveals microcytic hypochromic anaemia. She is described as a fussy eater by her mother, although she has a tendency to eat inappropriate items such as soil and paper. There is no history of medical problems.

3. A 15-year-old girl is found to be anaemic on her annual assessment. On examination, you notice that she is mildly jaundiced. Her haemoglobin is 9.2 g/dL, with a mean cell volume of 102 fL. She has been treated for Graves' disease in the past.

4. A 4-month-old boy presents with failure to thrive. You find hepatosplenomegaly on examination. A full blood count reveals haemoglobin 10.0 g/dL and mean cell volume 72 fL. A blood film confirms hypochromia.

5. A 6-year-old girl who was previously well presents to the paediatrics clinic with long-standing abdominal pain. Her parents have noticed her eating inappropriate substances such as paper and paint. A social history elicits that her performance at school has deteriorated recently. Routine investigations reveal hypochromic microcytic anaemia.

THEME 3: STRIDOR

Options

A. Inhaled salbutamol
B. Intramuscular adrenaline
C. Intramuscular and nebulized adrenaline
D. Intravenous (IV) broad-spectrum antibiotics
E. IV steroids
F. Intubation and ventilation
G. Intubation, ventilation and IV broad-spectrum antibiotics
H. Nebulized steroid
I. No management required
J. Oral antihistamine alone

K. Oral antihistamine and IV steroids
L. Oral antihistamine and nebulized steroids
M. Oral antihistamine and adrenaline
N. Oral antihistamine, IV steroids and intramuscular adrenaline
O. Oral antihistamine, nebulized steroids and intramuscular adrenaline
P. Oral steroid
Q. Rigid bronchoscopy

For each of the following children presenting with stridor, select the management steps that you would take after applying oxygen. Each option may be used once, more than once or not at all.

1. An 18-month-old girl presents with a cough and stridor. The cough is described as 'barking' in nature. She has a temperature of 38°C and is restless. She does not appear systemically unwell and is not cyanotic, but there is moderate stridor on exertion.

2. A 3-year-old girl presents with stridor of a few hours' duration. She has been well for the last few days. She has a temperature of 39.5°C. She sat on her mother's knee with her head leaning forward, is very quiet and is drooling. On examination, she is systemically unwell and has a quiet stridor and reduced air entry bilaterally.

3. A 16-month-old girl presents with stridor. She was with her family this afternoon at a picnic in the park. Since having lunch an hour ago, she developed swelling of her face and lips. She has a red rash over her trunk and limbs. On examination, she is pale, tachycardic and oedematous. She has a quiet stridor with reduced air entry bilaterally.

4. A 4-year-old girl presents with stridor of a few hours' duration. She has been unwell for a few days, complaining of a sore throat. She has a temperature of 39.5°C. She sat on her mother's knee, is very irritable, with her head tilted to one side and is drooling. On examination, she appears systemically unwell and has a quiet stridor but good air entry bilaterally.

5. A 21-month-old girl presents with a cough and stridor. This developed while she was having lunch with her family at home an hour ago. On examination, she is systemically well and has a quiet bilateral stridor with reduced air entry on the right.

THEME 4: DEVELOPMENTAL ASSESSMENT

Options

A. Newborn baby
B. 1 month
C. 6 weeks
D. 3 months
E. 6 months
F. 9 months
G. 12 months
H. 15 months
 I. 18 months
 J. 2 years
K. 2.5 years
L. 3 years
M. 4 years
N. 5 years

For each of the following stages, select the age at which you would expect to see this stage in development. Each option may be used once, more than once or not at all.

1. Can draw a triangle.
2. Can walk alone, feet apart, arms assisting balance.
3. Is able to babble loudly with repetitive syllables (e.g. 'dad-dad', 'adaba', 'agaga').
4. Can hop on one foot.
5. Is able to fix and follow an object through 180° in the horizontal plane.

THEME 5: OEDEMA

Options

A. Anaemia
B. Angioedema
C. Glomerulonephritis
D. Heart failure
E. Henoch–Schönlein purpura
F. Kwashiorkor
G. Liver failure
H. Marasmus
 I. Nephrotic syndrome
J. Protein-losing enteropathy
K. Renal failure
L. Thyrotoxicosis
M. Turner's syndrome

For each of the following cases, select the most likely diagnosis. Each option may be used once, more than once or not at all.

1. An 18-month-old boy presents with oedema. He has chronic diarrhoea and is listless and irritable. He had been breastfed until recently. On examination, despite being of African origin, he has hair with a red tinge. His skin is tight and cracked in places. A urine dipstick is negative for protein.

2. A 4-year-old boy presents with oedema. He is clinically unwell with severe abdominal pain, fever and guarding. Urine is positive for protein and his serum albumin level is low.

3. A 9-year-old boy presents with oedema, just 1 day after being diagnosed with tonsillitis by his GP. The oedema is most marked around his lips and face. He is clinically unwell with an urticarial rash and wheeze. A urine dipstick is negative for protein.

4. A 5-year-old girl presents with oedema. This is most marked over her lower lip, where she was hit by her brother. The oedema is not itchy and there is no inflammation. She has no wheeze audible. A urine dipstick is negative for protein.

5. A 6-month-old girl presents with oedema. She is failing to gain weight and appears very short of breath. Examination is normal except for peripheral oedema. A urine dipstick is negative for protein.

THEME 6: DIAGNOSIS OF ELECTROLYTE IMBALANCE

Options

A. Central diabetes insipidus
B. Diabetes mellitus
C. Glucocorticoid deficiency
D. Hypervolaemic hypernatraemia
E. Hypervolaemic hyponatraemia
F. Hypovolaemic hypernatraemia
G. Hypovolaemic hyponatraemia
H. Nephrogenic diabetes insipidus
I. Psychogenic polydipsia
J. Pyloric stenosis
K. Syndrome of inappropriate antidiuretic hormone secretion

For each of the following cases, select the most likely diagnosis. Each option may be used once, more than once or not at all.

1. A mother brings her 12-year-old son to the emergency department as she is concerned that he is drinking excessively. He drinks 4 L of water a day and passes a similar volume of urine. On examination, he looks clinically well and is not dehydrated. Blood tests reveal Na$^+$ 152 mmol/L (range 135–145 mmol/L). On restricting his fluid intake, his urinary-specific gravity remains low. On administration of desmopressin, concentration of the urine occurs.

2. A 5-year-old girl is admitted with gastroenteritis. She is passing five to ten loose stools a day and is not passing urine as frequently as normal. Her observations are pulse 100 beats/minute and capillary refill time <2 seconds. Her mucous membranes are dry and she reports feeling thirsty. The junior doctor in the emergency department takes bloods, which reveal a sodium concentration of 148 mmol/L.

3. A 6-year-old girl is admitted feeling acutely unwell. She has a temperature of 38.2°C and is tachypnoeic. Clinically, she appears well hydrated. A cannula is sited to commence IV antibiotics. Blood is sent for analysis, which reveals a serum sodium concentration of 128 mmol/L. Urea and creatinine are normal. A urine dipstick reveals a high specific gravity.

4. A mother brings her 14-year-old son to the emergency department as she is concerned that he is drinking excessively. He drinks 4 L of water a day and passes a similar volume of urine. On examination, he looks clinically well and is not dehydrated. You admit him for investigation. Blood tests reveal Na$^+$ 129 mmol/L (range 135–145 mmol/L). On restricting his fluid intake, his urinary-specific gravity increases.

5. A 3-week-old male infant presents with severe vomiting. On examination, he is shocked and hypotensive. You insert a cannula and send bloods for electrolytes, which reveal a normal pH, K$^+$ 5.9 mmol/L (range 3.5–4.5 mmol/L), Na$^+$ 118 mmol/L and glucose 5.8 mmol/L.

THEME 7: MANAGEMENT OF ELECTROLYTE IMBALANCE

Options

A. Fluid restriction
B. Hydrocortisone
C. IV furosemide
D. IV hypertonic saline
E. Low-sodium diet
F. Nasal desmopressin
   administration

G. Oral rehydration
H. Oral sodium supplementation
I. Pyloromyotomy
J. Stool-forming agent
K. Subcutaneous insulin

For each of the following cases, select the next most appropriate management of the electrolyte imbalance. Each option may be used once, more than once or not at all.

1. A mother brings her 12-year-old son to the emergency department as she is concerned that he is drinking excessively. He drinks 4 L of water a day and passes a similar volume of urine. On examination, he looks clinically well and is not dehydrated. Blood tests reveal Na$^+$ 152 mmol/L (range 135–145 mmol/L). On restricting his fluid intake, his urinary-specific gravity remains low. On administration of desmopressin, concentration of the urine occurs.

2. A 5-year-old girl is admitted with gastroenteritis. She is passing five to ten loose stools a day and is not passing urine as frequently as normal. Her observations are pulse 100 beats/minute and capillary refill time <2 seconds. Her mucous membranes are dry and she reports feeling thirsty. The junior doctor in the emergency department takes bloods, which reveal a sodium concentration of 148 mmol/L.

3. A 6-year-old girl is admitted feeling acutely unwell. She has a temperature of 38.2°C and is tachypnoeic. Clinically, she appears well hydrated. A cannula is sited to commence IV antibiotics. Blood is sent for analysis, which reveals a serum sodium concentration of 128 mmol/L. Urea and creatinine are normal. A urine dipstick reveals a high specific gravity.

4. A mother brings her 14-year-old son to the emergency department as she is concerned that he is drinking excessively. He drinks 4 L of water a day and passes a similar volume of urine. On examination, he looks clinically well and is not dehydrated. You admit him for investigation. Blood tests reveal Na$^+$ 129 mmol/L (range 135–145 mmol/L). On restricting his fluid intake, his urinary-specific gravity increases.

5. A 3-week-old male infant presents with severe vomiting. On examination, he is shocked and hypotensive. You insert a cannula and send bloods for electrolytes, which reveal a normal pH, K$^+$ 5.9 mmol/L (range 3.5–4.5 mmol/L), Na$^+$ 118 mmol/L and glucose 5.8 mmol/L.

THEME 8: CONGENITAL HEART DISEASE

Options

A. Atrial septal defect
B. Atrioventricular septal defect
C. Coarctation of the aorta
D. Critical aortic stenosis
E. Patent ductus arteriosus
F. Pulmonary atresia
G. Tetralogy of Fallot
H. Transposition of the great arteries
I. Truncus arteriosus
J. Ventricular septal defect

For each of the following scenarios, select the most likely congenital heart defect. Each option may be used once, more than once or not at all.

1. A 4-month-old girl presents with breathlessness. Her health visitor is concerned, as she is failing to thrive. Over the last 2 months, there have been intermittent episodes of her turning blue, especially when she is upset. These episodes resolve spontaneously. A chest X-ray reveals a boot-shaped heart.

2. You are asked to see a 2-day-old baby girl. She is tachycardic and cool to the touch. There is no murmur and no cyanosis. The femoral pulses are difficult to palpate.

3. A 4-month-old girl presents with breathlessness. Her health visitor is concerned, as she is failing to thrive. The parents deny any episodes of cyanosis. On examination, there is a moderate pansystolic murmur at the lower left sternal edge associated with a parasternal thrill. A chest X-ray reveals cardiomegaly.

4. You are asked to see a 2-day-old baby girl. She is tachycardic and cool to the touch. There is no murmur, but she looks blue. The femoral pulses are palpable.

5. A 4-month-old girl presents with breathlessness. Her health visitor is concerned, as she is failing to thrive. The parents deny any episodes of cyanosis. On examination, she has a loud murmur present throughout systole and diastole, heard best just inferior to the left clavicle. A chest X-ray reveals moderate cardiomegaly.

THEME 9: ORGANISMS ASSOCIATED WITH PAEDIATRIC PATHOLOGY

Options

A. *Campylobacter jejuni*
B. *Clostridium difficile*
C. *Mycobacterium tuberculosis*
D. *Mycoplasma pneumoniae*
E. *Neisseria meningitidis*
F. *Pneumocystis jiroveci*
G. *Salmonella typhi*
H. *Streptococcus pneumoniae*
I. *Treponema pallidum*

For each of the following descriptions, select the most appropriate organism. Each option may be used once, more than once or not at all.

1. A Gram-positive bacillus causing gastroenteritis
2. A spiral-shaped bacterium causing syphilis
3. A Gram-positive coccus causing respiratory infection
4. A Gram-negative comma-shaped bacterium causing gastroenteritis
5. A cell wall-deficient bacterium causing respiratory infection

THEME 10: THE CRYING BABY

Options

A. Constipation
B. Gastro-oesophageal reflux
C. Incarcerated inguinal hernia
D. Infantile colic
E. Intussusception
F. Maternal drug use
G. Non-accidental injury (shaken baby)
H. Sepsis
 I. Teething
 J. Urinary tract infection

For each of the following babies presenting with intractable crying, select the most likely diagnosis. Each option may be used once, more than once or not at all.

1. A 4-month-old baby presents with intractable crying for several months. His mother describes him as a very 'sicky baby' who has chronic hiccups. Examination is unremarkable.

2. A 4-week-old baby presents with intractable crying for the last 2 weeks. He was born at term with no risk factors for infection. He now presents as shocked and non-responsive. He is afebrile. There is bruising on his chest wall.

3. A 6-month-old baby presents with intractable crying for the last month. His mother says that he is also drooling excessively. The crying may occur at any time during the day. The baby is happy only when he has something in his mouth.

4. A newborn baby is admitted to the neonatal unit as he is small for gestation. After a number of days, he becomes very irritable. He has a high-pitched cry and has diarrhoea. He is difficult to settle to sleep, yet is persistently yawning. The observations are stable, with a temperature of 36.7°C.

5. A newborn baby is admitted to the neonatal unit from the maternity unit. His mother's waters broke more than 24 hours before delivery. Eighteen hours after delivery, he becomes very irritable, with a high-pitched cry. His temperature is 38.3°C.

Practice Paper 7: Answers

THEME 1: CONSTIPATION

1. F – Laxatives

This patient has an anal fissure. An anal fissure is a longitudinal tear at the anal margin that occurs after passing a constipated stool. Tears usually occur at the posterior margin, and multiple fissures may occur with Crohn's disease. Patients present with a stinging pain on defecation that can last up to 2 hours. This may be associated with small amounts of fresh bleeding and pruritus. On examination, the anal sphincter is in spasm and there may be a sentinel pile protruding from the anus (this represents a torn tag of the anal epithelium). Anal fissures cause a vicious cycle in constipation, because the child learns that it will be very painful to pass the hard constipated stools. This exacerbates the constipation as the stool is retained for longer, with more fluid being withdrawn from the already hard stool. As the constipation worsens, the hard stool reopens the fissure when it is passed. Small anal fissures heal spontaneously. Management options include treating the underlying constipation with laxatives. If this does not work, topical preparations that relax the anal sphincter can be used, such as glyceryl trinitrate or diltiazem pastes. Chronic recurring fissures may need excision.

2. D – Ethylenediamine tetraacetic acid chelation

This boy presents with features of encephalopathy, which are likely to be due to underlying lead poisoning given the history of pica (eating non-nutritive substances). Pica can be both a sign and a cause of lead poisoning. Lead poisoning affects the nervous, gastrointestinal and haematological systems. Affected children present with encephalopathic signs or behavioural problems. The diagnosis of lead poisoning can be confirmed definitively by measuring blood lead levels. Other blood tests will reveal hypochromic microcytic anaemia, and a blood film demonstrates basophilic stippling (the presence of granules within the cytoplasm of red blood cells). Treatment is with chelation of the lead using ethylenediamine tetraacetic acid (EDTA).

3. C – Bowel resection

This patient has Hirschsprung's disease. Hirschsprung's disease is a congenital absence of ganglion cells from the parasympathetic myenteric plexus of the large bowel, resulting in a narrowed, contracted segment. Without innervation, the bowel is spastic and has no peristalsis. This abnormally innervated bowel extends proximally from the rectum for a variable distance. Hirschsprung's disease often presents in neonates with abdominal distension, bile-stained vomiting or failure of passage of meconium. Rectal examination shows a narrowed segment, and removal of the examining finger is often followed by a gush of stools and flatus. Occasionally, a short-segment Hirschsprung's disease can present later in childhood with chronic constipation and abdominal distension without soiling. Confirmation of the diagnosis is by rectal biopsy, which demonstrates the absence of ganglion cells in the affected mucosa. Definitive management is by excision of the abnormal bowel with re-anastomosis to the anus (end-to-rectum anastomosis). Before surgery, temporary decompression of the colon can be brought about by rectal bowel washouts using physiological or 0.9% saline.

Harald Hirschsprung, Danish paediatrician (1830–1916).

4. J – Thyroxine

This child has congenital hypothyroidism (formerly known as cretinism). Congenital hypothyroidism has a number of causes, including embryological maldescent of the thyroid, maternal iodine deficiency and dyshormonogenesis (an autosomal recessive inborn error of thyroid hormone synthesis). Congenital hypothyroidism is now routinely screened for in neonates with the Guthrie test (along with phenylketonuria, sickle cell disease, cystic fibrosis [CF] and medium-chain acyl CoA dehydrogenase deficiency). Children with congenital hypothyroidism present with hypotonia, coarse facial features, delayed closure of the anterior fontanelle, a hoarse cry, dry skin, hypothermia, prolonged jaundice, umbilical hernia, short stature, developmental delay, constipation and learning difficulties. If thyroxine treatment is started early enough (usually within the first weeks of life), then learning difficulties can be minimized and sometimes entirely prevented. Bone age is used to monitor thyroxine therapy to ensure that there is no under- or over-treatment.

Robert Guthrie, American microbiologist (1916–1995).

5. E – Gastrograffin enema

Around 10% of infants with CF will present with meconium ileus, where a thick meconium plug causes intestinal obstruction. Affected babies will present with bile-stained vomiting and abdominal distension, and there will be no record of passage of meconium. Initial management is with a gastrograffin enema, which is both diagnostic and therapeutic. If the child is peritonitic, a gastrograffin enema is contraindicated and a laparotomy and bowel resection should be performed. In all cases, these children should be immediately started on prophylactic flucloxacillin to protect lung function, and a sweat test performed at 6 weeks of life to confirm the diagnosis of CF. See Rubin and Dale for a good review on chronic constipation.[*]

[*] Rubin G, Dale A. Clinical review: Chronic constipation in children. *BMJ* 2006; 333: 1051–5.

THEME 2: ANAEMIA

1. A – Blood film OR B – Haemoglobin electrophoresis

This is a case of sickle cell anaemia with dactylitis induced by low temperatures. The infection the week before may have been secondary to erythrovirus (formally known as parvovirus), which can cause an aplastic crisis (a reduction or total absence of haematopoietic cell lines of the marrow, leading to pancytopenia). Sickle cell disease is a homozygous inheritance of faulty β-globin genes that is most common in African, Mediterranean and Middle-Eastern countries. A single amino acid substitution (glutamine → valine) results in an abnormal haemoglobin that becomes insoluble in its deoxygenated state and causes sickling (crescentic shaping) of red blood cells. Sickled cells can become trapped in the microcirculation, leading to thrombosis and ischaemia. Such vaso-occlusive crises include dactylitis (swelling and pain in the digits) and priapism (prolonged erection). Management of acute painful crises is by analgesia, warmth and rehydration. Diagnosis of sickle cell disease can be made by several methods: blood film appearance, haemoglobin electrophoresis or using screening methods in which the blood is deoxygenated to induce sickling. Electrophoresis has two general applications. The first is the diagnosis of haemaglobinopathies, including sickle cell disease, by separating the abnormal haemoglobins at an alkaline pH. The second is in the investigation of myeloma to detect monoclonal immunoglobulins characteristic of the disease.

2. C – No investigation at this point

Investigation of iron-deficiency anaemia will reveal a hypochromic microcytic anaemia. However, this will not confirm the diagnosis, as there are other causes of hypochromic microcytic anaemia (e.g. thalassaemias and anaemia of chronic disease). Ferritin is a plasma protein that carries iron, and levels are reflective of total body iron stores. A low serum ferritin (in association with hypochromic microcytic anaemia) is the most useful test in confirming iron-deficiency anaemia. However, ferritin is an acute-phase protein and concentrations are raised in chronic inflammation or acute infection, such as here. Therefore, a normal ferritin level during this lower respiratory tract infection (LRTI) would not rule out iron deficiency and so should be delayed.

The question asks about which investigation you would perform at this point. This child is clinically unwell with pneumonia, and therefore the ferritin will most likely be high or normal. One should wait until the child has improved clinically before measuring the serum ferritin level. Oral iron is given to correct iron deficiency, and should produce a haemoglobin rise of 1 g/dL per week of therapy. Iron should be continued for a further 3–6 months after normal haemoglobin levels are attained to ensure that iron stores are replenished.

The girl in this question eats inappropriate foods. The compulsion to eat non-nutritive substances, such as paint, paper and soil, is called pica and is strongly associated with iron-deficiency anaemia.

Pica, from Latin *pica* = magpie (a bird that is reported to eat almost anything).

3. E – Schilling test

This patient has anaemia with macrocytosis (a high mean cell volume – the normal range being 80–90 fL). Considering her previous history of autoimmune disease, the likely cause of her features is pernicious anaemia. Pernicious anaemia is an autoimmune disease of the gastric parietal cells, which normally produce intrinsic factor (IF). IF is required for the absorption of vitamin B_{12} in the terminal ileum. In pernicious anaemia, because no IF is made, the serum vitamin B_{12} level is very low. Around 90% of patients demonstrate anti-parietal antibodies (but some normal people also have these), and 60% are found to have anti-IF antibody (which is a more specific marker). Although most patents with pernicious anaemia complain of lethargy and general malaise, specific features of vitamin B_{12} deficiency include peripheral neuropathy, smooth tongue, angular stomatitis, depression, dementia and subacute degeneration of the spinal cord. The blood film is likely to show macrocytic (increased mean cell volume) megaloblastic anaemia with hypersegmented neutrophil nuclei (>6 lobes). In addition, serum vitamin B_{12} levels are low and ferritin levels are normal, reflecting normal iron stores. Serum vitamin B_{12} levels can be measured directly, but this option is not provided.

The two-part Schilling test can be used to diagnose vitamin B_{12} deficiency. It can also help define whether this is due to pernicious anaemia or problems of the terminal ileum. Patients are initially given intramuscular vitamin B_{12}. This occupies all of the vitamin B_{12}-binding sites in the plasma, so any further absorbed vitamin B_{12} is immediately excreted via the kidneys. Oral vitamin B_{12} labelled with radioactive cobalt is then administered. If the patient starts excreting radiolabelled vitamin B_{12} in the urine, then they do not have a problem with vitamin B_{12} absorption. In those who do not excrete vitamin B_{12}, the second part of the test is performed. This time, oral radiolabelled vitamin B_{12} and IF are given. If the patient now starts excreting radiolabelled vitamin B_{12}, pernicious anaemia is confirmed. If there is still no excretion, an underlying bowel-related problem is the cause of poor vitamin B_{12} absorption. Pernicious anaemia is rare in this age group, and usually occurs in the female population aged over 50 years. There is an increased risk associated with autoimmune diseases such as vitiligo, thyroid disease and Addison's disease. Jaundice occurs due to haemolysis of the ineffective products of erythropoiesis by the spleen. Treatment of pernicious anaemia is with 3-monthly intramuscular injections of hydroxocobalamin, a vitamin B_{12} analogue.

Viktor Theodor Schilling, German haematologist (1883–1960).
fL = femtolitres. The prefix 'femto-' denotes 10^{-15} (a quadrillionth).
Femto-, from Danish and Norwegian *femten* = 15.

4. B – Haemoglobin electrophoresis

This child has thalassaemia. β-thalassaemia major is an autosomal recessive disorder in which there is a complete lack of production of the haemoglobin β-globin chain. It occurs mainly in Mediterranean and Middle-Eastern families and is due to a point mutation on chromosome 11. Because patients with β-thalassaemia major have mutations on both alleles and cannot synthesize any β-globin, they cannot produce functioning adult haemoglobin (HbA; $\alpha_2\beta_2$). This condition typically presents within the first year of life when the production of fetal haemoglobin (HbF; $\alpha_2\gamma_2$) begins to fall. Affected children become generally unwell and fail to thrive secondary to severe microcytic anaemia. Ferritin levels are normal, since there is no iron deficiency. A compensatory increase in the synthesis of HbF and haemoglobin A_2 (HbA$_2$; $\alpha_2\delta_2$) occurs, which can be detected on serum electrophoresis.

Clinical features include failure to thrive, lethargy, pallor and jaundice. On examination, there is often hepatosplenomegaly (secondary to extramedullary haematopoiesis), with bossing of the skull and long-bone deformity (due to excessive intramedullary haematopoiesis). The treatment of β-thalassaemia major is with regular blood transfusions, aiming to maintain the haemoglobin concentration above 10 g/dL, or with allogenic bone marrow transplantation. Regular iron-chelation therapy (with desferrioxamine) is required to prevent iron overload and deposition in vital organs such as the heart, liver and endocrine glands. If untreated, death is inevitable in the first years of life.

β-thalassaemia minor describes people heterozygous for the β-chain chromosomal mutation. Affected persons have only a mild anaemia and are usually asymptomatic.

α-thalassaemia is most common in Asian populations. There are four α-globin genes. The presence of defects in all four genes results in Hb Barts (tetramers of γ-chains), which does not carry oxygen effectively, and results in death *in utero*. The presence of defects in three of the four genes results in HbH (tetramers of β-chains), which causes chronic moderate haemolysis. Defects in only one or two of the four α-chain genes result in subclinical hypochromic microcytic anaemia. Treatment options are as for β-thalassaemia.

Leukaemia can also present with hepatosplenomegaly and anaemia. It would therefore be prudent to perform a blood film to identify blast cells.

Thalassaemia, from Greek *thalassa* = sea + *haima* = blood. It is so called as the disease is especially prevalent in 'countries by the sea' (i.e. the Mediterranean).

5. I – Serum lead levels

This girl has pica (the compulsive eating of non-nutritive substances). Of these, she is known to eat paint, which contains lead. Lead poisoning affects the brain, gut and blood. Children can present with a varied spectrum of symptoms ranging from abdominal pain to encephalopathy and behavioural problems. Examination may reveal a bluish line along the gums. Lead poisoning is not as common as it used to be, as household plumbing no longer uses lead pipes. A blood film may reveal basophilic stippling (multiple scattered granules throughout the cytoplasm of erythrocytes); however, this may also be seen in thalassaemia and other forms of anaemia. Diagnosis is made by measurement of serum lead levels. However, early lead poisoning can also be demonstrated by finding reduced concentrations of haem precursors (e.g. free protoporphyrin). Treatment is with chelating (binding) agents such as EDTA that speed up the excretion of lead.

Chelation, from Greek *chele* = claw.

THEME 3: STRIDOR

Stridor is a respiratory noise made on inspiration. Stridor implies extrathoracic airway obstruction. The intensity (volume) of the stridor is not a good clinical indicator of the degree of obstruction; indeed, a quiet stridor with reduced air entry is a very worrying sign. Any child with a stridor should never have their oropharnyx examined unless there is a consultant anaesthetist and ENT surgeon present to manage the airway (even if you think that it is croup). This is because examination can stimulate total obstruction of an already compromised airway in acute epiglottitis.

1. H – Nebulized steroid OR P – Oral steroid

Croup (laryngotracheobronchitis) typically follows a viral upper respiratory tract infection and accounts for 95% of laryngeotracheal infections in children. The main causative pathogen is the parainfluenza virus. It commonly affects children under the age of 2 years and can be very distressing for parents. These children often have a barking cough, harsh stridor and a low-grade fever (compared with the high-grade fever in epiglottitis). Various croup scores have been devised to assess the degree of stridor, cyanosis, respiratory distress, air entry and consciousness. Management options include steroids (nebulized or oral) to relieve the inflammation. In severe cases, the airway compromise can be significant enough to require nebulized adrenaline. Antibiotics are of no use.

2. G – Intubation, ventilation and intravenous (IV) broad-spectrum antibiotics

This is a case of acute epiglottitis, a bacterial infection caused by *Haemophilus influenzae* type b. Differentiating epiglottitis from a retropharyngeal abscess or bacterial tracheitis can be difficult clinically. In epiglottitis, the patient inevitably needs intubation to protect the airway. Antibiotics are required to treat this bacterial infection.

3. N – Oral antihistamine, IV steroids and intramuscular adrenaline

This girl is having a severe anaphylactic reaction. The treatment is not dependent on the cause (bee sting, food reaction, etc.). Anaphylaxis is an immunoglobulin E-mediated immunological reaction that is precipitated by allergen exposure (type I hypersensitivity). Release of inflammatory mediators, such as histamine and prostaglandins, results in vasodilatation and smooth muscle contraction, with symptoms ranging from mild irritation to anaphylactic shock and death. Such reactions are potentially life threatening and should be treated aggressively. Oxygen is required to prevent hypoxia, along with systemic administration of antihistamines, steroids and adrenaline. This girl may well need intubating and ventilating if the above steps are not rapidly successful.

4. D – IV broad-spectrum antibiotics

The child has a retropharyngeal abscess that presents with fever, drooling, dysphagia and stridor. (The relatively long history makes acute epiglottitis unlikely.) Occasionally, the head may be tilted to one side and the neck may be stiff (torticollis). A lateral X-ray of the neck shows an increase in the 'soft tissue' shadow between the vertebral column and the air in the pharynx. Invariably, the abscess will need incising with antibiotic cover.

5. Q – Rigid bronchoscopy

This girl has inhaled a foreign body, with typical presenting symptoms (cough, stridor and unilateral reduced air entry). A chest X-ray may locate the foreign object, but it will need to be removed by rigid bronchoscopy under anaesthesia. Foreign bodies that have been swallowed can also be removed by endoscopy, although those that have already passed through the lower oesophageal sphincter are managed conservatively with serial X-rays to ensure that they are moving along the gastrointestinal tract.

THEME 4: DEVELOPMENTAL ASSESSMENT

The assessment of development falls into four key areas:

1. Gross motor (including posture)
2. Fine motor and vision
3. Language
4. Social behaviour and play

An excellent and comprehensive description of child development can be found in, Sheridan MD, Frost M, Sharma A. *From Birth to Five Years, Children's Developmental Progress*, 4th edn. London: Routledge, 1997. The only way to learn how to assess development is to practise by seeing lots of normal children.

1. N – 5 years

At 5 years of age, one would expect a child to be able to walk on a narrow line and to stand on one foot with arms folded, to be able to build elaborate models when shown (e.g. three steps with six cubes) and to be able to colour pictures neatly and to draw squares and triangles. Their speech is fluent, and they will enjoy reading or being told stories that they act out later. They are able to give their full name, age and often their birthday.

2. H – 15 months

The stages one would expect a child to take to fully mobilizing are

- 6 months: take their own weight when held to stand
- 9 months: able to pull to stand, holding on to support for a few moments
- 12 months: crawling on hand and knees, shuffling on buttocks or 'bear-walking', cruising
- 15 months: walks alone, feet apart, arms assisting balance
- 18 months: walks well, carrying toy

3. F – 9 months

The language milestones at various ages are

- 6 months: vocalizes (e.g. a-a, muh, goo)
- 9 months: babbles with repetitive syllables (da-da), understands no and bye-bye
- 12 months: babbles loudly and incessantly in conversational cadences; vocalization contains most vowels and many consonants; waves goodbye, understands simple instructions (e.g. 'come to mummy')
- 18 months: uses 6–20 recognizable words; understands many more

4. M – 4 years

Hopping on one foot is a gross motor skill. Other gross motor skills expected by 4 years are climbing ladders and trees, the ability to stand, walk and run on tiptoe, sitting with knees crossed and showing increasing skill in ball games (throwing, catching, bouncing, kicking, etc.).

5. D – 3 months

At 6 weeks, the child can fix and follow 90° through the horizontal plane. This is increased to 180° by 3 months.

THEME 5: OEDEMA

Oedema is the accumulation of excess interstitial fluid. Its causes can be subdivided into those due to increased interstitial pressure and those due to low plasma protein concentrations. Low plasma protein levels can be caused by increased losses, decreased production or impaired lymphatic flow.

1. F – Kwashiorkor

Kwashiorkor is a clinical diagnosis. It is caused by severe protein deficiency due to poor nutrition – specifically protein–calorie malnutrition.

There is often adequate calorie intake but inadequate protein in the diet. Kwashiorkor is therefore more common in developing countries where carbohydrates are the staple diet. Oedema often masks the poor weight gain. Clinical features are chronic diarrhoea, irritability, listlessness, apathy and anorexia. Classically, these children have sparse discoloured hair, are oedematous, have tight skin and have abdominal distension. Marasmus is caused by total calorie malnutrition and does not cause oedema. Children with marasmus look emaciated and do not demonstrate abdominal distension.

Kwashiorkor, from Ghanaian = displaced child – so called as it affects children who have been newly displaced from breastfeeding.
Marasmus, from Greek *marasmos* = waste away, decay.

2. I – Nephrotic syndrome
Nephrotic syndrome is diagnosed if a patient has the triad of peripheral oedema, hypoalbuminaemia and proteinuria (such as in this case). About 85% of cases are caused by minimal-change glomerulonephritis. Loss of immunoglobulins in the urine puts these patients at high risk of pneumococcal and *Haemophilus* infections. In this case, the child is acutely unwell with abdominal pain associated with fever and guarding, which may be due to peritonitis. Treatment of nephrotic syndrome is prednisolone to induce remission. Salt restriction and replacement of fluids with human albumin solution is also occasionally required. Oral fluids often need to be restricted. Prophylactic penicillin should be started in all cases of nephrotic syndrome because of the risk of sepsis and peritonitis. This child will need IV antibiotics to treat the peritonitis.

3. B – Angioedema
This boy is having an allergic reaction, possibly from recently prescribed antibiotics. The swelling is caused by histamine release in response to a specific allergen. Management is with antihistamines (chlorphenamine), steroids and adrenaline, depending on the severity of the allergic/anaphylactic reaction.

4. B – Angioedema
Hereditary angioedema is a rare and potentially fatal autosomal dominant deficiency of the C1-esterase inhibitor. The C1-esterase inhibitor acts as a mediator of complement proteins of the immune system, and a lack of this protein allows the complement system to go unchecked, with an accumulation of vasoactive inflammatory mediators. This can result in intermittent itchy swelling of the face, lips, pharynx and limbs, along with abdominal pain, vomiting and diarrhoea. Attacks of hereditary angioedema can be mistaken for anaphylaxis, and repeated doses of antihistamine and adrenaline are given with no effect. There is often no identifiable trigger for attacks of hereditary angioedema, although recognized precipitators include minor trauma and strenuous exercise. Acute

attacks last 2 or 3 days, but can be treated with IV Cl-esterase inhibitor concentrate. Long-term management with anabolic steroids (e.g. danazol) helps promote synthesis of Cl-esterase inhibitor. Laryngeal oedema is the most concerning complication, and can be fatal.

5. D – Heart failure

This child has peripheral oedema, shortness of breath and failure to thrive. Differentials would include Turner's syndrome, anaemia and heart failure. Turner's syndrome is a chromosomal disorder (45XO), and these girls often present as neonates with oedema. It is the *in utero* oedema that causes the webbed neck that is classically seen. Anaemia has to be very severe to cause oedema, and is unlikely to cause such drastic symptoms. This child's oedema is thus most likely to be due to congenital heart disease. The most common congenital heart condition is a ventricular septal defect (VSD). If the VSD is large, it can cause heart failure, presenting with shortness of breath, which is worse on feeding, and failure to thrive. VSDs are usually associated with a pansystolic murmur, although large VSDs have an exceptionally quiet murmur or no murmur at all. This is because very little turbulent flow is created by such a large defect. Treatment of heart failure is complex, but diuretics are the first-line agents.

THEME 6: DIAGNOSIS OF ELECTROLYTE IMBALANCE

1. A – Central diabetes insipidus

This is a case of central diabetes insipidus (CDI). Diabetes insipidus (DI) presents with polyuria, polydipsia, frequency, nocturia and nocturnal enuresis. Differentials include nephrogenic DI (NDI), psychogenic polydipsia and diabetes mellitus. CDI is caused by a deficiency of antidiuretic hormone (ADH; also known as arginine vasopressin) secretion from the posterior pituitary. NDI is caused by insensitivity to ADH in the collecting ducts of the kidney. Causes of CDI include idiopathic, hypothalamic disease, head injury and meningoencephalitis.

The diagnosis of DI is confirmed using the water deprivation test. The patient is deprived of water, and the urine and plasma osmolalities are measured every 2 hours. If there is a raised plasma osmolality (>300 mmol/kg) in the presence of urine that is not maximally concentrated (i.e. <660 mmol/kg), then the patient has DI. At this point in the test, the patient is given an intramuscular dose of desmopressin (a synthetic analogue of ADH). If the patient now starts concentrating their urine, then they have cranial DI. If the urine osmolality remains <660 mmol/kg, then NDI is confirmed. Dipstick analysis of specific gravity allows for a bedside test for urinary osmolality. A low specific gravity indicates dilute urine and a high specific gravity indicates concentrated urine. The treatment of cranial DI is with desmopressin, although in mild cases hydration may be maintained orally. NDI is improved by thiazide diuretics.

2. F – Hypovolaemic hypernatraemia

This girl has gastroenteritis causing diarrhoea; however, she is not vomiting. She has become mildly dehydrated due to the loss of fluids in the diarrhoea. This loss of fluids has caused a hypovolaemic hypernatraemia. The clinical examination reveals a mild case of dehydration, and as the child is not vomiting, a trial of oral rehydration therapy is indicated. If this fails, then IV fluids could be used. Oral fluids are encouraged in such cases, as the electrolyte disturbance will be corrected naturally.

3. K – Syndrome of inappropriate antidiuretic hormone secretion

Syndrome of inappropriate antidiuretic hormone secretion is the inappropriate secretion of excess ADH. This causes retention of fluid by the kidneys, which results in hyponatraemia by diluting the serum (there is no absolute sodium loss). In children, the aetiology includes intracranial disease (head injury, meningitis, space-occupying lesions and haematomas), pulmonary disease and drugs. The diagnosis is one of exclusion, and should be made only if the child is not dehydrated or oedematous and there is no renal, adrenal, pituitary or thyroid dysfunction. Treatment is undertaken by restricting total intake of fluids. The patient should be monitored with daily weights, serial serum and urine osmolality and electrolyte analysis. In severe cases, if there are complications such as seizures, then more aggressive management may be required with hypertonic saline and concurrent furosemide. However, this should be done with extreme caution, as rapid correction of low sodium can result in central pontine myelinolysis (damage to the nerve sheath of the brainstem, resulting in paralysis, dysphagia, dysarthria or locked-in syndrome).

4. I – Psychogenic polydipsia

Psychogenic polydipsia is a relatively rare problem. It involves drinking excessive volumes of fluid without the physiological stimulus to do so. In children, it may be a sign of emotional difficulties – but it may well be an isolated problem in children who simply enjoy drinking a lot. Diagnosis is made using the water deprivation test, which assesses urinary concentration on restricting fluid intake. In psychogenic polydipsia, the previously dilute urine becomes concentrated. If the urine remains dilute, then DI is more likely. Treatment is with restriction of daily fluid intake.

5. C – Glucocorticoid deficiency

This baby has congenital adrenal hyperplasia (CAH) causing glucocorticoid (cortisol) and mineralocorticoid (aldosterone) deficiency. CAH is an autosomal recessive deficiency in the enzyme 21-hydroxylase. This enzyme is required to synthesize mineralocorticoids and glucocorticoids (but not adrenal androgens) from the hormone precursor 17-hydroxyprogesterone. Because there is a lack of mineralocorticoids and glucocorticoids, there is no negative feedback on the anterior pituitary, resulting in increased secretion of adrenocorticotropic hormone (ACTH). The high ACTH then causes an increased secretion of adrenal androgens, since this does not require the deficient hormone. The androgens result in the physical features of CAH, namely ambiguous genitalia (in girls), precocious puberty (in girls), accelerated growth in childhood and virilization. Patients who are steroid deficient can present with a salt-losing crisis. This presents with hypotension, features of dehydration, vomiting, shock and collapse. The aldosterone deficiency will result in high serum potassium and low sodium. Infants with CAH may present with genital hypertrophy and hypoglycaemia.

The treatment priority here is resuscitation with IV fluids, swiftly followed by IV hydrocortisone. Long-term treatment is with hydrocortisone and fludrocortisone to replace the deficient steroids.

THEME 7: MANAGEMENT OF ELECTROLYTE IMBALANCE

For explanations, see Theme 6: 'Diagnosis of electrolyte imbalance'.

1. **F – Nasal desmopressin administration**
2. **G – Oral rehydration**
3. **A – Fluid restriction**
4. **A – Fluid restriction**
5. **B – Hydrocortisone**

THEME 8: CONGENITAL HEART DISEASE

Approximately 1% of newborn babies will have some form of congenital heart disease. VSD is the most common, accounting for 25%–30% of lesions. Cardiac disease is commonly associated with chromosomal and genetic conditions.

Circulatory changes at birth: in the fetus, left atrial pressure is low, as little blood returns from the lungs. The pressure in the right atrium is much higher, as it receives all of the systemic venous blood and placental blood. Blood therefore passes from the right atrium to the left atrium via the flap valve of the foramen ovale. The ductus arteriosus connects the pulmonary artery to the aorta, so blood entering the pulmonary artery enters the aorta directly. Both the foramen ovale and ductus arteriosus help blood bypass the lungs. After birth, when the baby starts to breathe, resistance to pulmonary blood flow falls and the volume of blood passing through the lungs rises massively (leading to a high left atrial pressure). Conversely, the right atrial pressure falls, as there is no blood returning to the heart from the placental circulation. The immediate pressure differences that occur after birth between the right and left atria cause the flap valve of the foramen ovale to close (and become the fossa ovalis). The ductus arteriosus closes within a few hours of birth via a prostaglandin-mediated mechanism (becoming the ligamentum arteriosus). Some babies with congenital heart lesions rely upon the ductus arteriosus to maintain circulation. These babies deteriorate rapidly when the duct closes.

Foramen, from Latin *foramen* = hole or window.

1. G – Tetralogy of Fallot

Tetralogy of Fallot is the most common congenital cyanotic heart disease, the other being transposition of the great vessels (see below). The tetralogy comprises of the following:

1. Large VSD
2. Pulmonary stenosis
3. Aorta that overrides the VSD
4. Right ventricular hypertrophy

Patients with tetralogy have hypercyanotic spells, characterized by cyanosis, breathlessness and pallor. These can lead to myocardial ischaemia and death. Examination may reveal a loud, long ejection systolic murmur heard best in the third intercostal space with a single heart sound. Chest X-ray may reveal a 'boot-shaped' heart, where the normally convex-shaped pulmonary artery on the left heart border becomes a concavity. Congenital cyanotic heart conditions can result in clubbing.

Etienne-Louis Fallot, French physician (1850–1911).

2. C – Coarctation of the aorta

In coarctation of the aorta, the degree of stenosis of the aorta will affect the presentation. Severe stenosis will present soon after birth (when the ductus arteriosus closes). The femoral pulses are weak on examination due to reduced blood flow in the aorta distal to the stenosis. In addition, the blood pressures are higher in the arm than in the leg. Heart failure and a murmur (over the back) may or may not be present. Milder stenosis may not present until adulthood with heart failure, a murmur and hypertension. Chest X-ray in coarctation may demonstrate 'rib notching' due to the development of large intercostal collateral arteries running under the ribs posteriorly in an attempt to bypass the stenosis. Management is with surgical ligation or balloon dilatation of the stenosis. Critical aortic stenosis can also present with a shocked neonate with femoral pulses that are difficult to palpate. The difference clinically is that in critical aortic stenosis the radial/brachial pulses would also be difficult to palpate.

3. J – Ventricular septal defect

VSDs may be membranous (adjacent to the tricuspid valve: 80%) or muscular (completely surrounded by muscle: 20%). Small VSDs are usually asymptomatic. Large VSDs are almost always membranous. They present with heart failure (breathlessness, difficulty feeding, excessive sweating, recurrent upper and lower respiratory tract infections and failure to thrive) due to left-to-right shunting of blood. Examination may reveal either an ejection systolic murmur (small defect) or a loud pansystolic murmur (larger defect). If uncorrected, irreversible pulmonary hypertension ensues, with eventual reversal of the shunt (becoming right to left), known as Eisenmenger's syndrome. Surgical correction of the VSD should be performed prior to the development of Eisenmenger's syndrome. VSDs are often missed on examination soon after birth as there is little or no pressure gradient across the ventricles. There is therefore no shunting of blood that normally causes the murmur.

There are two types of atrial septal defect: ostium primum (deficiency of the atrioventricular septum) and ostium secundum (deficiency of the foramen ovale and the surrounding atrial septum). Examination features include a fixed, widely split second heart sound (due to the right ventricular stroke volume being equal in both inspiration and expiration) and an ejection systolic murmur heard best in the third left intercostal space (due to increased right ventricular outflow secondary to the left-to-right shunt). Increased flow across the tricuspid valve leads to a rumbling mid-diastolic murmur.

Victor Eisenmenger, Austrian physician (1864–1932).

4. H – Transposition of the great arteries

With these symptoms, sepsis is the most likely diagnosis, and so this child should be commenced on IV antibiotics until an echocardiogram can be performed to confirm transposition of the great arteries (TGA). This is a more difficult question, as pulmonary atresia could present in a similar fashion. However, this question tests your knowledge of incidences. Pulmonary atresia is less common, therefore TGA is the most likely diagnosis. In TGA, the great vessels are reversed (transposed), with the aorta coming off the right ventricle and the pulmonary artery off the left ventricle. Affected children are therefore dependent on the ductus arteriosus (duct dependent) to supply oxygenated blood to the systemic circulation. As the duct closes after birth, the baby will become profoundly cyanotic and acidotic. Chest X-ray shows a characteristic narrow mediastinum with an 'egg-on-side' appearance of the heart shadow. The 'switch operation' (surgical swapping of the pulmonary artery and aorta) is required as definitive management.

5. E – Patent ductus arteriosus

Normally, the ductus arteriosus will close in the first few days of life. This is caused by constriction of the vessel as the blood passing through it changes from deoxygenated to oxygenated. The vessel later fibroses. Patent ductus arteriosus (PDA) is more common in premature infants, but does occur in term babies. Features of PDA include a continuous machinery-sounding murmur inferior to the left clavicle. If the PDA is significant, massive left-to-right shunting of blood causes heart failure. Management is with indometacin (a prostaglandin synthetase inhibitor that closes the defect) or surgical ligation.

1. **B** – *Clostridium difficile*
2. **I** – *Treponema pallidum*
3. **H** – *Streptococcus pneumoniae*
4. **A** – *Campylobacter jejuni*
5. **D** – *Mycoplasma pneumoniae*

Medically important bacteria can be classified depending on their morphology and staining reactions. In clinical life, a microbiologist will be at hand to type organisms; however, organism classification comes up in exams. There is no easy way to overcome this – you just have to learn them.*

Gram-positive cocci
   Staphylococcus: S. aureus, S. epidermis
   Streptococcus: S. pneumoniae, S. pyogenes
Gram-positive bacilli
   Bacillus: B. anthracis, B. cereus
   Clostridium: C. difficile, C. tetani, C. perfringens
   Corynebacterium: C. diphtheriae
   Listeria: L. monocytogenes
Gram-negative diplococci
   Neisseria: N. meningitidis, N. gonorrhoeae
Gram-negative bacilli
   Escherichia: E. coli
   Klebsiella: K. pneumoniae
   Proteus: P. mirabilis
   Salmonella: S. typhi
   Shigella: S. sonnei
   Yersinia: Y. enterocolitica, Y. pestis
   Pseudomonas: P. aeruginosa
   Bordatella: B. pertussis
   Haemophilus: H. influenzae
   Legionella: L. pneumophila
Gram-negative comma-shaped/curved bacteria
   Vibrio: V. cholerae
   Campylobacter: C. jejuni
   Helicobacter: H. pylori
Spiral-shaped bacteria
   Treponema: T. pallidum
   Borrelia: B. burgdorferi
Acid-fast bacteria
   Mycobacterium: M. tuberculosis

---

* For more information, see Elliott T *et al. Lecture Notes: Medical Microbiology and Infection*, 5th edn. Oxford: Blackwell Science, 2011.

Cell wall-deficient bacteria
Mycoplasma: M. pneumoniae

Pneumocystis jiroveci (formerly *P. carinii*) is a yeast-like fungal infection and not a bacterium. *Pneumocystis* is responsible for infections (mainly pneumonia) in immunocompromised hosts.

THEME 10: THE CRYING BABY

Eliciting the cause of intractable crying in young infants poses a diagnostic challenge. It is thought that as many as 60% of afebrile children presenting with prolonged crying will have an underlying diagnosis.

1. B – Gastro-oesophageal reflux

Gastro-oesophageal reflux (GOR) is a common problem. Gastric contents reflux into the oesophagus and often into the mouth itself. It is caused by transient relaxation of the lower oesophageal sphincter and occurs most commonly after feeds when the stomach is full. Typical symptoms include regurgitation, vomiting, failure to thrive, irritability during and after feeds, arching, food refusal, excessive hiccups, iron-deficiency anaemia and aspiration pneumonia. Children can, however, present with more unusual symptoms such as wheeze, cough, apnoea, cyanotic episodes and sleep disturbance.

2. G – Non-accidental injury (shaken baby)

Looking after a child with intractable crying is draining. Good social networks are required to share the care of newborn infants. This infant is likely to have an intracranial pathology from a non-accidental injury. This is represented by a persistently crying baby who becomes acutely shocked and non-responsive despite no evidence or risk of infection.

3. I – Teething

Some babies are born with teeth (neonatal teeth). These are a third set of teeth, separate from milk teeth and adult teeth. Neonatal teeth are often removed, as there is a risk of aspiration and they can also cause problems with breastfeeding. The primary set of teeth (milk teeth) usually erupts at approximately 6 months, but this is variable. There is often an increase in salivation, and relief with chewing on various objects. The erupting teeth may be visualized on examination.

4. F – Maternal drug use

This is a case of opioid withdrawal in the infant of a heroin user. Maternal use of illicit drugs (e.g. cocaine, opiates and marijuana) is associated with infantile irritability. The key features of this scenario that make drug withdrawal more likely than meningitis or sepsis are the lack of fever, being small for gestation and frequent yawning.

5. H – Sepsis

Most cases of neonatal sepsis present in the first 48 hours of life (peak at 18 hours). Prolonged rupture of membranes (PROM) increases the risk of early sepsis. Prophylactic antibiotics should be commenced if PROM is associated with any other risk factors for sepsis, such as prematurity (<37 weeks), low birth weight (<2.5 kg), maternal fever, foul-smelling amniotic fluid or maternal colonization with group B streptococci. Differentiating clinically between neonatal sepsis and neonatal meningitis is difficult, although both are treated with the same antibiotics. Sepsis is ten-times more common than meningitis in newborns.

Note on infantile colic

Colic is a description and not a diagnosis. It is the description of a baby who cries for more than a total of 3 hours in any 3 days of 3 consecutive weeks (rule of threes). Because colic is a description, it does not have an individual underlying pathophysiology. For example, an infant who has reflux who cries for 3 hours in any 3 days over 3 weeks is a 'colicky' baby because of GOR. Treatment is supportive, and the baby with colic usually settles by the fourth month of life.

Practice Paper 8: Questions

THEME 1: SCROTAL PAIN AND SWELLING

Options

A. Epididymo-orchitis
B. Hydrocele
C. Incarcerated inguinal hernia
D. Non-strangulated inguinal hernia
E. Orchitis
F. Spermatocele
G. Strangulated inguinal hernia
H. Testicular torsion
 I. Testicular trauma
 J. Testicular tumour
K. Torsion of the hydatid of Morgagni
L. Varicocele

For each of the following scenarios, select the most likely diagnosis. Each option may be used once, more than once or not at all.

1. A mother brings her 15-month-old boy to the emergency department. She is concerned about a swelling in his scrotum. On examination, there is a smooth left-sided mass. You can feel above the mass, but are unable to feel the testicle behind it. The swelling transilluminates with a pen torch.

2. A 15-year-old boy presents to the clinic. He complains of a chronic ache in his scrotum. On examining the scrotum, you notice a large, soft, left-sided scrotal mass that feels like a collection of worms. You can get above the mass and it does not transilluminate with a pen torch. It does not exhibit a cough impulse.

3. A 16-year-old boy presents with a 10-hour history of scrotal pain and malaise. The pain is severe and radiates into the abdomen. On examination, the left testicle is tender and swollen. Lifting the left testicle results in relief of the pain.

4. A 12-year-old boy presents with sudden-onset scrotal pain. It first started when a football hit him in the groin at school in the last 4 hours. The pain is severe and radiates into the abdomen. On examination, the left testicle is tender and swollen. The cremasteric reflex of the left testicle is absent.

5. A 14-year-old boy presents with a 24-hour history of scrotal pain. His mother reports that he was ill 5 days ago with a temperature, when 'his glands were up'. On examination, his left testicle is tender and swollen.

THEME 2: ACID–BASE DISTURBANCES

Options

A. Diabetic ketoacidosis
B. Hypoxia
C. Metabolic acidosis with respiratory compensation
D. Metabolic acidosis without respiratory compensation
E. Metabolic alkalosis with respiratory compensation
F. Metabolic alkalosis without respiratory compensation
G. Normal blood gas
H. Pyloric stenosis
 I. Respiratory acidosis with metabolic compensation
 J. Respiratory acidosis without metabolic compensation
K. Respiratory alkalosis with metabolic compensation
L. Respiratory alkalosis without metabolic compensation

For each of the following scenarios, select the most appropriate description of blood gas. Each option may be used once, more than once or not at all.

Reference ranges (arterial): $Po_2 > 11.0$ kPa, Pco_2 4.6 – 6.0 kPa, bicarbonate 22–28 mmol/L, pH 7.35–7.45.

1. You see a 6-week-old baby with vomiting. The blood gas analyser has broken, so you cannot get a blood gas. You send some blood instead to the biochemistry laboratory for urea and electrolytes. The results are phoned through as Na^+ 138 mmol/L, K^+ 2.9 mmol/L, chloride 75 mmol/L, bicarbonate 34 mmol/L, creatinine 60 μmol/L and urea 5.9 mmol/L.

2. You are called to see a child with diabetes who has diarrhoea and vomiting. Her mother reports that she is drowsy and that her 'sugars' have been high. You take a venous blood gas. The results show pH 7.38, Pco_2 4.9 kPa, Po_2 3.9 kPa, bicarbonate 22 mmol/L and base excess −0.9.

3. You are called to see a child with diabetes who has diarrhoea and vomiting. Her mother reports that she is drowsy and that her 'sugars' have been high. Results of a venous blood gas are pH 7.24, Pco_2 3.2 kPa, Po_2 3.9 kPa, bicarbonate 14 mmol/L and base excess −8.5.

4. You are called to see a 5-year-old boy in the emergency department. You are told by the attending junior doctor that he has a fever of 39.8°C associated with a purpuric rash. His capillary refill time is 5 seconds. An arterial blood gas shows pH 7.3, Pco_2 4.9 kPa, Po_2 22.4 kPa, bicarbonate 16 mmol/L and base excess −4.5.

5. A 13-year-old girl attends the emergency department for treatment of a self-harm injury. The attending doctor notices pitting of the teeth. A venous blood gas shows pH 7.47, Pco_2 7.2 kPa, Po_2 4.6 kPa, bicarbonate 31 mmol/L and base excess +3.6.

THEME 3: SORE THROAT

Options

A. Acute epiglottitis
B. Candidal infection
C. Diphtheria
D. Gastro-oesophageal reflux
E. Infectious mononucleosis
F. Peritonsillar abscess (quinsy)
G. Retropharyngeal abscess
H. Streptococcal tonsillitis
I. Viral pharyngitis

For each of the following patients with a sore throat, select the most likely diagnosis. Each option may be used once, more than once or not at all.

1. A 7-year-old boy from India presents to the emergency department. He has been generally lethargic for a few days, with a mild sore throat. Over the last few hours, his sore throat has suddenly become much worse and he has a temperature of 39.6°C. There is no stridor, and examination of his throat shows a grey membrane covering his tonsils. He has a past medical history of asthma and has never been immunized.

2. A 7-year-old boy from India presents to the emergency department. He was lethargic and had a fever for 2 days before developing a sore throat. His GP diagnosed tonsillitis and commenced amoxicillin. The patient has now developed a widespread maculopapular rash. He has a past medical history of asthma and has never been immunized.

3. A 7-year-old boy from India presents to the emergency department. His mother describes that he has become very unwell very quickly. It started with a high fever and a sore throat. He is now very quiet and is drooling while sitting upright on the edge of the bed. You briefly examine him, and he appears shocked and tachypnoeic and has a very faint stridor. He has a past medical history of asthma and has never been immunized.

4. A 7-year-old boy from India presents to the emergency department. He has had a sore throat for 24 hours. He is drooling, as it is painful to swallow. On examination, he is systemically well and he is not shocked. There is no stridor, and examination of his throat demonstrates inflamed tonsils with a bulge from the right soft palate. His uvula is deviated to the left and his breath smells very bad. He has a past medical history of asthma and has never been immunized.

5. A 7-year-old boy from India presents to the emergency department. He complains of having a sore throat for the last 2 weeks. On examination, he is systemically well and he is not shocked. There is no stridor, and examination of his throat shows non-inflamed tonsils with white exudates. He has a past medical history of asthma and has never been immunized.

THEME 4: ILLNESSES PROTECTED AGAINST BY IMMUNIZATION

Options

A. Diphtheria
B. *Haemophilus* epiglottitis
C. *Haemophilus* meningitis
D. Measles
E. Mumps
F. Pertussis
G. Polio
H. Pneumococcal pneumonia
 I. Rubella
 J. Tetanus
K. Tuberculosis

For each of the following cases, select the most likely diagnosis. Each option may be used once, more than once or not at all.

1. A 5-year-old boy from Uganda presents to the GP with a sore throat. He has been generally unwell for the previous 3 days with a fever and a mild sore throat. Today, he has deteriorated. He is restless and febrile and his sore throat is severe. There is currently no stridor, and examination of the throat reveals a white membrane covering a red pharynx.

2. A 6-year-old boy from a travelling family presents to the emergency department having had what appeared to be a fit. He is very rigid, arching his body and hyperextending his neck. He is unable to speak, as his face is locked into a permanent smile. You notice a small wound on his leg, which his mother says has been there for a few days.

3. An 18-month-old boy, whose mother is a nurse, is admitted to the paediatric ward. He presents with a headache, mild fever and lethargy. A blood culture is taken and a lumbar puncture performed. The cerebrospinal fluid has a very high lymphocyte count, high protein and low glucose. Antibiotics are commenced but stopped when all the cultures come back negative. Despite treatment, the patient continues to deteriorate.

4. A 7-year-old boy from China presents with a history of headache, muscle pain and neck stiffness. Three days after the onset of these symptoms, his left leg becomes weak. On examination, he has a flaccid paralysis and loss of reflexes of the left leg. Sensation is normal in the limb.

5. A 5-year-old unimmunized boy presents to the GP with a chronic cough. His mother reports that he has had this cough for 3 months. It started with a normal 'cold and cough', but he has not managed to shake it off. For the first 4 weeks, the cough would occur in bursts and he would get very distressed, occasionally going blue and vomiting.

THEME 5: THE FEBRILE CHILD

Options

A. Bacterial endocarditis
B. Cat-scratch fever
C. Kawasaki's disease
D. Malaria
E. Malignancy
F. Meningitis
G. Pneumonia
H. Rheumatic fever
 I. Osteomyelitis
 J. Scarlet fever
K. Tuberculosis
L. Urinary tract infection

For each of the following children presenting with a fever, select the most likely diagnosis. Each option may be used once, more than once or not at all.

1. An 11-year-old girl who recently returned from Africa presents with a 6-week history of fever, which is worse at night. There are no other features, except that you notice that the girl has a painful purple rash on the lower limbs.
2. A 2-year-old girl from the UK presents with a fever for the last 6 days. Her eyes have been itchy and red, and her lips are sore. On examination, you note bilateral cervical lymphadenopathy and a widespread rash, and that the skin on her hands is peeling.
3. An 11-year-old girl who recently returned from Africa presents with a 6-week history of fever, which is worse at night. She reports being more tired than usual. There are no other features and there are no dermatological findings on examination.
4. An 11-year-old girl from the UK presents with a fever of 8 days' duration. On examination, she has a temperature of 38.7°C and has painful, hot lymph nodes in the left axilla. There is a small wound on the back of her left hand.
5. An 11-year-old girl who has recently returned from Africa presents with a 6-week history of fever. She reports being more tired than usual. On examination, she has widespread cervical and supraclavicular lymphadenopathy, which is not painful on palpation.

THEME 6: MODES OF INHERITANCE

Options
A. An acquired condition rather than an inherited one
B. Autosomal dominant
C. Autosomal recessive
D. Gene deletion syndrome
E. Mitochondrial
F. Uniparental disomy
G. X-linked dominant
H. X-linked recessive
I. Y-linked inheritance

For each of the following conditions, select the mode of inheritance. Each option may be used once, more than once or not at all.

1. Sickle cell disease
2. Prader–Willi syndrome
3. Marfan's syndrome
4. Duchenne muscular dystrophy
5. Williams' syndrome

THEME 7: HEADACHES

Options

A. Acute sinusitis
B. Alcohol intoxication
C. Febrile illness
D. Head injury
E. Idiopathic intracranial hypertension
F. Intracranial mass
G. Meningitis alone
H. Meningitis and septicaemia
 I. Migraine
J. Stress headache
K. Subarachnoid or intracerebral haemorrhage

For each of the following children with a headache, select the most likely diagnosis. Each option may be used once, more than once or not at all.

1. A 3-year-old girl presents with a 3-day history of a runny nose. For the last 24 hours, she has had a high fever and a severe frontal headache with toothache.

2. A 5-year-old girl presents with a 2-week history of moderately severe headache. The pain is present most mornings and is located on the crown of the head. Her mother has noticed that she has a fine tremor of the right hand on using cutlery. For the last month, the girl has become more clingy and withdrawn than usual.

3. A 6-year-old girl presents with acute-onset headache. She has been febrile since waking 3 hours ago. She is now resisting movement of her neck. On examination, she is cool peripherally and has a dark-red rash on her legs that does not disappear with pressure.

4. A 13-year-old girl is brought to the emergency department by her mother. She has had a severe headache since waking 3 hours ago. She has been vomiting. Yesterday afternoon, when she returned from her friend's house, her mother noticed that she was behaving oddly before going to bed early. On examination, her temperature is 37.2°C. She has no focal neurological signs and there is no neck stiffness or photophobia.

5. A 4-year-old girl presents to the emergency department with acute-onset headache. She avoids bright lights and has been vomiting since her arrival. She is unable to move the right side of her body and is unable to speak. On examination, her temperature is 36.8°C and there is no neck stiffness. She makes a full recovery within 48 hours.

THEME 8: DYSURIA

Options

A. Intravenous (IV) cephalosporin
B. IV amoxicillin
C. IV gentamicin
D. No treatment required
E. Oral cephalosporin
F. Oral ciprofloxacillin
G. Oral erythromycin
H. Oral metronidazole
 I. Oral oestrogen
J. Oral nystatin
K. Oral tetracycline
L. Surgical correction
M. Topical nystatin
N. Topical oestrogen

For each of the following cases, select the most appropriate first step in management. Each option may be used once, more than once or not at all.

1. A 15-year-old girl complains of pain on urinating associated with back pain. She has a temperature of 39.5°C, is haemodynamically stable and is tender in the right flank on examination. She is not vomiting. A urine dipstick is positive for leucocytes, blood and nitrites.

2. A 5-year-old girl complains of pain on urinating. On examination of the genitalia, the labia have the appearance of not being fully formed, with surrounding mild inflammation. A urine dipstick reveals no blood, nitrites or leucocytes.

3. A 5-year-old girl complains of pain on urinating, suprapubic abdominal pain and having to pass urine more frequently. She has a temperature of 37.8°C. She is otherwise systemically well and examination of the genitalia is normal. A urine dipstick is positive for leucocytes and nitrites.

4. A 15-year-old girl complains of pain on urinating. Her temperature is 37.0°C and she is otherwise systemically well. She is pregnant at 12 weeks' gestation. Cell culture reveals an intracellular organism.

5. A 2.5-year-old boy complains of infrequent penile pain on passing urine. His mother is concerned as his foreskin is non-retractile. There is no local inflammation or scar tissue and the microscopy, culture and sensitivity of urine are negative.

THEME 9: SHORT STATURE

Options

A. Chronic illness
B. Congenital hypothyroidism
C. Constitutional delay
D. Cushing's syndrome
E. Familial short stature
F. Growth hormone deficiency
G. Malnutrition
H. Prader–Willi syndrome
I. Trisomy 21
J. Turner's syndrome

For each of the following children who present with short stature, select the most likely diagnosis. Each option may be used once, more than once or not at all.

1. A 14-year-old boy who is overweight repeatedly attends hospital with severe exacerbations of his asthma. On examination, you notice that he is particularly short for his age.
2. A 16-year-old boy is concerned as he is the smallest in his class. He has not yet entered puberty. His father tries to be reassuring, mentioning that he was also late beginning puberty.
3. A 15-year-old girl is concerned as she is the smallest in her class. She has not yet entered puberty. There is no family history of delayed puberty. On examination, you hear a systolic murmur that radiates to the back.
4. An 18-month-old boy with a cleft palate presents with short stature. He had frequent episodes of hypoglycaemia as a neonate.
5. A 9-month-old boy is admitted to the ward for investigation of his failure to thrive. On examination, he has a large tongue and an umbilical hernia.

THEME 10: PETECHIAE AND PURPURA

Options

A. Aplastic crisis
B. Disseminated intravascular coagulation
C. Drugs
D. Henoch–Schönlein purpura
E. Idiopathic thrombocytopenic purpura
F. Increased superior vena cava pressure
G. Malignancy
H. Meningococcal septicaemia
 I. Non-accidental injury
J. Thrombotic thrombocytopenic purpura
K. Wiskott–Aldrich syndrome

For each of the following children presenting with a non-blanching rash, select the most likely diagnosis. Each option may be used once, more than once or not at all.

1. A 2-year-old boy presents acutely unwell. He has a temperature of 39.5°C and is shocked. Examination of the lower limbs and trunk reveals widespread purpura. Broad-spectrum antibiotics are commenced, and blood cultures reveal Gram-positive cocci.

2. You are asked to see a 3-year-old boy in the emergency department. The referring doctor is worried about physical abuse, as this boy has presented three times in the last 2 months with 'viral-sounding illnesses' and on two occasions bruising was noticed. Today, he presented with a fever and coryzal symptoms. His mother also reports that he 'just hasn't been himself' recently, as he is lethargic during the daytime. On examination, there is widespread bruising over his upper and lower limbs and there is a ring of petechiae around this wrist where his mother says 'his brother grabbed him this morning'. His full blood count shows a platelet count of 30×10^9/L (range $200–400 \times 10^9$/L) and a white cell count of 54×10^9/L (range $4–11 \times 10^9$/L).

3. A 4-year-old boy presents with a long history of coughing. Over the last 2 days, he has been having paroxysms of coughing followed by an inspiratory 'whoop' with occasional vomiting. His mother is worried that he has developed meningitis. On examination, he is afebrile and has petechiae on his upper chest and face.

4. You are asked to see a 3-year-old boy who has a ring of petechiae around his wrist where his mother says 'his brother grabbed him this morning'. He had a viral illness 5 days ago, but has now recovered. Blood tests are performed that reveal normal haemoglobin and renal

function. The platelet count is 30×10^9/L and the white cell count is 9×10^9/L.

5. A 4-year-old boy is unable to weight bear because of pain in his joints. He reports having abdominal pain. He has a temperature of 38.7°C, and examination of the lower limbs demonstrates an urticarial rash that in places is becoming purpuric.

Practice Paper 8: Answers

THEME 1: SCROTAL PAIN AND SWELLING

1. B – Hydrocele

Hernias and hydroceles are the most common causes of inguinal masses in boys. To differentiate between a hydrocele and an inguinal hernia:

- A hernia will transmit a cough impulse; hydroceles will not.
- You cannot 'get above' a hernia, but you can with a hydrocele.
- The testis can be palpated separately with a hernia; it cannot with a hydrocele.
- A hernia does not transilluminate with a pen torch; a hydrocele will.

A hydrocele is a collection of serous fluid in the tunica vaginalis, a membrane that covers the testis. Hydroceles can be primary or secondary to an underlying cause. Primary hydroceles (as in this case) are tense, painless, fluctuant swellings that transilluminate. Because the fluid surrounds the testicle, the underlying testis is often not palpable; however, the epididymis above can be felt as a separate structure. Primary hydroceles are benign, but can be surgically excised if desired. (Simple aspiration of the cyst will result in re-accumulation of fluid.) A secondary hydrocele can occur when the membranous sac around the testis becomes filled with exudates secondary to tumours or inflammation of the underlying testis or epididymis. Secondary hydroceles are usually small and lax. An ultrasound scan should be performed in all adults presenting with a hydrocele to exclude an underlying tumour. Secondary hydroceles require treatment of the underlying condition.

2. L – Varicocele

The differential diagnoses here would be a varicocele or a testicular tumour. An inguinal hernia is ruled out as you can get above the lesion, and hydrocele and spermatocele are ruled out as the mass does not transilluminate. Testicular tumours are usually painless, and this boy is relatively young for such a diagnosis.

The term varicocele describes varicosities in the pampiniform venous plexus, the network of veins that drains the testicle. It usually occurs on the left side and is present in 10% of males. Patients present with a scrotal swelling on standing that feels like a 'bag of worms', and they may experience a heavy, dragging sensation. Varicoceles are usually harmless, but have been associated with defective spermatogenesis, rendering some patients subfertile (although this is a contentious issue). Varicoceles can be diagnosed by ultrasound, which shows venous dilatation greater than 2 mm. Management is by reassurance and wearing supportive underwear. If a patient desires treatment, then radiological embolization of the left testicular vein, or ligation and division of the testicular veins, can be performed.

3. A – Epididymo-orchitis
In the final three cases, including with semi-acute-onset scrotal pain, your first action should be to provide adequate analgesia and organize an urgent testicular ultrasound. Epididymo-orchitis (inflammation of the epididymis and testis) presents with a painful swelling of the epididymis with constitutional symptoms, such as pyrexia and malaise. Patients may also exhibit a secondary hydrocele. Because epididymo-orchitis is usually a consequence of ascending infection (e.g. from a urinary tract infection [UTI] or sexually transmitted urethritis), there may also be a history of dysuria or urethral discharge. Prehn's sign (relief of pain on elevation of the testes) can help clinically diagnose epididymo-orchitis. However, when someone presents with a painful, swollen testicle, it is important to rule out testicular torsion – if in doubt, the patient should be referred for urgent surgical exploration. Treatment of epididymo-orchitis is with bed rest and a long course of antibiotics (e.g. 6 weeks of oral ciprofloxacin). If an abscess develops, it requires drainage.

Douglas Prehn, American urologist (1901–1974).

4. H – Testicular torsion
The development of sudden-onset pain and swelling in the testicle strongly suggests torsion of the testicle, which is a surgical emergency. Torsion accounts for 30% of cases of a painful scrotum. Patients may also suffer referred pain in the lower abdomen and groin (due to the T10 nerve, which supplies the lower abdomen as well as the testes) along with nausea and vomiting. The torsion occurs around the spermatic cord when there is an anatomically abnormal testicle, often following a history of mild trauma. An example of an anatomical anomaly is the 'bell-clapper' testis, where the testicle is not anchored to the scrotum by the gubernaculum ligament (as it should be normally), leaving it to swing freely like the clapper of a bell.

In testicular torsion, the testis may be riding high within the scrotum, although a normal lie of the testicle does not exclude torsion. Prehn's sign is negative and the cremasteric reflex may be lost. Irreversible infarction of a torsioned testicle occurs within 6–12 hours, so affected patients should be taken to theatre for surgical exploration without further investigation. (Generally, to preserve spermatogenesis, torsion should be relieved within 4 hours.) Surgical management includes untwisting of the testicle and bilateral fixation of the testes to the tunica vaginalis to prevent further torsion. Bilateral fixation is required because anatomical abnormalities of the testes that predispose to torsion usually occur on both sides.

The hydatid of Morgagni is an embryological remnant on the upper pole of the testis. Torsion of this structure may affect boys just prior to puberty. It usually presents with pain that increases in intensity over 1–2 days. Sometimes, it can be seen as a blue dot on the superior aspect of the scrotal skin (the blue-dot sign). Torsion of the hydatid requires surgical excision.

Giovanni Battista Morgagni, Italian anatomist (1682–1771).

5. E – Orchitis
This boy's febrile episode with 'the glands up' is the parotid swelling of mumps infection. Mumps is caused by a paramyxovirus infection that is spread by saliva droplets and affects preadolescents. As well as constitutional symptoms, patients develop inflammation of the parotid glands (parotitis). Recognized complications of mumps include meningitis, pancreatitis and orchitis. Around 20% of postpubertal males with mumps will develop orchitis. Treatment is with bed rest, scrotal support and analgesia. Testicular atrophy is common, occurring in 50% of cases. If bilateral, this can cause infertility. The incidence of mumps has been drastically reduced by routine administration of the measles, mumps and rubella vaccine.

THEME 2: ACID–BASE DISTURBANCES
The body normally controls serum pH within a tight range. One must always remember that pH is a logarithmic scale (base 10) and so a change from 8 to 7 is a tenfold increase in H^+ concentration. A normal intracellular pH is required for the functioning of many enzyme systems. When blood becomes profoundly acidotic (pH < 7), cellular function becomes impossible and death ensues.

Simple interpretation of arterial blood gases is usually all that is required in final EMQs. Any blood gas can be interpreted through three simple questions:

1. What is the pH? The pH value shows whether the gas is acidotic (<7.35) or alkalotic (>7.45).
2. What is the Pco_2? Carbon dioxide becomes acidic when mixed with water (Henderson–Hasselbalch). If the pH corresponds with the Pco_2 then this is a 'respiratory picture' (i.e. a low pH with a raised Pco_2 is a respiratory acidosis).
3. Does the bicarbonate (or base excess) suggest a metabolic disease, component or compensation?

In some cases of blood gas disturbance, the body has time to compensate. In other words, whichever chemical is causing the imbalance is counteracted by the opposite one. For example, if there is high bicarbonate and high pH (metabolic alkalosis), then Pco$_2$ starts to increase to bring in some acidity and counteract the alkalosis. If compensation is successful, the pH will return to within the normal range (7.35–7.45), even if the bicarbonate and Pco$_2$ levels are abnormal. It is important to know that the body can never overcompensate (i.e. if there is an initial acidosis, the body can never make that into an alkalosis, and the pH will always remain on the acidic side of normal [<7.40]). Similarly, a compensated alkalosis will always have a pH > 7.40, on the alkalotic side of normal.

1. H – Pyloric stenosis

This is difficult. Without a blood gas analyser, it would be difficult to say whether this was definitely metabolic alkalosis with respiratory compensation. However, the history and results are strongly suggestive of pyloric stenosis. Pyloric stenosis is hypertrophy of the circular muscle of the pylorus, causing gastric outflow obstruction. It presents in the first few weeks of life and it most commonly affects first-born males. The presentation of non-bile-stained projectile vomiting soon after feeds in a hungry baby is characteristic of pyloric stenosis. A characteristic hypochloraemic, hypokalaemic, metabolic alkalosis results from vomiting stomach acid. Pyloric stenosis is diagnosed by giving the baby a 'test feed': When the baby is given milk, visible gastric peristalsis may be seen over the epigastrium, and the pylorus is felt as an olive-shaped mass in the upper abdomen. If the diagnosis is in doubt, an ultrasound scan can be performed. After initial rehydration, management is by Ramstedt's pyloromyotomy (in which the muscle of the pylorus is cut longitudinally down to the mucosa). The baby can tolerate milk feeds a few hours after the operation.

2. G – Normal blood gas

The only abnormal result here is the Po$_2$; however, this is a venous blood gas, so a low Po$_2$ is expected. This is therefore a normal blood gas. It is important to rule out diabetic ketoacidosis (DKA) in children with diabetes who are unwell with high blood sugars. The learning point here is that blood gas analysis does not just have to be performed on arterial blood. A lot can be established from venous or capillary samples.

3. C – Metabolic acidosis with respiratory compensation

This gas here demonstrates a metabolic acidosis with respiratory compensation. However, you do not have a result for ketones, so you cannot technically diagnose DKA. She will need aggressive management, as DKA is a life-threatening complication of type 1 diabetes.

4. D – Metabolic acidosis without respiratory compensation

This boy has meningococcal sepsis causing metabolic acidosis. In this case, the acidosis is relatively mild and there is no respiratory compensation. He will need intravenous (IV) fluids to correct his poor perfusion, as well as IV antibiotics, such as penicillin or a cephalosporin. Note the high oxygen level. This is because the emergency department doctor correctly approached this case in an ABC manner and commenced oxygen therapy.

5. E – Metabolic alkalosis with respiratory compensation
This history and acid–base disturbance are suggestive of bulimia. The teeth are pitted due to chronic acid exposure. Chronic vomiting is associated with metabolic alkalosis. The CO_2 is mildly elevated, suggesting a degree of compensation.

THEME 3: SORE THROAT
Most sore throats are simply viral infections that are self-limiting. It is always important to consider group A streptococcal infections because of the complications associated with scarlet fever and rheumatic fever.

1. C – Diphtheria
Diphtheria is a rare cause of sore throat, especially now with the uptake of the DTaP vaccine. Characteristically, there is a grey slough covering the mucosa of the tonsils and pharynx. Culture of the organism *Corynebacterium diphtheriae* and demonstration of its toxin are required to confirm the diagnosis.

2. E – Infectious mononucleosis
Infectious mononucleosis (glandular fever) is caused by Epstein–Barr virus (EBV). Symptoms are varied and include fever, malaise, pharyngitis, tonsillitis and lympadenopathy. Other features are petechiae on the soft palate, jaundice, splenomegaly and hepatomegaly. Symptoms may persist for as long as 3 months. Infectious mononucleosis can be diagnosed using the monospot test or the Paul Bunnell test. Treatment is symptomatic.

In this case, the GP incorrectly prescribed antibiotics. Administration of ampicillin or amoxicillin in infectious mononucleosis causes a widespread maculopapular rash. This rash can scar. This makes treatment of any form of tonsillitis or pharyngitis with these antibiotics difficult, as EBV cannot be ruled out clinically. Penicillin is difficult to administer due to its bitter taste, although it is better to use this than potentially to cause a drug reaction with amoxicillin or ampicillin.

3. A – Acute epiglottitis
Acute epiglottitis is a life-threatening emergency caused by *Haemophilus influenzae* type b. A toxic-looking child with stridor, drooling and fever is strongly suggestive of acute epiglottitis. The child sits upright and immobile in order to optimize the airway. Do not be reassured by a quiet stridor or a quiet wheeze. This is often a sign that the airway is almost closed and very little air can be moved. Examination of the throat should be performed only by an ENT surgeon in an intensive care unit with facilities to intubate and protect the airway. Do not attempt to examine the throat yourself or make the child lie down, as this may precipitate airway

obstruction. Treatment is with IV antibiotics (e.g. a cephalosporin), with rifampicin prophylaxis given to all contacts.

A differential diagnosis in this case would be a retropharyngeal abscess. A retropharyngeal abscess is often preceded by an upper respiratory tract infection. The child with a retropharyngeal abscess presents with a fever, drooling, dysphagia and stridor. Occasionally, the head may be tilted to one side and the neck may be stiff.

4. F – Peritonsillar abscess (quinsy)

Quinsy (peritonsillar abscess) is a collection of pus outside the tonsil usually seen in older children as a complication of tonsillitis. Affected patients are unwell and may develop severe dysphagia, earache and trismus (lockjaw). As you inspect the pharynx, there will be a unilateral bulge of the soft palate, with deviation of the uvula to the opposite side. The tonsils will be inflamed and there is associated halitosis. Rupture of the abscess can result in aspiration pneumonia. Treatment is with penicillin. There may be as many as five organisms in the pus found in the abscess. Six weeks after quinsy, it is conventional to perform tonsillectomy.

5. B – Candidal infection

This boy with white oral lesions and a sore throat has probably developed oesophageal candidiasis. Infection of the oesophagus by *Candida albicans* occurs most often in patients who are immunosuppressed (e.g. with AIDS) or who have recently used antibiotics. Inhaled steroids can cause a candidal infection at the back of the mouth due to local immunosuppression. Asthmatic patients on inhaled steroids should be advised to keep their inhaler by their toothbrush. This will remind them to take their steroids but also to rinse their mouth out afterwards. Patients often complain of dysphagia, odynophagia and a hoarse voice. Oesophageal candidiasis can be treated with antifungals such as fluconazole, nystatin or amphotericin.

THEME 4: ILLNESSES PROTECTED AGAINST BY IMMUNIZATION

The illnesses protected against by immunizations are now becoming rare. This has resulted in a significant reduction in morbidity and mortality. However, cases do still present, and so a knowledge of the clinical features is required. Also, to counsel a family effectively regarding the protection given by immunization, one needs to be aware of the effects that these infections cause.

1. A – Diphtheria

Diphtheria is caused by the Gram-positive anaerobe *Corynebacterium diphtheriae*. It is a highly contagious droplet-borne infection. Affected children present with a flu-like illness, pharyngitis and neck swelling. The diphtheria toxin released by the bacterium can also cause severe hypotension. On examination, a greyish membrane can be seen to cover the tonsils and pharynx.

Diphtheria, from Greek *diphtheria* = leather, alluding to the leathery membrane that covers the pharynx.

2. J – Tetanus

Tetanus is caused by wound contamination by the Gram-positive anaerobe *Clostridium tetani*. It is not the organism itself but its neurotoxic exotoxin, tetanospasmin, that acts on the motor cells in the central nervous system to cause muscle spasm. Signs of tetanus include

- Trismus: lock jaw
- Risus sardonicus: grinning face due to facial muscle spasm
- Opisthotonus: arched body, hyperextended neck
- Autonomic dysfunction: tachycardia/arrhythmias, low blood pressure and sweating

Death is eventually caused by aspiration, respiratory failure, cardiac failure or exhaustion. Treatment is with anti-tetanospasmin immunoglobulins.

Risus sardonicus, from Latin *risus* = smile + *sardonicus* = sardonic (mocking, scornful).
Trismus, from Greek *trismos* = grinding of teeth.

3. K – Tuberculosis

Tuberculous meningitis is rare, but does occur. The onset of symptoms is gradual, with lethargy, irritability, a low-grade fever and a change in personality. Headache, confusion and neck stiffness may then follow. The priority is to rule out pyogenic meningitis caused by more common bacteria and treat with broad-spectrum antibiotics. However, if there is no growth and the child continues to deteriorate, then one must consider tuberculosis (TB) as a possible organism.

4. G – Polio

Poliomyelitis is an acute disorder of the anterior horn cells caused by the highly contagious RNA poliovirus. It affects lower motor neurones. Features include a flu-like illness associated with muscle pain, flaccid paralysis and areflexia. The infection can also cause cranial nerve dysfunction, resulting in deafness, blindness, dysarthria and dysphagia. Paralysis of the respiratory muscles historically warranted management in a non-invasive negative-pressure ventilator (iron lung). Although polio is now rare in the UK and other developed countries, it should still be included in your differential diagnosis for any patient presenting with an acute onset of flaccid paralysis of a single limb.

Poliomyelitis, from Greek *polios* = grey + *myelos* = spinal cord.

5. F – Pertussis

Whooping cough is caused by the bacterium *Bordetella pertussis*. The illness usually begins with coryza, and a dry cough develops a few days later. This cough becomes more pronounced and occurs in paroxysms.

Repeated episodes of coughing classically then end with an inspiratory 'whoop'. Another name for pertussis is the '100-day cough', as the symptoms often continue for that duration. There is no treatment that will change the course of the illness, although erythromycin is said to reduce the period of infectivity. Complications are uncommon, but include pneumonia and bronchiectasis. Immunization does not give total protection, and protection is not necessarily lifelong.

Pertussis, from Latin *per* = throughout + *tussus* = cough ('intensive coughing').

THEME 5: THE FEBRILE CHILD

1. K – Tuberculosis

TB is the most common infection worldwide, occurring most often in poorer areas, in people with poor nutrition and in those infected with HIV. It is caused by *Mycobacterium tuberculosis*. Primary infection is often asymptomatic and occurs through droplet inhalation. Re-infection or re-activation of TB causes postprimary disease, which presents with cough, haemoptysis, dyspnoea, fever, night sweats and anorexia. Skin lesions of TB are erythema nodosum (see below) and lupus vulgaris (nodular, painful, disfiguring lesions, predominantly on the face). Chest X-ray may show lesions in the upper lobes. Infection may be confirmed by skin tuberculin testing: either the Heaf test (multipuncture method, read at 5–7 days) or the Mantoux test (intradermal tuberculin injection, read at 2–4 days). Drug management is with anti-tuberculous therapy for 6 months (four drugs for 2 months, then two drugs for 4 months). Common drugs include rifampicin, isoniazid, pyrazinamide and ethambutol.

In this case, recurrent fever without a source of infection along with erythema nodosum (a painful, inflamed rash on the lower limbs) suggest TB. Other causes of erythema nodosum include streptococcal throat infection, drug reactions (sulphonamide antibiotics or the oral contraceptive pill), inflammatory bowel disease, sarcoidosis and idiopathic.

2. C – Kawasaki's disease

Kawasaki's disease is an acute febrile systemic vasculitis affecting children. It is most common in Japanese boys. The diagnosis is made clinically as follows: patients must have a fever for 5 or more days plus four of the following:

- Cervical lymphadenopathy
- Oral mucosal erythema (red lips, strawberry tongue)
- Conjunctivitis without exudates
- Rash
- Extremity changes such as oedema and desquamation (peeling)

There may also be thrombocytosis. Treatment is with anti-inflammatories and IV immunoglobulins. The main complication of

Kawasaki's disease is the development of coronary aneurysms (which can result in heart attack and sudden death), and patients conventionally undergo coronary angiography after recovery to rule this out.

Tomisaku Kawasaki, Japanese paediatrician (described the condition in 1967).

3. D – Malaria
Malaria remains endemic in many parts of the world where the *Anopheles* mosquito that transmits the disease is present. Four species of the parasite *Plasmodium* are responsible: *P. falciparum, P. vivax, P. malariae* and *P. ovale. P. falciparum* and *P. vivax* cause the most severe illness. *P. vivax* and *P. ovale* can also remain dormant in the liver, with recurrence later in life (remember: 'V and O do not go').

4. B – Cat-scratch fever
The wound on the back of this girl's hand is an infected cat scratch. Cat-scratch fever is caused by infection with the Gram-negative bacterium *Bartonella henselae,* which lives in cats' blood. The original scratch is followed 7–14 days later by painful, hot, regional lymphadenitis and flu-like symptoms. Some patients may suffer altered mental state and convulsions. Treatment is with antibiotics.

5. E – Malignancy
This child presents with widespread painless lymphadenopathy that is typical of lymphoma. Many children (30%) will also have systemic symptoms such as fatigue, weight loss, itching, fevers and night sweats. These are known as 'B' symptoms and indicate a worse prognosis.
Causes of generalized lymphadenopathy include

- Viral infection: EBV, cytomegalovirus, HIV
- Bacterial infection: brucellosis, syphilis
- Protozoal infection: toxoplasmosis
- Malignancy: lymphoma, leukaemia
- Inflammatory conditions: rheumatoid arthritis, systemic lupus erythematosus, sarcoidosis

THEME 6: MODES OF INHERITANCE
The inheritance of various conditions, diseases and syndromes comes up in exams time and time again. These have to be learnt. The mode of inheritance can be the key exam clue in determining which of two possible answers is correct, and so marks are there to be gained or lost.

1. C – Autosomal recessive
Sickle cell disease is an autosomal recessive condition. These patients have defective globin genes. When exposed to hypoxia or acidaemia, the abnormal globin causes sickling of the red blood cells, resulting in a painful crisis. Other autosomal recessive conditions include: cystic fibrosis,

congenital adrenal hyperplasia, oculocutaneous albinism, thalassaemia, Tay–Sachs disease and galactosaemia.

2. F – Uniparental disomy

Children with Prader–Willi syndrome are hypotonic as infants and go on to develop learning difficulties and obesity (due to hyperphagia) in childhood. Angelman's syndrome (happy disposition, little speech, severe learning disabilities, poor attention span and epilepsy) is also inherited by uniparental disomy. Both these conditions are caused by 'imprinting', whereby the gene required for normal function comes from only one parent. If this gene is deleted (*de novo* deletion) or both genes come from the other parent (uniparental disomy), then the syndrome will ensue. In Prader–Willi syndrome, only the paternal copy of the Prader–Willi gene is active (chromosome 15q11–13). Therefore, either the paternal copy is deleted or both copies come from the mother.

Harry Angelman, British paediatrician (described the condition in 1965). Andrea Prader and Heinrich Willi, Swiss paediatricians (described the condition in 1956).

3. B – Autosomal dominant

Marfan's syndrome is characterized by tall stature, high arched palate, mitral valve disease, lens dislocation, joint laxity and arachnodactyly. Other autosomal disorders include achondroplasia, Huntington's disease, neurofibromatosis, Noonan's syndrome and tuberous sclerosis.

Antoine Marfan, French paediatrician (1858–1942).

4. H – X-linked recessive

Duchenne muscular dystrophy is an X-linked recessive condition, though approximately 30% of cases are due to a new mutation. Children present in the first 5 years of life with delayed walking, frequent falling, difficulty climbing stairs, Gower's sign and pseudohypertrophy of the calves. Gower's sign describes a patient who uses their hands to 'walk up' their own body when standing from a sitting position. Other X-linked recessive conditions include colour blindness, fragile X syndrome, haemophilia A and B and glucose-6-phosphate dehydrogenase deficiency.

Guillaume Benjamin Amand Duchenne, French neurologist (1806–1875).

5. D – Gene deletion syndrome

Williams' syndrome is a form of microdeletion syndrome. It is caused by a loss of chromosomal material at chromosome 7q11. Affected children characteristically have a short stature, elf-like faces, transient hypercalcaemia as infants, supravalvular aortic stenosis and mild-to-moderate learning difficulties. Other conditions arising from microdeletions include cri-du-chat and DiGeorge's syndromes.

J.C.P. Williams, New Zealand cardiologist (described the condition in 1961).

Other forms of inheritance include X-linked dominant (e.g. vitamin D-resistant rickets) and mitochondrial disorders, which are inherited from the mother (e.g. Leber hereditary optic neuropathy).

THEME 7: HEADACHES

1. A – Acute sinusitis

Acute sinusitis is inflammation of the paranasal sinuses, which usually occurs following a bacterial or viral upper respiratory tract infection. Common bacterial causes are streptococci, staphylococci and *Haemophilus* spp. The main features are pain and headache. The pain of acute sinusitis is worse on bending and coughing, and percussion or palpation over the affected area will elicit tenderness. The site of the pain depends on which sinus is affected. Acute maxillary sinusitis causes pain over the cheek, which may be referred to the teeth. Acute frontal sinusitis causes pain above the eyes. Acute ethmoid and sphenoid sinusitis can result in pain between or behind the eyes. In reality, however, the site of sinusitis may be very difficult to distinguish. In maxillary sinusitis, a skull X-ray may show a fluid level on the affected side. Treatment is with antibiotics (if bacterial infection is suspected, as in this case where the child is systemically unwell) and analgesia. Vasoconstricting nose drops (1% ephedrine) aid drainage of the sinus.

2. F – Intracranial mass

This girl has an intracranial mass until proven otherwise (which requires neuroimaging by computed tomography [CT] or magnetic resonance imaging). The warning signs here are the focal neurological signs (tremor) and the behavioural changes. The right-sided tremor indicates a left-sided tumour. Headaches associated with intracranial masses tend to be worse in the morning, and are worse with coughing, bending and straining (these actions cause raised intracranial pressure). Examination may reveal papilloedema.

3. H – Meningitis and septicaemia

This is a case of meningitis with meningococcal septicaemia. The likely causative organism is *Neisseria meningitidis*. Rapid treatment of shock with IV fluids and the administration of IV antibiotics are required. Always administer oxygen (ABC) in cases such as this, as much of the damage caused is due to hypoxia.

4. B – Alcohol intoxication

This girl has a hangover, although encephalitis, meningitis and subarachnoid haemorrhage would certainly be differential diagnoses. A good history would prevent expensive and invasive investigations.

5. I – Migraine

This girl has a hemiplegic migraine associated with dysphasia. The headache associated with migraines is profound and disabling. Migraines are frequently associated with ataxia, nausea, vomiting and visual aura. Migraine, however, is a diagnosis of exclusion, and other causes of hemiplegia should be ruled out before making a formal diagnosis.

Features of concern when assessing headaches include an acute onset, exacerbation on lying supine, associated vomiting, changes in personality, unilateral pain, developmental regression, hypertension, papilloedema, increasing head circumference and focal neurological signs.

Idiopathic intracranial hypertension (previously known as benign intracranial hypertension) usually occurs in young women and is associated with obesity. There is raised intracranial pressure in the absence of a mass lesion. This can be idiopathic or precipitated by drugs (tetracyclines, oral contraceptive pills and steroid withdrawal). Features include headache, transient diplopia and bilateral papilloedema. A CT scan is normal and a lumbar puncture will confirm a raised cerebrospinal fluid pressure. Management options include weight loss, avoidance of precipitating drugs and repeated lumbar puncture. The aim of treatment is to prevent permanent visual loss.

THEME 8: DYSURIA

1. E – Oral cephalosporin

This girl has an upper UTI – pyelonephritis – involving the right kidney. Some patients can have pyelonephritis with a negative urine dipstick, but in this case, the blood, nitrites and leucocytes confirm a UTI. This question is testing your knowledge of management (i.e. Should the antibiotics be IV or oral, and which antibiotic should be used?). As she is not vomiting, she can tolerate oral antibiotics. A 7- to 10-day course of oral antibiotics should be used in patients with pyelonephritis once a culture has been sent. If the patient is septic or cannot tolerate oral antibiotics (due to vomiting), then IV antibiotics are given instead. In pyelonephritis, antibiotics that have a low resistance pattern should be used such as a cephalosporin or co-amoxiclav. The antibiotic of choice may depend on local guidelines/resistance patterns.

2. N – Topical oestrogen

Labial adhesions are relatively common in prepubertal girls. They are caused by recurrent irritation, trauma or infection. The prepubescent labia are prone to adhesions due to the lack of oestrogenized epithelium. Bleeding and dysuria are common with these adhesions. This condition has a high enough incidence to require all physicians in paediatrics and general practice to be familiar with and comfortable in diagnosing and managing it in their patients. Most cases will require no treatment. Treatment is required only if the patient is symptomatic with dysuria or frequent vulval or vaginal infections. Most cases respond with topical oestrogen therapy. If unsuccessful, symptomatic cases need surgical intervention.

3. E – Oral cephalosporin

This patient has a lower UTI – cystitis. A midstream urine should be sent to obtain microscopy, culture and sensitivity to ensure that any organism found is sensitive to the empirical antibiotic that you have started. A dipstick positive for nitrites and leucocytes confirms the diagnosis of UTI. A 3-day course of relevant antibiotics (e.g. a cephalosporin, trimethoprim or co-amoxiclav) should be completed. Ciprofloxacin offers good antibiotic cover in community-acquired UTIs, but should be avoided in children and growing adolescents due to the risk of arthropathy (unless the benefit of using this drug outweighs the risk).

4. G – Oral erythromycin

This girl is pregnant and is therefore having unprotected sex. As a result, she is at risk of sexually transmitted infections (STIs). UTIs are also more common in pregnancy. In this case, she is systemically well and has grown an intracellular organism. *Chlamydia trachomatis* is an obligate intracellular organism that is sexually transmitted. (*Neisseria gonorrhoeae*, another common STI organism, is a Gram-negative diplococcus.) Oral ciprofloxacin or cephalosporins are used to treat gonorrhoea. Oral tetracyclines (e.g. doxycyline) can be used to treat chlamydial infection, but is contraindicated in this scenario as it is teratogenic in the first trimester and causes dental discolouration in the second and third trimesters. Erythromycin is therefore the drug of choice here. STIs should be treated in specialist GUM clinics to enable screening for further STIs and contact tracing.

5. D – No treatment required

Phimosis is the inability to retract the prepuce. 90% of boys will have a retractile prepuce by the age of 3 years. Phimosis should be diagnosed only at an age when one would expect the foreskin to be retractile. In this case, the non-retractile foreskin is causing a degree of pain on micturition. As it is infrequent, no management should be performed in this case. Only if the prepuce remains non-retractile, or if he has a UTI/balanitis secondary to the phimosis, should surgical correction be performed.

Paraphimosis is caused by retraction of a tight foreskin over the glans. The foreskin then acts as a tight band, impeding venous outflow from the glans and resulting in oedema, making it more difficult to reduce the skin. The management of paraphimosis is by administering a local anaesthetic ring block to the glans followed by simultaneous squeezing of the glans and reduction of the foreskin. After paraphimosis, formal circumcision should be performed to prevent recurrence.

THEME 9: SHORT STATURE

1. D – Cushing's syndrome
This boy has a chronic illness which in itself can be a cause of short stature. However, he is obese, suggesting that his chronic illness is not causing a hypercatabolic state. Rather, he is having repeated exacerbations of asthma that require treatment with oral steroids, resulting in iatrogenic Cushing's syndrome.

2. C – Constitutional delay
Constitutional delay is a normal variant, which is seen more frequently in boys. Puberty is delayed, as is the growth spurt associated with it. Bone age would also be delayed, and mid-parental height will be achieved later than in peers. Laboratory tests will be normal. There is often a family history of delayed puberty.

3. J – Turner's syndrome
This girl is likely to have Turner's syndrome (45XO), as she is short, is in pubertal failure and has a murmur suggestive of coarctation of the aorta. Turner's syndrome needs to be excluded in all girls whose height is below that expected of their mid-parental height, as not all affected girls will show the classic phenotype of a webbed neck, widely spaced nipples, wide carrying-angle, etc.

4. F – Growth hormone deficiency
Growth hormone deficiency can be either congenital or acquired. Acquired causes include head injury, irradiation and tumours. Congenital deficiencies can be inherited, idiopathic or associated with midline defects such as cleft palate. Babies with congenital growth hormone deficiency tend to have episodes of hypoglycaemia and/or prolonged jaundice in the neonatal period. Treatment is with growth hormone supplementation.

5. B – Congenital hypothyroidism
Most cases of congenital hypothyroidism are now diagnosed on screening with the Guthrie card, which looks for an elevated thyroid-stimulating hormone (TSH) level (found in >90% of cases). Early treatment is required to prevent learning difficulties. Treatment is with lifelong oral thyroxine (T_4), titrating the dose to maintain normal hormone levels (TSH and T_4) and normal growth.

THEME 10: PETECHIAE AND PURPURA

Petechiae are pinpoint, flat, red lesions that do not blanch on pressure. They are caused by capillary bleeding into the skin. Purpura comprises larger lesions that are red, brown or purple. They do not blanch with pressure, are raised and may be palpable.

1. B – Disseminated intravascular coagulation

This child is septic and the culture has grown Gram-positive cocci, which could be either staphylococci or streptococci. Meningococcal sepsis can present in a very similar manner, but this would have grown the Gram-negative coccus *Neisseria meningitidis* on culture. Disseminated intravascular coagulation (DIC) is a generalized consumption of clotting factors, platelets and anticoagulant proteins. This process can be triggered by severe illness, hypoxia, acidosis, tissue necrosis or endothelial damage. Clinical findings may include generalized bleeding, purpura and thromboembolism. Investigations may reveal fever, hypotension, proteinuria and hypoxia, with low platelets, increased prothrombin time and activated partial thromboplastin and reduced fibrinogen. Fibrinogen correlates most closely with the severity of the event. DIC is often accompanied by shock.

2. G – Malignancy

The emergency department doctor is right to be concerned about physical abuse. Petechiae forming a ring around a limb can be a sign of a twisting injury. To make a diagnosis of non-accidental injury, one has to rule out pathological causes. In this case, the key symptoms are lethargy, bruising, frequent infections and petechiae. The blood tests confirming a thrombocytopenia with a very high white cell count are indicative of underlying haematological malignancy.

3. F – Increased superior vena cava pressure

This boy has pertussis, which can often produce violent coughing and vomiting. Both coughing and vomiting can cause increased pressure in the superior vena caval region, resulting in bleeding from the superficial capillaries into the skin. The petechiae will be restricted to the drainage distribution of the superior vena cava (upper limbs, face and trunk above the nipple line).

4. E – Idiopathic thrombocytopenic purpura

Causes of thrombocytopenia in a well child are idiopathic thrombocytopenic purpura (ITP), systemic lupus erythematosus, HIV, drugs and congenital disorders (TAR syndrome (thrombocytopaenia with absent radius), Wiskott–Aldrich syndrome and Fanconi's anaemia). ITP is the most common of these. It is characterized by autoantibody formation to platelets (specifically to the IIb/IIIa glycoprotein). Children present 2–3 weeks after a viral infection with sudden-onset purpura and epistaxis. The platelet count is low, but bleeding is only usually a problem if it is $<20 \times 10^9$/L. Management is symptomatic. The most severe complication of ITP is intracranial bleeding, which occurs in less than 1% of cases. Half the cases of ITP will re-establish a normal platelet count within 2 months.

Wiskott–Aldrich syndrome is an X-linked recessive disorder characterized by thrombocytopenia, immunodeficiency, eczema and a predisposition to haematological malignancies. Fanconi's anaemia is an autosomal recessive condition characterized by short stature, aplastic anaemia, skeletal anomalies and a predisposition to haematological malignancies.

5. D – Henoch–Schönlein purpura

Henoch–Schönlein purpura is an immunologically mediated diffuse vasculitis, often preceded by an upper respiratory tract infection (especially β-haemolytic streptococci). It usually occurs at between 3 and 10 years of age, and is twice as common in boys. The child characteristically presents with a non-thrombocytopenic palpable purpura (usually on the buttocks and extensor surfaces of the lower limbs), arthralgia, periarticular oedema, colicky abdominal pain and glomerulonephritis. The rash is initially urticarial, rapidly becoming purpuric. Treatment is symptomatic.

Eduard Heinrich Henoch, German paediatrician (1820–1910).
Johann Lukas Schönlein, German paediatrician (1793–1864).

Practice Paper 9: Questions

THEME 1: DEMENTIA

Options

A. Alzheimer's disease
B. Creutzfeldt–Jakob disease
C. Depression
D. HIV dementia
E. Huntington's disease
F. Lewy body dementia
G. Normal-pressure hydrocephalus
H. Parkinson's disease
I. Pick's disease
J. Vascular dementia
K. Wernicke–Korsakoff syndrome

For each of the following scenarios, select the most appropriate cause of dementia. Each option may be used once, more than once or not at all.

1. A 73-year-old man presents with a 6-month history of worsening forgetfulness and intellectual decline. He has, however, had frequent episodes of relative lucidity during this period. He tries to chase soldiers that he thinks he sees in the garden, but his gait has markedly slowed down. His sleeping pattern is now irregular.

2. A 58-year-old woman presents to the emergency department following her first-ever seizure. Her husband said that she had to leave her job because, over a period of 2 months, she has rapidly lost the ability to cope with its intellectual demands. A previous cryptic crossword fanatic, she cannot even fill out the simplest tabloid grid. On further questioning, she admits to muscle weakness and difficulty walking.

3. A 75-year-old man who is a lifelong smoker presents with a mild but sudden-onset loss of concentration and problem-solving ability. This has become progressively more severe on three separate occasions without recovery in between.

4. A 45-year-old man has been arrested by the police for stealing furniture and verbally abusing his neighbours. They took him to the hospital because he appeared confused. His family are concerned that he is behaving strangely and is unable to cope with his work and finances. His general demeanour is apathetic.

5. A 66-year-old woman presents with a fall, having been unsteady on her feet for some time. She has severe memory loss, but is relatively well orientated. She has recently developed urinary incontinence. On examination, she has a wide-based gait.

THEME 2: FIRST-RANK SYMPTOMS

Options

A. Delusional perception
B. Made actions
C. Made feelings
D. Made impulses
E. No first-rank symptoms
F. Running commentary
G. Somatic passivity
H. Third-person auditory hallucinations
 I. Thought broadcast
 J. Thought insertion
K. Thought withdrawal
L. Voices repeating the patient's thought

For each of the following scenarios, select the most appropriate first-rank symptom. Each option may be used once, more than once or not at all.

1. An 18-year-old man sees someone being given a parking ticket and, as a result, at that moment he realizes that it is the right time to begin his mission of revolutionizing the world of fashion.

2. A 27-year-old woman complains to her university lecturer that a fellow art student was deleting the ideas from her head before she had time to say them or write them down.

3. A 45-year-old man experiencing hallucinations quotes the voice as saying "and he's calling a cab while he's having a smoke, and he's taking a drag, now he's going to bed."

4. A 21-year-old woman has been acting out of character for several days. She is spending all the money available to her because she feels invincible and capable of anything.

5. A 38-year-old man has not slept for 3 days. He says that he is being kept awake by aliens incessantly poking and pinching him.

THEME 3: CAUSES OF WEIGHT LOSS

Options

A. Anorexia nervosa
B. Bulimia nervosa
C. Depression
D. Hyperthyroidism
E. Hypothyroidism
F. Malignancy
G. Mania
H. Obsessive–compulsive disorder
I. Patient does not meet criteria for any of the above conditions

For each of the following scenarios, select the most likely cause of weight loss. Each option may be used once, more than once or not at all.

1. A 21-year-old woman presents to the GP complaining that her periods have stopped. She has lost 14 kg from her normal healthy weight over the past few months and is now 42 kg. She admits to restricting her eating and running for 2 hours a day in an attempt to reduce her weight. Her motivation is to change the way that she looks; she says that she is embarrassed by her obesity.

2. A 28-year-old man reluctantly visits his dentist with dental caries. He admits to stealing his grandmother's Senna tablets, and feels that his eating is out of control. Sometimes, he will not eat all day in order to lose weight and at other times, when he is alone, he eats two large pizzas in one go, followed by a family-size tub of ice-cream.

3. A 55-year-old woman presents to her GP with weight loss and tiredness. She has lost 10 kg in the last month, although she denies any desire to lose weight. She has not used any laxatives, but has noticed an increase in frequency of bowel movements over the last 6 months, with occasional blood.

4. An 18-year-old woman presents to her GP complaining of weight loss, and admits to not eating proper meals. She also complains of insomnia, but denies any worry about her weight. She does mention that she no longer takes pleasure dining out and visiting her friends, activities that she previously enjoyed, as she does not see the point.

5. A 19-year-old woman presents to her GP with her mother, complaining of gradual weight loss over 1 year. Her weight is now 69 kg, around what is expected of someone her size. She admits to thinking that she still needs to lose some more weight and is disgusted by her body shape. She eats very little, and occasionally makes herself vomit. She has not noticed any other symptoms and has no medical history. Her only medication is the oral contraceptive pill.

THEME 4: MOOD DISORDERS

Options

A. Atypical depression
B. Bipolar affective disorder
C. Cyclothymia
D. Depression – mild
E. Depression – moderate
F. Depression – severe
G. Dysthymia
H. Hypomania
 I. Mania
J. Masked depression
K. Schizophrenia
L. Seasonal affective disorder
M. Somatic syndrome
N. This does not meet the criteria for any of the above

For each of the following scenarios, select the most appropriate diagnosis. Each option may be used once, more than once or not at all.

1. A 24-year-old man asks his GP for a sick note from work. He says that he feels down, is lethargic and has stopped enjoying playing the piccolo (his main hobby). He was admitted to a psychiatric hospital last year following an episode of mania.

2. A 19-year-old man has been happier and more positive than usual, with more energy than he has ever felt before for no particular reason. He has been getting more work done at the office today and has been socializing with his friends as usual.

3. A 60-year-old woman is admitted to hospital after a fall. She is noted to maintain poor eye contact. When asked how she is feeling, she admits to feeling low in mood, having very little energy and losing enjoyment in all her usual hobbies. She has also found it difficult to concentrate, feels that she is no good at anything, feels guilty over minor issues and feels very negative about the future.

4. A 55-year-old woman who attends the clinic has recently been diagnosed with a depressive episode. She complains of unintentionally waking early in the morning, a recent disinterest in sex and a loss of appetite, losing 5 kg in weight in the last month. She feels that her mood improves as the day wears on.

5. A 40-year-old woman presents to the GP with low mood. Of note, she has an increased appetite and has gone up two dress sizes. She also complains that she cannot get out of bed until the afternoon as she is so tired.

THEME 5: DESCRIPTIVE PSYCHOPATHOLOGY 1

Options

A. Circumstantiality
B. Coprolalia
C. Delusion
D. Egomania
E. Eidetic image
F. Flight of ideas
G. Hypnagogic hallucination
H. Hypnopompic hallucination
 I. Knight's move thinking
 J. Neologism
K. Obsession
L. Overvalued idea
M. Pareidolia
N. Perseveration
O. Word salad

For each of the following scenarios, select the most appropriate description. Each option may be used once, more than once or not at all.

1. A 20-year-old man with mania is difficult to understand. He is declaring, "I want to become a shawalawam maker. Shawalawams can help you all!"
2. A 69-year-old man being investigated for confusion asks, "When can I go for a cigarette … ette … ette … ette … ette … ette … ette?"
3. A 25-year-old woman says that her mind is racing and that no one is intelligent enough to keep up with the speed of her thoughts. She speaks rapidly, frequently changing the subject without explaining her meaning.
4. A 45-year-old man with severe depression feels that he is a despicable human being because he ran over a cat in his car in the dark by mistake. The worry and guilt that surround this incident are dominating his thoughts and conversation. He occasionally reluctantly accepts that it could have happened to anyone, but he still continues to think that what happened is unforgiveable.
5. A 31-year-old woman who has no previous psychiatric history fell asleep on a train. She said that as she woke up she saw a scuba diver momentarily swimming through the carriage.

THEME 6: SLEEP DISORDERS

Options

A. Hypersomnia
B. Insomnia
C. Narcolepsy
D. Night terrors
E. Nightmares
F. Non-organic disorder of the sleep–wake cycle
G. Physical problem causing sleep disturbance
H. Psychiatric/psychological problem causing sleep disturbance
 I. Psychoactive substance causing sleep disturbance
J. Sleep apnoea
K. Somnambulism

For each of the following scenarios, select the most likely sleep disturbance. Each option may be used once, more than once or not at all.

1. A 3-year-old girl wakes suddenly during the night screaming and seems very distressed. She is unable to explain why she is upset, and returns to sleep after 10 minutes. The next morning, she cannot remember any of it.

2. A 5-year-old boy wakes from his sleep after a terrifying dream, and he explains to his parents that he was being chased by a monster. He had a similar dream once before.

3. A 36-year-old woman presents with daytime tiredness and difficulty getting to sleep at night. Her mood is not affected, and she is usually fit and well.

4. A 55-year-old woman presents with difficulty sleeping, particularly waking up around 5 a.m. and being unable to get back to sleep. She also has a decreased appetite and, on examination, she is less well-groomed than usual and difficult to engage with.

5. A 12-year-old girl on a residential school trip is found wandering the corridors during the night. She appears disorientated when questioned, but goes back to bed. In the morning, she cannot remember the events.

THEME 7: SUICIDE

Options

A. 1 in 1,000,000
B. 1 in 10,000
C. 3 in 1000
D. 1%
E. 10%
F. 66.6%
G. 90%
H. 100%

For each of the following description, select the most appropriate proportion. Each option may be used once, more than once or not at all.

1. The likelihood that any member of the population will die as a result of suicide in the next year (taking no other factors into consideration)
2. The likelihood that a person who presents with deliberate self-harm will go on to complete suicide during the next year
3. The proportion of people with completed suicide who have seen a GP in the last month
4. The proportion of people with completed suicide who have a psychiatric illness
5. The likelihood that any member of the population will present with an episode of self-harm in the next year (taking no other factors into consideration)

THEME 8: PSYCHIATRIC DISORDERS RELATING TO WOMEN'S HEALTH

Options

A. Couvade syndrome
B. Cyclic psychosis
C. Dysmenorrhoea
D. Maternity blues
E. Not a psychiatric condition
F. Postnatal depression
G. Perimenstrual syndrome
H. Premenstrual syndrome
I. Postmenstrual syndrome
J. Pseudocyesis
K. Puerperal psychosis

For each of the following scenarios, select the most likely diagnosis. Each option may be used once, more than once or not at all.

1. A 30-year-old woman gave birth to her first child 3 days ago. It was a planned pregnancy and there were no physical problems with the delivery or baby. She has no past psychiatric history, but has become inconsolably tearful, anxious and low in mood today.

2. A 32-year-old man presents to his GP with abdominal distension, insomnia, urinary frequency, constipation and cravings for beetroot with ice-cream. His wife is pregnant at 39 weeks' gestation.

3. A 22-year-old woman complains of abdominal bloating, headache and breast tenderness accompanied by irritability and low mood for at least 1 week every month.

4. A 28-year-old woman who is 2 weeks postpartum was brought to the emergency department by her partner and parents. She is confused and upset, and is complaining of hearing voices telling her to kill her baby. Over the last few days, she has been having difficulty sleeping, despite the baby sleeping well.

5. A 25-year-old woman is pregnant for the first time. Her husband has noticed her walking around the house talking to her unborn baby. This began 3 days ago. She has no previous psychiatric history.

THEME 9: SUBSTANCE USE

Options

A. Alcohol use
B. Alcohol withdrawal
C. Amphetamine use
D. Amphetamine withdrawal
E. Cannabis use
F. Cannabis withdrawal
G. Cocaine use
H. Cocaine withdrawal
 I. Opiate use
 J. Opiate withdrawal
K. Sedative use
L. Sedative withdrawal

For each of the following scenarios, select the most likely cause. Each option may be used once, more than once or not at all.

1. A 76-year-old woman is an inpatient on a surgical ward following a hip replacement. The nursing staff said that she vomited earlier and she has been unresponsive since her operation 12 hours ago. On examination, you notice that her pupils are small and she has a respiratory rate of 7 breaths/minute.

2. An 18-year-old man presents to his GP complaining of a dry cough and tiredness. His mother said that he has become very suspicious of those around him. She adds that he has withdrawn himself socially and has not been the same since he met a new group of friends at university.

3. A 34-year-old man presents to the emergency department complaining of the sensation of insects crawling over his skin. He is tachycardic and hypertensive, and his pupils are noted to be large.

4. A 74-year-old woman has recently changed GPs and has moved into a nursing home. The doctor is called because she became unwell; she was sleeping poorly, complaining of nausea and sweating, and went on to have a seizure.

5. A 63-year-old man was admitted for an elective cholecystectomy. On the second postoperative day, he complains of sweating and tremor. On examination, he is confused, anxious and tachycardic, and appears to be responding to visual hallucinations. He says that he can see thousands of miniature country dancers running around the floor.

THEME 10: SYNDROMES IN PSYCHIATRY

Options

A. Capgras' syndrome
B. Cotard's syndrome
C. Couvade syndrome
D. de Clerambault's syndrome
E. Ekbom syndrome
F. Folie à deux
G. Fregoli's syndrome
H. Ganser's syndrome
I. Munchausen's syndrome
J. Othello syndrome
K. Rett's syndrome
L. Pickwickian syndrome
M. Tourette's syndrome

For each of the following descriptions, select the most appropriate syndrome. Each option may be used once, more than once or not at all.

1. A 19-year-old man presents to the emergency department having been at a cocaine party. He complains that he has 'little parasites, like ants' running around inside his body.

2. A 2-year-old girl is brought to the GP by her parents. They say that her behaviour has changed drastically over the last 3 months; she is screaming and has stopped interacting with those around her. She is also finding it increasingly difficult to walk and feed herself. Previously, her developmental milestones were all normal.

3. A 34-year-old woman works in a sandwich bar near Downing Street. She is convinced that the Prime Minister is in love with her, which is why he lives so close to her place of work. (It is well known that the current Prime Minister does not eat sandwiches.)

4. A 28-year-old woman is in court charged with benefit fraud. When asked how many children she has, she replies 'seventy-three'. When asked to confirm her name, she says 'Mary Queen of Scots'. (This is not her real name!)

5. A 42-year-old woman who is estranged from her physically abusive former husband attends the GP in tears. She is upset because she thinks that her former husband is following her, in disguise as her sister.

Practice Paper 9: Answers

THEME 1: DEMENTIA

Dementia is defined as a progressive, irreversible decline in cognitive function without impaired consciousness. It can affect all aspects of higher brain function: concentration, memory, language, personality and emotional control.

Dementia, from Latin *de* = away + *mens* = mind.

1. F – Lewy body dementia

Lewy body dementia is the third most common dementia after Alzheimer's disease and vascular dementia. Characteristic features of Lewy body dementia include day-to-day fluctuating levels of cognitive functioning, visual hallucinations, sleep disturbance, transient loss of consciousness, recurrent falls and Parkinsonian features (tremor, hypokinesia, rigidity and postural instability). Although people with Lewy body dementia are prone to hallucination, antipsychotics should be avoided, as they precipitate severe Parkinsonism in 60% of cases. Lewy bodies are abnormalities of the cytoplasm found within a neurone, containing various proteins and granular material. They are found in the cerebral cortex in patients with Lewy body dementia, and are also found in patients with Parkinson's disease.

Frederick Lewy, German neurologist (1885–1950).

2. B – Creutzfeldt–Jakob disease

Creutzfeldt–Jakob disease (CJD) is a rapidly progressive dementia caused by prions (infectious agents composed only of protein). The prion proteins can be transmitted by neurosurgical instruments and human-derived pituitary hormones. Features of CJD include rapid cognitive impairment, which may be preceded by anxiety and depression. Eventually, physical features become prominent, including muscle disturbance (rigidity, tremor, wasting, spasticity, fasciculations, cyclonic jerks and choreoathetoid movements). Convulsions may also occur. The EEG is characteristic (showing stereotypical sharp-wave complexes). Death occurs within 6–8 months.

New variant CJD (nvCJD) occurs secondary to ingestion of bovine spongiform encephalopathy-infected beef. It is more common in younger adults. The features are as for CJD, but decline is slower, with mortality occurring within 18 months. There are no typical electroencephalogram (EEG) changes in nvCJD, although there is a characteristic feature on magnetic resonance imaging (MRI; symmetrical hyperintensity in the posterior nucleus of the thalamus – the pulvinar sign).

Other prion diseases include kuru (in Papa New Guinea, transmitted by cannibalistic consumption of human neural tissue) and Gerstmann–Straussler syndrome (an autosomal dominant mutation of the prion protein gene on chromosome 20).

Hans Gerhard Creutzfeldt, German neuropathologist (1885–1964).
Alfons Maria Jakob, German neurologist (1884–1931).

3. J – Vascular dementia
Vascular dementia is an ischaemic disorder characterized by multiple small cerebral infarcts in the cortex and white matter. When >100 mL of infarcts have occurred, dementia becomes clinically apparent. Vascular dementia begins in the 60s with a stepwise deterioration of cognitive function. Other features include focal neurology, fits and nocturnal confusion. Risk factors for vascular dementia are as for any atherosclerotic disease (male sex, smoking, hypertension, diabetes and hypercholesterolaemia). Life expectancy in vascular dementia is shorter compared to Alzheimer's dementia and is usually around 3–5 years following the diagnosis due to ischaemic heart disease or stroke.

4. I – Pick's disease
Pick's disease is a form of frontotemporal dementia (it can only be differentiated from other forms at post mortem, so 'frontotemporal dementia' is the preferred term). Clinical features include disinhibition, inattention, antisocial behaviour and personality changes. Later on, apathy, akinesia and withdrawal may predominate. Memory loss and disorientation only occur late. Postmortem examination shows atrophy of the frontal and temporal lobes (knife-blade atrophy) and Pick's bodies (cytoplasmic inclusion bodies of tau protein) in the substantia nigra. In advanced cases, the atrophy may be seen on MRI.

Arnold Pick, Czechoslovakian neurologist and psychiatrist (1852–1924).

5. G – Normal-pressure hydrocephalus
Normal-pressure hydrocephalus is characterized by the triad of dementia (mainly memory problems), gait disturbance and urinary incontinence. It is caused due to an increase in volume of cerebrospinal fluid (CSF), but with only a slightly raised pressure (as the ventricles dilate to compensate). There is an underlying obstruction in the subarachnoid space that prevents CSF from being reabsorbed but allows it to flow from the ventricular system into the subarachnoid space. Diagnosis is by lumbar puncture (to demonstrate a normal CSF opening pressure) followed by head computed tomography/MRI (showing enlarged ventricles). Treatment is with ventriculoperitoneal shunting.

HIV-related dementia (also known as AIDS dementia complex) occurs years after initial infection. It presents with reduced cognitive function, low energy and libido, general apathy and eventually muscle spasticity with hyper-reflexia, incontinence and ataxia. The virus itself causes it, rather than an opportunistic infection. Diagnosis is based on clinical probability.

Pseudodementia is recognized in people with severe depression. Their apparent cognitive dysfunction is heavily affected by their lack of motivation. The mood disturbance precedes the cognitive impairment, and patients may not try during formal assessments, often providing 'don't know' responses to questions asked. They are more likely to complain of memory loss, whereas someone with true dementia is more likely to confabulate and try to hide it. Depressive pseudodementia is a diagnosis of exclusion in someone with depression, and management aims to treat the underlying mood disorder.

Huntington's disease is an autosomal dominant disorder with excess CAG trinucleotide repeats on chromosome 4. Onset is usually in mid-adulthood. Features include choreiform movements, with an increased rate of depression, schizophrenia and suicide. Seizures may be a late feature. Insight tends to be maintained for much of the early course. Diagnosis is clinical, but can be confirmed by DNA analysis. Treatment is symptomatic.

George Huntington, American physician (1850–1916).
Choreiform, from Greek *chorea* = dance.

Alzheimer's disease is the most common type of dementia. There is global brain atrophy, with deposition of β-amyloid protein in the brain. Features include gradual progressive cognitive decline, apathy/lability of mood, personality deterioration, paranoia and Parkinsonian features. The diagnosis is made by excluding other causes of dementia. The mainstay of treatment is acetylcholinesterase inhibitors (donepezil, galantamine and rivastigmine), which increase concentrations of the neurotransmitter acetylcholine, although these may only be effective in a select proportion of cases. Early-onset Alzheimer's disease (<65 years) can occur in people with Down's syndrome and in those who inherit the amyloid precursor or presenilin proteins.

Wernicke's encephalopathy is a reversible condition caused by a severe deficiency of thiamine (vitamin B₁). It is often associated with alcohol abuse, the processes being the lack of adequate oral intake, hyperemesis and malabsorption caused by gastrointestinal lesions. The triad of features in Wernicke's syndrome is confusion, ataxia and nystagmus. Ophthalmoplegia is also an important feature. If untreated, Wernicke's encephalopathy can lead to the irreversible Korsakoff's syndrome, characterized by confusion, anterograde and retrograde amnesia and confabulation.

Alois Alzheimer, German psychiatrist (1864–1915).
Sergei Korsakoff, Russian neuropsychiatrist (1854–1900).
Karl Wernicke, German psychiatrist (1848–1905).

THEME 2: FIRST-RANK SYMPTOMS

Kurt Schneider described the 'first-rank symptoms' as being highly suggestive of schizophrenia in the absence of organic brain disease. However, they are absent in 20% of people with schizophrenia and can be present in other psychiatric disorders, such as depression and mania. The presence of first-rank symptoms in schizophrenia is not an indicator of prognosis.

Kurt Schneider, German psychiatrist (1887–1967).

1. **A – Delusional perception**
2. **K – Thought withdrawal**
3. **F – Running commentary**
4. **E – No first-rank symptoms (more indicative of mania)**
5. **G – Somatic passivity**

The first-rank symptoms can be categorized as follows:

- Auditory hallucinations: third-person, running commentary, repeating thought
- Thought alienation: thought insertion/withdrawal/broadcast
- Influences on the body: made feelings/actions/impulses
- Other: somatic passivity and delusional perception

In third-person auditory hallucinations, the patient hears the voices of more than one person discussing matters between themselves. A running commentary is one voice describing the patient's every action. Finally, the patient can experience thought sonorization (hearing their thoughts out aloud). These 'audible thoughts' can occur either at the same time as the real thoughts (gedankenlautwerden) or just afterwards (écho de la pensée).

In thought insertion, the patient believes that thoughts are being put into their mind by an outside agency. In thought withdrawal, they feel as if their thoughts are being removed. Thought broadcasting is where the patient feels that their thoughts are being made accessible to others (i.e. others can hear them).

Made feelings, actions or impulses describe when the patient feels that their feelings/actions/impulses are under the control of a third party and that their free will is being taken away. In delusional perception, a real perceived event leads to a different idea or incorrect conclusion without logical reasoning. Somatic passivity is where the patient feels that they are receiving bodily sensations from an outside agency (e.g. an alien is twisting their intestines).

THEME 3: CAUSES OF WEIGHT LOSS

1. **A – Anorexia nervosa**

A diagnosis of anorexia nervosa requires all four of the following:

- Body weight 15% below expected, or body mass index <17.5 kg/m^2

- Self-induced weight loss (by dieting, exercising, vomiting, etc.)
- Morbid fear of being fat (an overvalued idea rather than a delusion)
- Endocrine disturbance (e.g. amenorrhoea, pubertal delay or lanugo hair)

The incidence of anorexia is 4 per 100,000, with a peak at age 18 years. Around 10% of cases of anorexia occur in males. Risk factors include being Caucasian, high social class, academic prowess and interests such as ballet or modelling. Other common features are anaemia, expressing a high interest in preparing or buying food, feeling tired and cold, bradycardia and hypotension. Treatment options include cognitive-behavioural therapy/supportive therapy and raising calorie intake. Hospitalization is indicated if there is a weight loss of over 35%. Around 50% of people with anorexia nervosa eventually recover completely. The mortality rate is 5%, usually from starvation or suicide.

Anorexia, from Greek *an* = without + *orexe* = appetite.

2. B – Bulimia nervosa
A diagnosis of bulimia nervosa requires all three of the following:

- Binge eating
- Methods to prevent gaining weight (e.g. vomiting, purging, laxatives, etc.)
- Morbid fear of being fat (overvalued idea, not a delusion)

The incidence of bulimia is 12 per 100,000, with females being affected ten-times more commonly than males. Individuals tend to be of a normal or above-normal weight. Complications are caused by starvation and vomiting, and include hypokalaemia, dehydration, enlargement of the parotid glands, dental caries, Mallory–Weiss tear, osteoporosis and Russell's sign (thick skin on the dorsum of the hands due to repeated induced vomiting by digitally stimulating the gag reflex with the fingers). Treatment is similar to that of anorexia, but selective serotonin reuptake inhibitors may improve bingeing behaviour. 70% of cases recover within 5 years and there is no increase in mortality.

Bulimia, from Greek *bous* = ox + *limos* = hunger.

3. F – Malignancy
Malignancy is a common cause of weight loss and should always be considered, particularly in older people who complain of tiredness and a reduced appetite. A full examination and systems review should be carried out to determine a possible site of malignancy.

Thyroid dysfunction is associated with weight change. Hyperthyroidism can lead to weight loss despite a good appetite, and hypothyroidism can cause weight gain without increased intake.

4. C – Depression
Many psychiatric conditions may indirectly result in weight loss. The woman in this scenario complains of weight loss, insomnia and anhedonia,

features suggestive of biological depression. Other features of biological depression are early morning wakening, decreased libido and psychomotor retardation/agitation. It should be noted that atypical depression is associated with reverse neurovegetative symptoms, namely hypersomnia, hyperphagia and weight gain.

Patients with obsessive–compulsive disorder may present with weight loss. This may be influenced by large periods of time taken up by the repetitive rituals. Additionally, if there is a preoccupation with cleanliness and a fear of contamination, this may affect eating habits. People with mania can lose weight with overactivity. They may also neglect eating for fear of wasting time.

5. I – Patient does not meet criteria for any of the above conditions

This girl presents with weight loss, induced vomiting and a poor body image. Although she may be on the slippery slope to an eating disorder, she does not quite meet the criteria for anorexia or bulimia.

THEME 4: MOOD DISORDERS

1. B – Bipolar affective disorder

Bipolar affective disorder is usually characterized by two or more episodes in which mood and activity levels are significantly disturbed. This should include at least one episode of elevation of mood and increased energy and activity (hypomania or mania), although on other occasions there may be a lowering of mood and decreased energy and activity (depression). Some would consider a single episode of mania alone as sufficient for a diagnosis of bipolar disorder. There is a 1% lifetime risk, with the average age of onset being in the mid-20s. Males and females have equal risk of developing bipolar disorder, and higher social classes have a greater risk.

Manic episodes present with elevated mood in 70% of cases and irritable mood in 80% of cases. Biological symptoms of mania are decreased sleep, increased energy and psychomotor agitation. Cognitive symptoms are decreased concentration, flight of ideas and lack of insight. Manic patients often display thought disorders, such as circumstantiality (where the speaker eventually gets to the point in a very roundabout manner) and tangential speech (where the speaker digresses further and further away from the initial topic via a series of loose associations). Psychotic features include grandiose or persecutory delusions, hyperacusis and hyperaesthesia. First-rank symptoms occur in 20% of cases. In extreme cases, there is manic stupor, in which the patient is unresponsive, akinetic, mute and fully conscious, with elated facies.

Acute episodes of mania are managed with neuroleptics drugs (e.g. olanzapine or haloperidol), with benzodiazepines for agitation. Long-term prophylaxis (mood stabilization) is most often given in the form of lithium. (Carbamazepine and sodium valproate may also be effective.)

Mood stabilizers are prescribed only if there has been more than one episode of mania. Lithium causes sustained remission in 80% of cases. Psychotherapies have a supportive role and can improve concordance with therapy. Electroconvulsive therapy (ECT) is used for manic stupor and resistant mania, but if used during a depressive episode in a patient with bipolar disorder, there is a risk of switching to mania.

2. H – Hypomania

Hypomania is distinguished from mania in that the mood elevation is mild and does not disrupt social activity, nor is there psychosis. In rapid cycling bipolar disorder, there are at least four affective episodes in a 12-month period. This is more common in women and is associated with a poor prognosis.

3. F – Depression – severe

The three core symptoms of depression are low mood, anhedonia (loss of pleasure) and anergia (low energy). The diagnostic criteria require there to be a history of two out of three core symptoms for at least 2 weeks. In addition, there should be at least two of the following seven symptoms:

- Decreased concentration
- Reduced self-esteem
- Guilt
- Pessimism about the future
- Self-harm ideation
- Disturbed sleep
- Reduced appetite

The severity of depression is classified as mild (four symptoms in total), moderate (five or six symptoms in total) and severe (seven symptoms in total, including all three core symptoms).

Beck's cognitive triad describes types of negative thought that occur in depression. These are a negative view of oneself, a negative view of the world and a negative view of the future.

The lifetime risk of depression is 10%–25% in females and 5%–12% in males. Marital status affects the risk of depression: The highest-risk group are those who are divorced, followed by people who are separated, then single, then married. Other risk factors are having three or more children below the age of 14, unemployment, maternal death below the age of 11 and a lack of confiding relationships. An adverse life event in the previous 6 months, personality disorders and a family history of bipolar disorder predispose to depression. Coexisting medical conditions are a risk factor – some specific examples are discussed in 'Psychiatric signs of physical illness' (Paper 10 Answers, Theme 8). Examples of medications that increase the risk of depression include β-blockers, steroids, anticonvulsants, benzodiazepines, antipsychotics, opiates and non-steroidal anti-inflammatory drugs.

Aaron Beck, American psychiatrist (born 1921).

4. M – Somatic syndrome

Biological features of depression include

- Anhedonia
- Decreased emotional reactivity
- Early morning wakening
- Diurnal variation
- Psychomotor retardation/agitation
- Decreased appetite
- Weight loss (>5% in 1 month)
- Reduced libido

If a patient displays at least four of these eight biological symptoms, this constitutes the somatic syndrome.

5. A – Atypical depression

Atypical depression is characterized by reverse neurovegetative biological symptoms; that is, hyperphagia, weight gain and hypersomnia. Seasonal affective disorder presents with depressive episodes in the autumn and winter months, with an improvement in spring. It tends to be associated with symptoms of atypical depression. In masked depression, the patient does not present with low mood. Some patients present with somatization of symptoms; others do not complain of any symptoms, and maintain a cheerful exterior despite having significant symptoms affecting their life.

Persistent mood disorders (dysthymia and cyclothymia) last longer than 2 years and usually start in early adulthood. Dysthymia is a mild reduction in mood, and cyclothymia is a mild reduction in mood alternating with mild elevations of mood. 'Double depression' is when a depressive episode occurs in an individual with dysthymia.

THEME 5: DESCRIPTIVE PSYCHOPATHOLOGY 1

1. J – Neologism
2. N – Perseveration

Speech disorders

A neologism is a new word, or a known word used in a new way. In perseveration, mental operations are continued beyond when they are relevant. It is highly suggestive of organic brain disease. Examples are palilalia, which is repeating a whole word (e.g. 'knife … knife … knife …') and logoclonia, which is repeating the last syllable of a word (e.g. 'pass the Yorkshire pudding … ding … ding … ding'). Word salad, or schizophasia, is an incomprehensible mish-mash of words and phrases. Dysprosody is loss of the normal melody of speech. Logorrhoea describes fluent, rambling speech – an extreme version of verbal diarrhoea!

Expressive aphasia is a difficulty verbalizing thoughts, although comprehension is intact. It is seen in patients after a stroke. In receptive aphasia, there is difficulty understanding and, although the patient feels that they are speaking fluently, it is not usually possible to make out any words in their voice. In global aphasia, both expressive and receptive aphasias are present. Dysarthria is physical difficulty in controlling movements of the mouth in order to articulate words.

Mutism is complete loss of speech. Poverty of speech is reduced/restricted speech (e.g. monosyllabic answers). Pressure of speech is increased quantity and rate of speech. Stammering is when the flow of speech is broken by pauses and repetition. Echolalia is the imitation of another person (even if it is in a foreign language). Coprolalia is the explosive exclamation of obscenities, seen in Tourette's syndrome.

Coprolalia, from Greek *kopros* = dung + *lalein* = talk.

The following forms of speech give the examiner insight into the form of the patient's thoughts. Knight's move thinking is demonstrated when speech jumps from one subject to another with no link. Flight of ideas is accelerated thoughts with abrupt incidental changes of subject and no central direction. The connections between topics are based on chance relationships, such as rhyming words or alliteration. Circumstantiality is the incorporation of unnecessary trivial details into speech, but the eventual goal is reached.

3. F – Flight of ideas
4. L – Overvalued idea
Thought disorders

Schneider's three features of normal thought are constancy, organization and consistency. There are five features of Schneider's formal thought disorder:

- Derailment: a thought derails on to a subsidiary thought
- Drivelling: a disordered intermixture of constituent parts of a thought
- Fusion: heterogeneous thoughts are interwoven
- Omission: part of a thought is omitted
- Substitution: a major thought is substituted with a subsidiary thought

A delusion is a belief held with absolute conviction, such that it is not changeable, even by compelling counterargument or proof to the contrary. A primary delusion has no obvious cause considering the patient's circumstances. Secondary delusions are more closely linked with the rest of the clinical picture; for example, grandiose delusions (the belief of inflated self-worth) are common in mania, and a persecutory delusion may be seen in paranoid schizophrenia. A bizarre delusion is one that would be seen as totally implausible within the patient's culture.

An overvalued idea is an unreasonable, sustained, intense preoccupation that is maintained with less than delusional intensity; that is, the patient may accept that it might not be true. An obsession is a repetitive senseless thought that is recognized as irrational but is unsuccessfully resisted by the person. The motor equivalent of an obsessional thought is a compulsion – a repetitive, stereotyped, seemingly purposeful behaviour that is not actually useful and is recognized as such by the patient. Ideas of reference are thoughts that the events or objects in one's immediate environment have a particular or unusual significance. Monomania is a pathological preoccupation with a single subject, and egomania is a pathological preoccupation with oneself.

5. H – Hypnopompic hallucination
Sensory disorders

A hallucination is a false perception in the absence of a real external stimulus. It can be visual, auditory or tactile. Examples of hallucinations include autoscopy (the person sees their own image in front of them as if looking in a mirror), extracampine hallucinations (hallucinations that occur beyond what would be reasonably expected of the sensory field; e.g. able to see someone who is standing directly behind the person or hearing voice coming from a neighboring city), functional hallucinations (precipitated by another stimulus; e.g. a hearing a voice every time the tap is turned on), reflex hallucinations (a stimulus in one sensory modality causes a hallucination in a different sensory field; e.g. a green monster is seen at the sound of a flushing toilet), formication (the sensation of insects crawling over or under the skin) and the trailing phenomenon (when moving objects appear as a series of pictures). Hypnagogic and hypnopompic hallucinations can occur in any modality (more commonly auditory or visual) and happen while one is falling asleep or waking up from sleep, respectively. They can be normal phenomena.

A pseudohallucination is an image seen in subjective space, as if within the person's mind. One form is an eidetic image, which is the vivid reproduction of a previous memory (much like a photographic memory). Another form is pareidolia, which describes the phenomenon in which one can make out images while looking at a poorly structured background; for example, seeing someone's face in a camp fire. An illusion is a false perception of a real external stimulus; for example, thinking that a shadow of a post box is a person in the distance.

Sensory distortions are abnormal sensory experiences that are altered experiences of a real stimulus. Examples include hyper-/hypo-aesthesia (a non-organic increase or decrease in sensation), dysmegalopsia (the inability to judge the size of objects), chloropsia/erythropsia/xanthopsia (where all objects appear green, red or yellow, respectively) and macropsia and micropsia (objects seem much larger or smaller than normal).

THEME 6: SLEEP DISORDERS

Sleep disorders can be divided into primary and secondary. Secondary problems are further subdivided depending on whether they are caused by a physical or psychiatric illness, or whether they are caused by psychoactive substances.

1. D – Night terrors
Night terrors are seen in children, affecting 6% of 4–12-year-olds, and resolve by adolescence. The child usually awakes suddenly during the first third of the night in a state of panic and tearfulness. There are associated autonomic responses; for example, tachycardia and dilated pupils. Affected children are not easily comforted, but when they fully awake (usually the next morning), they have no recollection of the event.

2. E – Nightmares
Nightmares are frightening dreams in which the individual awakes suddenly and is then fully alert and can remember the dream very well. They usually occur during the second half of the night. Nightmares affect up to 50% of adults occasionally, while 3–5-year-olds are more likely to experience repeated nightmares.

3. B – Insomnia
Insomnia is a condition describing a reduced quantity or quality of sleep for a prolonged period. This may involve difficulty getting to sleep/staying asleep and early morning wakening. It is a common symptom of other conditions, but if it dominates the clinical picture, it can be considered a condition in its own right. Assessment involves a careful history for causes, including other illnesses and substances (e.g. caffeine). Factors in the daily routine that may be unhelpful should be identified and advice given about sleep hygiene. This involves going to bed and getting up at the same time each day, doing relaxing tasks such as bathing, reading, drinking hot milk before bed, using the bed for sleep only (except for sex) and not watching television. If there is an underlying cause, this should be treated. Drug treatments are limited and include short-acting benzodiazepines such as temazepam (which have less of a hangover effect than longer-acting ones such as diazepam) or zopiclone (which is similar). However, these drugs should have a limited duration, and their use for longer than 2 weeks increases the risk of addiction. Ideally, they should not be taken every day. The diagnosis of insomnia can be made at any age, but it is more common in the elderly.

Hypersomnia is a condition defined as either excessive daytime sleepiness with sleep attacks or an abnormal length of time taken to reach full arousal after sleeping (in the absence of an organic disorder). It affects 0.3%–4% of the population. The management includes looking for a physical cause, improving sleep hygiene and occasionally stimulants such as dexamphetamine and methylphenidate.

4. H – Psychiatric/psychological problem causing sleep disturbance
This woman presents with insomnia, early morning wakening and a blunted affect. This could be indicative of underlying depression.

5. K – Somnambulism

Somnambulism (sleepwalking) is a state of altered consciousness in which there are some features of wakefulness and some of sleep. The individual usually arises from bed (during the first third of nocturnal sleep) and begins walking, but with reduced awareness, reactivity and motor skill. Upon awakening, there is usually no recollection of the event. It is more common in children. Management is by reassurance, simple safety measures and gentle encouragement to return to bed by the family.

Narcolepsy forms a part of the differential diagnosis. It is less common, affecting <0.1% of the population. It is a neurological condition caused by a loss of inhibition of rapid eye movement sleep. It has four main features: irresistible attacks of sleep at inappropriate times, cataplexy (sudden loss of muscle tone when intense emotion occurs, leading to collapse), hypnogogic/hypnopompic hallucinations (hallucinations that occur on falling asleep and waking, respectively) and sleep paralysis. Not all cases of narcolepsy have all four features. When forming the diagnosis, factors that point to hypersomnia are sleeps that have a gradual onset, are worse in the mornings and rarely occur in unusual places. Factors that suggest narcolepsy are a short duration of sleep (10–20 minutes), the inability to control sleep attacks and interrupted night-time sleep, as well as the four main features. Management falls under the remit of neurologists.

Sleep apnoea is a physical condition in which the upper respiratory tract becomes partially occluded during sleep. This can cause transient cessation in breathing, which causes the patient to wake repeatedly during the night, reducing the quality of sleep. Sleep apnoea results in daytime tiredness. It is more common in overweight males who snore. Treatment is by continuous positive airway pressure via facemask during sleep.

Non-organic disorder of the sleep–wake cycle is caused by a lack of synchrony with the desired sleep–wake pattern. The problem is often perceived as either insomnia or hypersomnia. Management is by attention to sleep hygiene.

THEME 7: SUICIDE

Suicide is important to consider because it is one of the most extreme negative outcomes in psychiatry. It is important to assess and be aware of risk factors in order to identify and prevent suicide in those at risk. A thorough assessment of an individual's risk should be made in the psychiatric history; this involves frank questioning about suicidal ideation, particularly after an act of self-harm. Discussing suicidal ideation with a patient does not increase their risk of suicide (as is sometimes feared). Past history of attempted suicide or self-harm is also an important indicator of future risk. Whilst various risk assessment tools exist, there is no substitute for a comprehensive overall history. Obtaining collateral history is equally important. Despite best efforts, it may sometimes not be possible to accurately predict future risk.

Risk factors for suicide include

- Male sex
- Age >45 years
- Being divorced, single or widowed
- Unemployment
- Social classes I and V
- Psychiatric illness
- Previous episodes of self-harm
- Chronic physical illness
- Recent adverse life events

Protective factors include having children and being religious. In populations, the rate of suicide increases in summer months and decreases during times of war.

1. B – 1 in 10,000
The annual incidence of suicide is 1 in 10,000.

2. D – 1%
After an act of self-harm, the risk of completed suicide within the next year is 1%; that is, 100-times more than the risk in the general population. The following features of self-harm are indicators of strong suicidal intent: a more violent/dangerous action, careful planning and preparation, making precautions to avoid being discovered, failing to seek help afterwards and final acts (e.g. making a suicide note or a will). It should be ascertained whether or not they intended to die at the time and, if so, what their reaction is to still being alive (do they regret being alive and still wish to die?). There is a high rate of recurrence in people who self-harm, with the majority of those who go on to commit suicide having sought help following an episode of self-harm in the preceding 12 months.

3. F – 66.6%
Two-thirds of people who have completed suicide have seen a GP within the last month. Around 25% are psychiatric outpatients and half of those who are under current psychiatric care will have seen their psychiatrist during the previous week.

4. G – 90%
90% of those who self-harm have a psychiatric illness; the most common of these are depressive episodes, alcohol dependence, other substance use, personality disorders, chronic neuroses and schizophrenia.

5. C – 3 in 1000
The annual incidence of self-harm is 3 in 1000. The nomenclature and definitions of self-harm are contentious. The term 'parasuicide' is now outdated, and use of the word 'deliberate' before self-harm is out of favour, because it implies blame or judgement (as does using the term to 'commit'

suicide). Self-harm describes either self-injury (10%) or self-poisoning (90%) that is non-fatal. If a drug or poison is ingested that is not actually harmful, or at a dose that is not harmful, the term self-harm is still used if the patient believed it to be harmful. Risk factors for self-harm include female sex, age 15–25 years, lower social class, unemployment and living in an urban area. Individual risk factors are psychiatric illness, learning disability, death of a parent at a young age and childhood neglect/abuse. Predisposing factors at a particular time include physical illness (in the patient or a family member), relationship loss/difficulties and criminal proceedings. Additionally, in severe depression with psychomotor retardation, a recent improvement in symptoms is a risk factor for suicide, because patients gain enough motivation and energy to do it.

THEME 8: PSYCHIATRIC DISORDERS RELATING TO WOMEN'S HEALTH

1. D – Maternity blues

Maternity blues affects two-thirds of women postpartum. It begins 3–5 days after birth, and lasts no longer than 10 days. It is characterized by low mood and tearfulness, and usually recovers spontaneously. Management is by reassurance. Postnatal depression starts within 3 months of giving birth, and usually lasts less than 6 months. It affects 10% of women. Features are similar to those of depressive episodes, but some symptoms of depression (insomnia, tiredness and low libido) are normal postpartum. There may be obsessional thoughts, particularly intrusive thoughts about harming the baby. There may be an excessive concern about the baby's health and the mother's own adequacy as a parent. Treatment may be solely supportive or include antidepressants.

2. A – Couvade syndrome

Couvade syndrome occurs in males around the time of the birth of their child. They experience symptoms similar to those of pregnancy, such as nausea and dyspepsia. They may even suffer abdominal distension and labour-like contraction pains. The cause is not well understood, but symptoms usually resolve soon after birth. Pseudocyesis is the presence of the signs and symptoms of pregnancy (e.g. amenorrhoea, breast enlargement and significant abdominal distension) in a non-pregnant woman.

Couvade, from Old French _couver_ = to hatch.
Pseudocyesis, from Greek _pseudes_ = false + _kyesis_ = pregnancy.

3. H – Premenstrual syndrome

Premenstrual syndrome (PMS) describes the emotional and physical symptoms during the second half of the menstrual cycle, which increase in intensity until menstruation. Around 40% of women report symptoms at some time. Symptoms affecting mood include irritability, low mood, tiredness, tension and emotional lability. Management is supportive, and aims to identify and avoid psychological stressors. Antidepressants can be effective in reducing the psychological symptoms, and the oral contraceptive pill is effective at alleviating the physical symptoms. Cyclic psychosis can be seen as a rare complication of extreme PMS, with psychotic symptoms that are absent for most of the cycle. Dysmenorrhoea relates to pain during menstruation itself (or very slightly before).

Neither 'perimenstrual syndrome' nor 'postmenstrual syndrome' are recognized medical conditions, although there are outrageous allegations that these concepts exist!

4. K – Puerperal psychosis
The puerperium is defined as the first 6 weeks after childbirth. This is a high-risk period for developing psychiatric illness. Puerperal psychosis affects one pregnancy in 500 and has a rapid onset during the first 3 weeks after birth. There may be a prodrome of insomnia and irritability, followed by acute confusion and psychosis. It should be treated as a medical emergency in a specialist centre, because there is a suicide risk of 5% and an infanticide risk of 4%. 70% of cases recover fully. The aims of treatment are to keep the mother and child together in a safe environment, and ECT is sometimes required.

Puerperium, from Latin *puer* = child + *parere* = to give birth.

5. E – Not a psychiatric condition
Although this behaviour may be seen as eccentric, there is nothing in the history that suggests an underlying psychiatric disorder.

THEME 9: SUBSTANCE USE

1. I – Opiate use
This woman is likely to be suffering the effects of opiate use. Examples of opiates include morphine, heroin, methadone and codeine. Effects of opiates (in addition to analgesia) include euphoria, nausea and vomiting, constipation, anorexia, hypotension, respiratory depression, tremor, pinpoint pupils and erectile dysfunction. The treatment of overdose (after ABC) is with the antidote naloxone. This is ideally given intravenously (but can be given intramuscularly or by inhalation). An infusion of naloxone may be necessary, as the half-life is short. The effects of opiate withdrawal can be very extreme. They include dilated pupils, lacrimation, sweating, diarrhoea, insomnia, tachycardia, abdominal cramp-like pains, nausea and vomiting. Opiate withdrawal symptoms are managed by using drugs such as methadone (opiate agonist) or buprenorphine (partial opiate agonist). Longer-term management of opiate dependence may include maintenance doses of methadone or naltrexone (an opiate antagonist) for those wishing to achieve complete abstinence, in addition to other psychosocial interventions.

2. E – Cannabis use

The psychoactive component of cannabis is Δ^9-tetrahydrocannabinol, which has the following effects: dry cough, increased appetite, conjunctival injection and fatigue. Psychological effects include euphoria, relaxation, altered perception of time, social withdrawal and paranoia.

3. G – Cocaine use

Cocaine intoxication may present with tachycardia, mydriasis, hypertension, nausea and vomiting, euphoria, increased interest in sex and formication (a tactile hallucination described as insects crawling over the skin). Cocaine withdrawal results in a dysphoric mood, cravings, irritability and paranoia. Cocaine use is a risk factor for cardiovascular disease.

4. L – Sedative withdrawal

This woman may be on long-term sedatives (benzodiazepines or barbiturates) that stopped being prescribed when she moved location. Symptoms of sedative withdrawal include nausea and vomiting, autonomic hyperactivity, insomnia, delirium and seizures. Features of sedative use include loss of coordination, slurred speech, decreased attention and memory, disinhibition, aggression, meiosis, hypotension and respiratory depression.

Amphetamines are available illegally, but are also prescribed in narcolepsy, hyperkinetic syndromes (e.g. attention-deficit hyperactivity disorder) and as appetite suppressants. Features of intoxication include euphoria, insomnia, agitation, hallucinations, hypertension and tachycardia. Symptoms of the withdrawal state include dysphoric mood, fatigue and agitation. Methamphetamine (street names: crystal meth or ice) is similar in structure to amphetamines and increases dopamine levels in the brain, leading to symptoms that mimic schizophrenia.

5. B – Alcohol withdrawal

Alcohol withdrawal usually occurs if the blood alcohol concentration falls in someone with alcohol dependence. Symptoms usually start approximately 12 hours after the last intake and include anxiety, insomnia, sweating, tachycardia and tremor. Seizures may occur after 48 hours. Treatment is supportive with a reducing dose of regular benzodiazepines (e.g. chlordiazepoxide) and vitamin B supplements (intravenous or oral). The mortality rate is approximately 5%.

Delirium tremens may also be a feature of alcohol withdrawal, and occurs after 48 hours, lasting for 5 days. There is tremor, restlessness and increased autonomic activity, fluctuating consciousness with disorientation, a fearful affect and hallucinations. Hallucinations may be auditory, tactile or visual, and delusions may also be present. Lilliputian hallucinations (seeing little people) are characteristic.

Lilliputian, named after the island of Lilliput in Jonathan Swift's novel *Gulliver's Travels*, in which the inhabitants were 'not six inches high'.

Alcohol intoxication presents with mood changes, loss of inhibition, cerebellar signs (dysdiadochokinesis, ataxia, nystagmus, intention tremor, slurred speech, hypotonicity and hyporeflexia) and decreased conscious level.

Alcohol consumption is measured in units, calculated using the formula: Strength (ABV) × Volume (mL) ÷ 1000. ABV – or 'alcohol by volume' – is expressed as a percentage, and is defined as the number of millilitres of ethanol present in 100 mL of the beverage at 20°C. One unit is equal to 10 g of alcohol. Recommended limits are not more than 21 units/week for men and 14 units/week for women, with not more than 4 and 3 units per day, respectively, and having at least two alcohol-free days a week.

Excessive drinking can lead to alcohol-dependence syndrome, which is characterized by the following seven features:

- Increased tolerance (the drug produces less effect per gram ingested)
- Repeated withdrawal symptoms
- Subjective awareness of compulsion to drink, and cravings if resistance is attempted
- Prioritization of alcohol over other aspects of life (e.g. career and family)
- Avoidance of withdrawal by continued drinking
- Narrowing of the drinking repertoire (habits develop, including the preference of one particular drink, often as part of a daily routine)
- Rapid reinstatement of alcohol if a period of abstinence is successfully achieved

The CAGE questionnaire is a sensitive screening tool for alcohol dependence. There are four questions:

- Have you ever felt that you should **C**ut down?
- Have you ever been **A**nnoyed by criticism of your drinking?
- Have you ever felt **G**uilty about your drinking?
- Have you ever had an **E**ye-opener (morning drink)?

Examples of physical morbidity from alcohol use are vomiting, peptic ulcer disease, Mallory–Weiss tears, oesophageal varices, hepatic cirrhosis and liver failure, pancreatitis, repeated trauma, endocrine disturbances and aspiration pneumonia. Fetal alcohol syndrome is seen in children whose mothers had drunk excessive amounts of alcohol during pregnancy. Features include microcephaly, small nose, low IQ (mean 70), strabismus and a long philtrum.

THEME 10: SYNDROMES IN PSYCHIATRY

1. E – Ekbom syndrome
Ekbom syndrome is a delusional psychosis that one is infected with parasites. It may be accompanied by a physical sensation of parasites crawling

around or burrowing into the skin (formication). Cotard syndrome is a nihilistic delusion that one is dead, has lost all one's possessions, does not exist or is decaying, etc. It can be a feature of severe depression.

Formication, from Latin *formica* = ant.
Jules Cotard, French neurologist (1840–1889).
Karl Axel Ekbom, Swedish neurologist (1907–1977).

2. K – Rett's syndrome

Rett's syndrome is a neurodevelopmental disorder, similar to autism, in which developmental decline occurs after 1–2 years of age following a normal initial development. Typical behaviours include screaming attacks, avoidance of eye contact, poor social interactions, loss of fine motor skills, development of stereotyped hand movements (especially hand-wringing) and ataxia. It occurs almost exclusively in girls.

The Pickwickian syndrome is the association of obesity with sleep apnoea and hypersomnia. It is named after a character in Charles Dickens' novel *The Pickwick Papers* who was extremely obese and often fell asleep during the day. Tourette's syndrome is characterized by multiple vocal and motor tics.

Andreas Rett, Austrian neurologist (1924–1997).
Georges Gilles de la Tourette (1859–1904).

3. D – de Clerambault's syndrome

de Clerambault's syndrome (erotomania) is a delusional belief that someone of higher social status is in love with them. It is more common in women.

Gaetan Gatian de Clerambault, French psychiatrist (1872–1934).

4. H – Ganser's syndrome

Ganser's syndrome is a factitious disorder in which people give approximate answers to simple questions that show that they understand the underlying theme of the questions asked. Individuals mimic what they believe to be psychotic behaviours; for example, when asked how many legs a donkey has, they will answer 'twelve' as opposed to 'chicken wing'. Ganser's syndrome was first described in prison inmates awaiting trial.

Munchausen's syndrome is a factitious disorder in which people repeatedly feign illness or self-inflict pathology for the sole purpose of seeking medical attention (e.g. injecting faecal matter into the skin). In Munchausen by proxy, a different person is used for the same purpose (e.g. saying that a child has been repeatedly fitting).

Sigbert Ganser, German psychiatrist (1853–1931).
Karl Munchausen, German baron (1720–1797). He acquired a reputation for telling exaggerated tales about his adventures in other countries, including travelling to the moon.

5. G – Fregoli's syndrome

Fregoli's syndrome is a delusion that a persecutor is able to change into many forms and disguise themselves to look like different people, much like an actor. It is named after Leopold Fregoli, an Italian actor (1867–1936) who was famous for being able to make quick changes of appearance during stage acts.

Othello syndrome (delusional jealousy) is a feeling of delusional intensity that one's partner is being unfaithful. It is named after Shakespeare's character Othello, who murdered his wife based on false beliefs of her disloyalty. Capgras' syndrome is a delusional belief that a close acquaintance has been replaced by an identical double. It is most commonly seen in schizophrenia. Folie à deux is when a delusion in one person becomes shared by someone close to them. A similar effect can occur in three or more people (folie à trois and folie à plusieurs, respectively).

Folie à deux, from French *folie* = madness.
Joseph Capgras, French psychiatrist (1873–1950).

Practice Paper 10: Questions

THEME 1: NEUROTIC DISORDERS

Options

A. Acute stress reaction
B. Agoraphobia
C. Dissociative (conversion) disorder
D. Generalized anxiety disorder
E. Grief reaction
F. Obsessive–compulsive disorder
G. Panic disorder

H. Posttraumatic stress disorder
I. Social phobia
J. Somatization disorder
K. Specific phobia
L. Undifferentiated somatoform disorder

For each of the following scenarios, select the most likely diagnosis. Each option may be used once, more than once or not at all.

1. An 18-year-old woman prefers to spend time at home. She has started doing all her shopping online, and insists that her friends visit her at her own house, where she is quite happy. When she absolutely must go out anywhere, she dreads it for days, occasionally gets palpitations and finds the whole situation unbearable. The most frightening place is her busy college common room.
2. A 45-year-old man attends the GP with his wife because he is never able to relax. He worries excessively over trivial daily issues, with no obvious pattern, and his muscles always feel tense.
3. A 61-year-old woman presents to her GP, and appears very concerned about the cause of her abdominal pains. They have been present for 3 years, and fluctuate in intensity and exact position. She has had a gastroscopy, colonoscopy, ultrasound and computed tomography scans and has also seen consultants privately.
4. A 21-year-old man presents to the emergency department with shortness of breath and chest pain. His symptoms started very suddenly while at a bus station, and were associated with light-headedness, dizziness and a fear that he was going to die. His symptoms resolved after 10 minutes. He has had four previous similar episodes.
5. A 22-year-old woman who describes herself as having always been generally anxious admits to having unpleasant thoughts over the past 6 months. She cannot control them, but recognizes that they are her own. She also admits to spending 3 hours a day packing and repacking her bag before leaving the house to avoid forgetting anything.

THEME 2: SIDE EFFECTS OF PSYCHIATRIC MEDICATION

Options

A. Acute dystonia
B. Agranulocytosis
C. Akathisia
D. Cheese reaction
E. Hyperprolactinaemia
F. Lithium toxicity
G. Neuroleptic malignant syndrome
H. Parkinsonism
I. Serotonin syndrome
J. Tardive dyskinesia
K. Weight gain
L. Weight loss

For each of the following descriptions, select the most appropriate side effect. Each option may be used once, more than once or not at all.

1. A 42-year-old man with paranoid schizophrenia has been taking chlorpromazine. He has developed symptoms of restless legs and is requesting treatment for this.
2. A 65-year-old man has been taking haloperidol for many years. On examination, he had unusual facial movements that look as though he is chewing or sucking his tongue.
3. A 40-year-old woman with schizophrenia has recently had an increase in her dose of clozapine. She presented to the emergency department unconscious with a temperature of 39.8°C and muscle rigidity. Initial blood tests revealed a raised white cell count and a creatine kinase of 5000 IU/L.
4. A 23-year-old woman presents to her GP because she and her partner are concerned about a noticeable change in her body habitus. She has been taking olanzapine for 6 months.
5. A 30-year-old woman was seen by her GP with symptoms of sweating and fever, which was thought to be caused by a viral infection. She later presents to the emergency department with agitation and confusion. On examination, she is shocked and has overactive reflexes. Routine observations reveal a heart rate of 130 beats/minute and a blood pressure of 210/110 mmHg. She denies illicit drug use, but has recently started taking an over-the-counter preparation for depression. Her repeat prescription includes lansoprazole, salbutamol inhaler and fluoxetine.

THEME 3: DESCRIPTIVE PSYCHOPATHOLOGY 2

Options

A. Agitation
B. Amnesia
C. Depression
D. Dysphoria
E. Echopraxia
F. Echolalia
G. Euphoria
H. Fugue state
 I. Hyperamnesia
 J. Hyperkinesia
K. Stupor
L. Paramnesia

For each of the following scenarios, select the most appropriate descriptive term. Each option may be used once, more than once or not at all.

1. A 36-year-old woman has had a difficult day at work. She is now in an unpleasant mood.
2. An 80-year-old woman is asked about the events leading up to a fall she had earlier in the day. She explains exactly what she can remember, but the description that she gives is significantly different from the account of her carers who were present at the time.
3. A 60-year-old man with schizophrenia is copying the exact movements of his social worker during a multidisciplinary team meeting.
4. A 26-year-old woman is very unhappy that she has just been sectioned. She appears restless and is not keeping her hands still. She is also intermittently striding around the room.
5. A 55-year-old man with severe depression was found in his flat by police. He was sitting on the floor, absolutely still, not speaking at all.

THEME 4: PSYCHOTIC DISORDERS

Options

A. Antisocial personality disorder
B. Catatonic schizophrenia
C. Delusional disorder
D. Hebephrenic schizophrenia
E. Organic psychotic disorder
F. Psychotic depression
G. Schizoaffective disorder
H. Schizoid-type personality disorder
 I. Simple schizophrenia
 J. Substance-induced psychotic disorder
K. Transient psychosis

For each of the following scenarios, select the most appropriate diagnosis. Each option may be used once, more than once or not at all.

1. A 45-year-old man presents with a 4-week history of low mood, lack of enjoyment in his usual activities and reduced energy. He feels unhappy with his own abilities and appearance. He says that he is also worried about how to keep his thoughts clean, 'especially as they have been all over the BBC website for the past 6 weeks'.

2. A 60-year-old woman with a long history of recurrent depression is complaining that she can smell rotting flesh and that it is coming from her legs. Peripheral vascular examination is normal.

3. A 54-year-old man with a 30-year history of mental health problems is found to be standing on one leg with his arm in the air. He did not move for 30 minutes until a nurse pulled his arm down. It then stayed in the new position. He has not said anything for an hour, but yesterday was noted to be repeating the same word incessantly.

4. A 19-year-old male student is admitted to a psychiatric ward after hearing voices and behaving strangely. He admits to spending half of his weekly food budget on 'skunk'.

5. A 21-year-old woman has always preferred to be by herself. She has no hobbies and finds it difficult to share her feelings with others. She was referred to a psychiatrist, and a thorough mental state examination revealed a blunted affect. There were no specific abnormalities of thinking.

THEME 5: PSYCHIATRY OF SEXUALITY

Options

A. Exhibitionism
B. Fetishism
C. Loss of sexual desire
D. Male erectile disorder
E. Masochism
F. Non-organic dyspareunia
G. Premature ejaculation
H. Sadism
 I. Sexual aversion
 J. Transsexualism
K. Transvestic fetishism
L. Vaginismus
M. Voyeurism

For each of the following scenarios, select the most appropriate diagnosis. Each option may be used once, more than once or not at all.

1. A 45-year-old man has begun to gain sexual excitement from shiny materials such as PVC. He is now relying on it in order to become aroused.
2. A 19-year-old man was arrested after flashing his genitals to a group of teenage girls at a fairground.
3. A 35-year-old man has felt for a long time that he is a woman trapped in a man's body. He has changed his name from Fred to Freda and is saving money for an operation to change his anatomy. He usually wears a pink pinafore dress and says that he feels 'much more comfortable dressed like this'.
4. A 45-year-old woman is married but says that she has never enjoyed sex. She has no specific physical problems with the process of it, but she dreads it and feels emotionally uncomfortable during intercourse itself, as well as while talking and thinking about it.
5. A 27-year-old man has a new sexual partner, but has been finding it increasingly difficult to achieve an erection. The more he worries about it, the less likely he is to be successful.

THEME 6: MANAGEMENT OF DEPRESSION

Options

A. Amitriptyline
B. Cognitive-behavioural therapy
C. Diazepam
D. Electroconvulsive therapy
E. Fluoxetine
F. Imipramine
G. Lithium
H. Moclobemide
I. Phenelzine
J. Psychodynamic psychotherapy

For each of the following scenarios, select the most appropriate step in the management. Each option may be used once, more than once or not at all.

1. A 25-year-old woman presents to her GP with a 3-month history of low mood. She feels that her self-esteem has suffered since stopping her usual hobbies and social activities after the breakdown of a relationship.

2. A 64-year-old man had been an inpatient for 3 months with severe depression. His symptoms have been resistant to selective serotonin reuptake inhibitors, lithium and the supportive environment of the hospital itself. He has deteriorated further to the point that he is not communicating and not adequately feeding himself.

3. A 36-year-old woman presents to her GP with a 4-month history of low mood, poor appetite and tearfulness. She has had a previous episode of depression, which responded to a 6-month course of first-line drug treatment.

4. A 45-year-old man with severe depression is managed by a community psychiatry team. His depression has not responded to three different antidepressants and, although he and his wife are fairly reliable and are coping at the moment, they are very keen to see some improvement. The only food that he likes to eat is pizza.

5. A 59-year-old woman with depression had started a course of fluoxetine, but was forced to discontinue it due to side effects. Poor sleep is a prominent feature of her illness.

THEME 7: TRANSCULTURAL PSYCHIATRIC DISORDERS

Options

A. Amok
B. Depressive episode
C. Dhat
D. Generalized anxiety disorder
E. Koro
F. Latah
G. Piblokto
H. Susto
I. Windigo

For each of the following scenarios, select the most appropriate diagnosis. Each option may be used once, more than once or not at all.

1. A 28-year-old man living in Malaysia took a knife and ruthlessly murdered nine of his family members and neighbours in a 30-minute rampage before finally killing himself. He had no previous psychiatric history and there was no obvious motive.
2. A 19-year-old man of Chinese origin has developed symptoms of severe anxiety and has become preoccupied with the fear that his penis is going to disappear inside him. He has tried to clamp it to prevent this happening.
3. A 38-year-old woman living in the Arctic Circle had a sudden-onset episode of bizarre behaviour. She cannot remember it, but her family say that she began screaming and crying hysterically and started throwing furniture and eating the broken splinters. She had to be physically restrained when she became violent.
4. A 22-year-old Indian man presented to his doctor complaining of extreme fatigue and anxiety. On questioning about his ideas regarding the cause, he admitted to excessive guilt about masturbation, and felt that he was losing semen in his urine.
5. A 26-year-old woman living in Tunisia is involved in a road traffic collision. Soon after the accident, she appears very on-edge, with a markedly exaggerated startle response. She has started repeating the words of everyone around her.

THEME 8: PSYCHIATRIC SIGNS OF PHYSICAL ILLNESS

Options

A. Cushing's syndrome
B. Delirium
C. Hyperthyroidism
D. Hypothyroidism
E. Multiple sclerosis
F. Neurosyphilis
G. Pellagra
H. Punch-drunk syndrome
I. Space-occupying lesion
J. Systemic lupus erythematosus

For each of the following scenarios, select the most likely underlying physical cause. Each option may be used once, more than once or not at all.

1. A 58-year-old woman presents to the emergency department hearing voices. Her partner has noticed increased irritability, restlessness, change in behaviour and loss of libido over the past 2 months. On examination, she has a fine tremor, is underweight and has an irregular pulse.
2. A 45-year-old woman presents with low mood and tearfulness. She is upset about severe pains in her knees and hands and an embarrassing red rash over her face. She also complains of worsening shortness of breath.
3. A 42-year-old man presents with memory loss, and his wife says that he has been pointing at things in the room that are not there. He has also had a headache for over a month, which is worse in the mornings.
4. A 77-year-old woman was found by her carers confused and disorientated. She is usually lucid. The carers notice that she has been incontinent of urine.
5. A 34-year-old woman presents to her GP complaining of feeling sad all the time, difficulty sleeping and weight gain. She has a history of Crohn's disease and is taking medication regularly for frequent exacerbations.

THEME 9: THE MENTAL HEALTH ACT

Options

A. Section 2
B. Section 3
C. Section 4
D. Section 5(2)
E. Section 5(4)
F. Section 12
G. Section 17
H. Section 35
I. Section 36
J. Section 37
K. Section 135
L. Section 136

For each of the following scenarios, choose which section of the Mental Health Act is most likely to be used. Each option may be used once, more than once or not at all.

1. A 46-year-old woman is detained by the police after a member of the public alerted them to her strange behaviour. She has been playing on the swings all day and singing to the birds in her pyjamas, despite it being December. The police decide that it is best to take her to hospital.

2. A 19-year-old man presents with his first episode of psychosis and is seen by a consultant psychiatrist. He needs to be admitted for formal assessment, but the man is adamant that he wants to go straight home.

3. A 36-year-old woman, who is an inpatient on a psychiatry ward with depression, had agreed to her admission 1 week ago. She is now trying to leave. She has told a care assistant that she is following the devil's instructions to her, and will jump off a bridge once she has left. The psychiatry medical team are all away on a conference.

4. A 55-year-old man with known chronic severe depression is being managed in the community. He has recently deteriorated and is not currently safe at home. The community psychiatrist decides that he needs admission for treatment, although it is against the patient's wishes.

5. A 25-year-old man presents to the emergency department on a Saturday night, behaving strangely. His only speech is an impersonation of a rap artist, which he does while breakdancing. He has a history of bipolar affective disorder. His mother is concerned that he has stopped sleeping, and thinks that this is a manic episode. His usual consultant will be available on Monday morning, but the attending doctor decides that he needs to be admitted until then.

THEME 10: PERSONALITY DISORDERS

Options

A. Anankastic
B. Antisocial
C. Anxious (avoidant)
D. Dependent
E. Emotionally unstable (borderline type)
F. Emotionally unstable (impulsive type)
G. Histrionic
H. Paranoid
I. Schizoid

For each of the following scenarios, select the most appropriate personality disorder. Each option may be used once, more than once or not at all.

1. A 19-year-old factory worker has no friends and has been experiencing difficulty with relationships at work. People have complained that he has aggressive outbursts and has no regard for anyone else's feelings. He himself does not feel guilty, but blames those around him who have made him feel frustrated. At school, he was diagnosed with conduct disorder.

2. An 18-year-old woman agrees to have a baby with her boyfriend, because he is extremely keen to do so and she wants to make him happy. She fears that he will leave her if she does not. She hates spending time alone and has difficulty making her own decisions.

3. A 35-year-old woman presents to the emergency department following an overdose. She has had 17 similar presentations this year, usually after an argument, and this time it was an attempt to stop her boyfriend from leaving her. They have an intense relationship, but her attitude towards it is variable, and sometimes she does not want to be a part of it.

4. A 50-year-old man is known as the local 'loner'. He has no interest in other people, nor does he enjoy any activities. If directly addressed, he appears detached and shows little emotion.

5. A 45-year-old woman has racked up enormous debt buying clothes and make-up. Her teenage children cringe at how she wears excessively revealing clothes and makes uninhibited advances towards male strangers. She behaves dramatically and can become very upset if she is not the centre of attention.

Practice Paper 10: Answers

THEME 1: NEUROTIC DISORDERS

Generally, neurotic disorders in childhood do not lead to neurosis in later life. Neuroses in children are more common in males, but are dominant in females after adolescence.

1. B – Agoraphobia

Agoraphobia is an example of a phobic anxiety disorder. The other two types are social phobias and specific phobias. Phobias usually relate to specific situations or triggers. There is anxiety even in anticipation of the trigger (anticipatory anxiety), and avoidance behaviour ensues. The fear in a phobia is out of proportion to the actual risk, but is not relieved by rational reasoning. Avoidance behaviour is reinforced because it temporarily relieves the anxiety.

Agoraphobia is the general term for fear of situations such as public places, open spaces, crowds, shops and public transport. It is often seen as a fear of the inability to escape. The fear is usually worse when the person is alone. The condition can be disabling, because severe avoidance can lead to the patient being housebound, and there is a predisposition to developing panic attacks.

Social phobia is the fear of scrutiny and criticism from others. It usually coexists with low self-esteem and may cause problems especially with speaking to strangers, answering the phone and public speaking. There may be problems with tremor, blushing and urinary urgency.

Specific phobias relate to one specific trigger. Examples include animals (zoophobia), small spaces (claustrophobia), heights (acrophobia), strangers (xenophobia) and inanimate objects such as buttons (koumpounophobia).

Management of phobic anxiety disorders is by graded exposure therapy, which involves gradually increasing the intensity and proximity of the source of phobia. Antidepressants also have a role.

Phobia, from Greek *phobos* = fear.
Agoraphobia, from Greek *agora* = a place of gathering, marketplace.

2. D – Generalized anxiety disorder

Generalized anxiety disorder is defined as generalized, excessive worry for more than 6 months. It is twice as common in females and occurs frequently in early adulthood. Sufferers of generalized anxiety disorder feel anxious or nervous most of the time. There is no single particular trigger, and it can be described as 'free-floating'. There is an underlying worry that 'something bad may happen'. Physical symptoms include trembling, sweating, light-headedness, palpitations, dizziness, abdominal discomfort and muscle tension. Genetic predisposition overlaps with the predisposition to depression. Management options include psychological therapies, selective serotonin reuptake inhibitors (SSRIs), benzodiazepines for rapid anxiolysis and β-blockers for autonomic symptoms. The disease course is usually chronic and fluctuating.

3. J – Somatization disorder
The patient has somatization disorder. This is characterized by the following:

- Over 2 years of multiple, variable physical symptoms of no underlying cause
- Refusal to accept doctors' reassurance
- Impairment of social function
- Symptoms not intentionally produced

Patients often see doctors of several different specialties and undergo investigations with negative outcomes. There is often social/family disruption. There is some evidence that somatization disorder is more common in people who experienced parental physical illness as children. Management is difficult, and the development of a physical illness needs to be excluded. In undifferentiated somatoform disorder, the diagnostic criteria for somatization disorder are not met. Symptoms may last less than 2 years and they are likely to be even more generalized and varied. Somatization disorders are much more common in females.

4. G – Panic disorder
Panic disorder is characterized by sudden-onset, spontaneous severe panic attacks that are not limited to one particular situation. Panic attacks last a few minutes and are often accompanied by a fear of going mad or dying. Physical symptoms include nausea, hyperventilation, palpitations, chest pain, sweating and lightheadedness. Affected people are symptom free between attacks. Panic disorder is diagnosed only if there is no other underlying disorder such as depression. First-line management is with cognitive-behavioural therapy (CBT). Panic disorder is most common in young female adults.

5. F – Obsessive–compulsive disorder
Obsessive–compulsive disorder (OCD) is characterized by persistent obsessional thoughts and compulsive acts despite conscious resistance. Obsessions are images or ideas that are recognized as the patient's own thoughts, but are recurrent, intrusive and not pleasurable. Attempts to resist them are usually unsuccessful. Compulsions are the irresistible

urges to perform tasks or rituals that are stereotyped behaviours from which the patient derives no pleasure. They may appear to have the purpose of preventing harm, but are objectively useless (and recognized as such by the patient). OCD is associated with simultaneous anxiety. OCD is equally common in males and females. Psychological therapies include response prevention (learning how to cope with tension), mass practice (where the patient is forced to repeat their rituals) and thought-stopping (blocking the undesired thoughts). OCD may respond to antidepressants, although severe, intractable cases with major life disruption may respond to psychosurgery (cingulotomy).

Acute stress reaction is a transient phenomenon that occurs secondary to exceptional physical or mental stress in people without a preexisting psychiatric disorder. It can start a few minutes after the trigger and may last for a few days. The typical features are an initial 'daze' followed by disorientation and the inability to process external stimuli. There may later be amnesia of the event. If the duration exceeds 3 days, an alternative diagnosis should be considered.

Posttraumatic stress disorder ('shell shock') occurs secondary to a traumatic stressor (i.e. one that any 'normal' person would find stressful). Diagnostic features include

- Experience of a major traumatic event
- Re-experiencing the trauma (nightmares or flashbacks)
- Avoidance behaviour
- Increased arousal (hypervigilance, insomnia or enhanced startle reaction)
- Onset is delayed (but within 6 months) and the features should last ≥1 month

The usual course is recovery, but occasionally symptoms become chronic. An adjustment disorder is defined as a state of emotional distress that interferes with social functioning occurring within 1 month of a significant life event.

The stages of normal grief (described by the Swiss-born psychiatrist Elisabeth Kubler-Ross in 1969) are denial, anger, bargaining, depression and acceptance. This process usually lasts less than 6 months. Complicated grief is suggested by duration above 6 months, suicidal ideation, hallucinations and functional impairment.

Dissociative disorders are characterized by a loss of normally integrated concepts such as self-identify, memories of the past, awareness of the present and even control of bodily movements. There must be some form of traumatic or interpersonal stress and the absence of a preexisting physical or psychiatric disorder in order to make the diagnosis. The term conversion describes the unconscious change of intrapsychic anxiety into physical symptoms of symbolic significance.

THEME 2: SIDE EFFECTS OF PSYCHIATRIC MEDICATION

1. C – Akathisia
2. J – Tardive dyskinesia

Typical antipsychotics block dopamine D_2 receptors in the central nervous system (CNS) in various pathways. This accounts for both their therapeutic activity and their side effects. The effect on the mesolimbic pathway improves psychotic symptoms, but action on the mesocortical pathway worsens negative symptoms. The effect on the tuberoinfundibular pathway causes the side effect of hyperprolactinaemia (leading to gynaecomastia, galactorrhoea, reduced sperm count, amenorrhoea and reduced libido). Action on the chemoreceptor trigger zone has an antiemetic property.

Extrapyramidal side effects are a consequence of nigrostriatal pathway blockade. These include Parkinsonism (rigidity, bradykinesia and tremor, which can begin within 1 month and are treated with anticholinergics; e.g. procyclidine), acute dystonias (which occur within 72 hours of treatment and include trismus, tongue protrusion, spasmodic torticollis, opisthotonus, oculogyric crisis and grimacing), akathisia (which occurs within 60 days and features a subjective feeling of inner tension and restless leg syndrome, but can be treated with β-blockers and benzodiazepines) and tardive dyskinesia (which affects 20% in the long term and presents with chewing, grimacing, sucking and a darting tongue). Treatment of tardive dyskinesia can be difficult and, following a gradual reduction in dose, other options such as benzodiazepines and tetrabenazine could be tried.

Other side effects of typical antipsychotics are anticholinergic effects, which cause an increased QT interval, arrhythmias and cardiac arrest. α-adrenoreceptor blocking action causes postural hypotension, and antihistamine activity causes sedation and weight gain. Chlorpromazine specifically causes greying of the skin in response to sunlight and a reduced seizure threshold.

3. G – Neuroleptic malignant syndrome

Neuroleptic malignant syndrome is a life-threatening neurological condition that can occur with the use of typical and atypical antipsychotics, particularly after an increase in dose. Symptoms include pyrexia, fluctuating consciousness, muscle rigidity and autonomic dysfunction. Investigations may reveal a raised creatine kinase, raised white cell count and abnormal liver function tests. Treatment is to stop the offending drug in the first instance, along with fluid resuscitation. Adjunctive drugs such as dantrolene (to treat muscle spasm) and bromocriptine (to reverse dopamine blockade) can also be helpful in more severe cases.

4. K – Weight gain

Two examples of atypical antipsychotics are clozapine and olanzapine. These act on dopamine D_1 and D_4 receptors. They generally have fewer extrapyramidal side effects and cause less worsening of negative symptoms. Olanzapine does cause weight gain, diabetes and sedation. Clozapine causes agranulocytosis in 1% of cases, and must be withdrawn if the leucocyte or neutrophil count falls significantly. Risperidone and amisulpride are other examples of atypical antipsychotics.

5. I – Serotonin syndrome

This woman has taken an over-the-counter preparation for depression, which is likely to be St John's wort. The combination of this herb with SSRIs (fluoxetine in this case) is associated with the development of serotonin syndrome. Signs include severe hypertension, tachycardia, high pyrexia, myoclonus, sweating and hyper-reflexia. Management is initially symptomatic, followed by removal of the offending drugs.

THEME 3: DESCRIPTIVE PSYCHOPATHOLOGY 2

1. D – Dysphoria
Description of mood and feeling

The affect refers to a snapshot of a patient's emotional state. It tends to be used to describe the observer's impression of a patient's mood at one particular time. A blunted/flattened affect describes reduced emotional reactivity. Inappropriate affect is emotion that is inappropriate to the associated speech or thought; for example, laughing when talking about death.

Mood refers to a patient's sustained emotional state. Dysphoria is an unpleasant mood and elation is an abnormal exaggeration of the feeling of well-being. Euphoria is the feeling of contentment and lack of concern. It can be caused by opiates and is a late complication of head injury. Apathy is the loss of emotional tone (detachment or indifference) and alexithymia is difficulty in understanding and describing one's emotions.

Anxiety is apprehension and tension due to anticipation of an internal or external danger. In phobic anxiety, there is a clear focus on the danger and it is avoided. In free-floating anxiety, the anxiety is pervasive and unfocused. Fear is anxiety due to a realistic danger at a conscious level. Tension is an unpleasant increase in psychological stress. Agitation describes the excess motor activity associated with feelings of inner tension. Depressive retardation is psychomotor retardation in depression. Hyperchondriasis is the fear of a serious illness that is not based on any real organic pathology, but on unrealistic interpretations of physical signs. Depersonalization is the feeling that you are not real, or are altered in some way. Derealization is the feeling that the surroundings do not seem real.

2. L – Paramnesia
Description of memory, intellect and attention

Amnesia is an inability to recall past experiences. Hypermnesia is exaggerated retention of detail about past experiences. Paramnesia is a distorted recall of events, such that falsification of memory occurs. Confabulation is verbal evidence of unconscious filling of gaps in memory with false memories. A fugue state is an abandonment of personal identity and a loss of memory, often associated with travel/wandering to unexpected locations. It is important to determine a patient's insight into their psychiatric condition, because it has a high impact on their concordance with treatment. This can be done by asking: 'Are you ill? Is it psychiatric? Do you need treatment?'

Learning difficulty is categorized according to IQ. Mild retardation is defined as an IQ between 50 and 70, moderate retardation is defined as an IQ between 35 and 49, severe retardation is defined as an IQ between 20 and 34 and profound retardation is defined as an IQ less than 20. Distractibility is a state in which the patient's attention is drawn to unimportant stimuli. In selective inattention, anxiety-provoking stimulants are ignored.

3. E – Echopraxia
4. A – Agitation
5. K – Stupor

Description of movement

Stupor describes the state of being unresponsive, akinetic and mute, but fully conscious. Stupor can occur in depression, mania, catatonia, epilepsy and hysteria. Obsessional slowness is a reduced rate of activity due to repeated doubts and compulsive rituals in OCD. Hyperkinesis is often seen in children and teenagers. It comprises overactivity, distractibility, impulsivity and excitability. Motor tics are repeated involuntary movements involving a group of muscles. Parkinsonism describes a group of characteristic movements that occur in Parkinson's disease and other conditions. These include resting tremor, cogwheel rigidity, festinant gait (an involuntary tendency to making short, accelerated steps when walking) and posture abnormalities.

Movements seen in schizophrenia

Ambitendency involves making tentative incomplete movements, apparent when shaking hands. Echopraxia is copying of another person's movements, even when asked to stop. Mannerisms are repeated involuntary movements that appear goal directed (e.g. flicking hair). Stereotypies are repeated patterns of movement that are not goal directed (e.g. moving the head from side to side). Negativism is a motiveless resistance to commands and attempts to be moved. Posturing is where a bizarre body position is adopted for an inappropriately long time. Waxy flexibility is when the patient remains motionless, but allows their limbs to be moved by someone else. The limbs will remain in the new posture.

THEME 4: PSYCHOTIC DISORDERS

Schizophrenia is characterized by distortions in thought and perception, with a blunted, inappropriate affect. Intellect and clear consciousness are usually maintained. The most important features are first-rank symptoms, thought disorder and negative symptoms. Example of negative symptoms include apathy, poverty of thought, reduced speech, blunted affect, psychomotor retardation, social isolation, poor self-care and cognitive deficit.

There is a lifetime risk of 1%, with a peak age of onset of 18–25 years in both males and females, but a second peak in females during the perimeno-pausal years. There is a slightly higher incidence in males. Risk factors for relapse include low socioeconomic status and exposure to a high level of expressed emotion (over 35 hours/week). There is also a higher incidence in those with a family history, winter/spring birthdays, maternal influenza infection during the second trimester of pregnancy, decreased brain volume and increased ventricle size, adverse life events and lack of social interactions. The dopamine hypothesis is a theory regarding the mechanism of schizophrenia. Briefly, it says that the symptoms are caused in part by central dopaminergic hyperactivity in the mesolimbic–mesocortical system.

Psychosis should lead to the diagnosis of schizophrenia only if symptoms have been present for 1 month and there is an absence of significant mood disorder, overt brain disease and drug intoxication/withdrawal. Important differential diagnoses are organic psychotic disorder, substance-induced psychotic disorder, delusional disorder, schizoaffective disorder, transient psychosis and schizotypal disorder.

First-line management of schizophrenia is with an atypical neuroleptic (e.g. olanzapine). Response takes 3–4 weeks. Monthly depot injections can improve compliance. All antipsychotics are similar in efficacy, except for clozapine, which is used in treatment-resistant cases (i.e. two different antipsychotics, at least one of which is an atypical, have been tried for an adequate dose and duration). Benzodiazepines are given for aggression. In cases in which clozapine is not appropriate or there has been an inadequate response to clozapine, antidepressants and lithium are used for augmentation. Electroconvulsive therapy (ECT) is used for catatonic schizophrenia only.

Schizophrenia, from Greek *schitz* = split/shattered + *phrenes* = mind/heart.

1. G – Schizoaffective disorder
Schizoaffective disorder is diagnosed when the patient meets the full criteria for both a mood disorder and schizophrenia. It can be divided into manic-type and depressed-type.

2. F – Psychotic depression
This woman is having a nihilistic delusion – the delusion that parts of her body are rotting away. This is a recognized psychotic symptom associated with severe depression.

3. B – Catatonic schizophrenia
Catatonic schizophrenia has a prominence of catatonic symptoms. These are stupor, excitement, posturing, negativism, rigidity, waxy flexibility, perseveration of words and mutism.

The most common subtype of schizophrenia is the paranoid subtype, in which there are predominantly positive symptoms (delusions and hallucinations) with an increased suicide risk. Paranoid schizophrenia has the best prognosis. Hebephrenic schizophrenia has an earlier age of onset and a worse prognosis, and the main features are negative symptoms, thought disorders and an incongruent affect. Simple schizophrenia is a gradual decline in functioning. There are negative symptoms without positive symptoms. Chronic schizophrenia can be diagnosed if negative symptoms persist 1 year after positive symptoms. In delusional disorder, it is delusions alone that make up the clinical picture, although very occasional and transient hallucinations do not exclude the diagnosis. It usually starts in middle age. Transient psychotic disorder usually reaches a crescendo of symptoms within 2 weeks, with complete resolution within 3 months. It may be precipitated by a stressful life event.

4. J – Substance-induced psychotic disorder
If there is a potential organic or drug-related cause for someone's psychotic symptoms, this should be suspected above a true psychiatric condition. In this case, it is likely that excessive cannabis consumption has resulted in psychotic symptoms.

5. H – Schizoid-type personality disorder
Schizoid personalities have a preference for their own company over that of others. They lack emotional expression and may consequently be perceived by others as cold and disinterested. They may not gain pleasure from many activities, and have little interest in forming sexual or confiding relationships. Thought disorders and psychoses, which are features of schizophrenia, are not present in schizoid personalities. However, people with schizoid personalities are not exempt from developing schizophrenia.

THEME 5: PSYCHIATRY OF SEXUALITY
Psychosexual disorders are non-organic problems preventing an individual from participating in a satisfactory sexual relationship. However, there is frequently a combination of physical and psychological factors contributing to an impairment of function.

1. B – Fetishism
2. A – Exhibitionism
Paraphilias are defined as disorders of sexual preference. Fetishism focuses on inanimate objects as a source of sexual stimulation; for example, shoes or leather. Transvestic fetishism is the use of cross-dressing in order to gain sexual excitement. Exhibitionism is the tendency to expose genitalia to strangers in public places with subsequent gratification,

particularly if there are reactions of shock or horror. Type 1 exhibitionism (80% cases) occurs often in young men, showing a flaccid penis. There is often remorse afterwards. Type 2 exhibitionism is the exposure of an erect penis. This is more common in those with dissocial personality types and there is often a lack of remorse. Voyeurism is the tendency to watch other people engaging in sexual activity. Sadism involves gaining pleasure from inflicting pain or humiliating someone else. Masochism involves gaining sexual excitement from having pain or humiliation inflicted on oneself by another. Sadomasochism is a term comprising both sadism and masochism.

> Sadism, from the French novelist Marquis de Sade, whose writings describe it.
> Masochism, from the Austrian writer Leopold von Sacher-Masoch, whose stories describe it.

3. J – Transsexualism

Transsexualism, a gender identity disorder, is the persistent desire to live and be accepted as a member of the opposite sex. There is a feeling that the physical body is inconsistent with the sense of self. There may be a desire to have surgery or hormonal treatment in order to change it. Dual-role transvestism is the intermittent desire to dress as the opposite sex that is not for the purpose of arousal or for any permanent change. The male-to-female ratio is approximately 3:1. Management is usually by specialists, and surgery/hormone treatments can be given, although the long-term outcome is uncertain. There is usually a requirement to live as the opposite sex for a year before starting treatment.

4. I – Sexual aversion
5. D – Male erectile disorder

Sexual aversion is an example of sexual dysfunction. There are four stages of sexual arousal – desire, excitement, orgasm and resolution – and problems with each will be dealt with in order. Loss or lack of sexual desire can be diagnosed when it is the principal problem, not caused by another factor (e.g. pain). Sexual aversion is the tendency to avoid sex due to negative feelings or associations. There may not be a specific problem with one of the four stages of the cycle, but there is an overall lack of enjoyment. Dyspareunia is pain during intercourse. It can occur at any stage, in either party. It may be caused by organic pathology or may be psychogenic in origin. Vaginismus describes spasm of muscles in the outer third of the vagina making intercourse painful or impossible. Failure of the genital response interferes with the excitement stage. This includes male erectile disorder – a difficulty in achieving or maintaining an erection – or a lack of lubrication in women. Problems at the stage of orgasm can be premature ejaculation in men, and anorgasmia, which is more common in women.

THEME 6: MANAGEMENT OF DEPRESSION

In recent-onset mild depression, an acceptable first step is 'watchful waiting' with review in approximately 2 weeks. This is particularly appropriate if the patient is reluctant to have any intervention and if it appears likely that it might resolve spontaneously.

1. B – Cognitive-behavioural therapy

In mild depression, antidepressants are not the first-line intervention, because the risk–benefit ratio is poor. The first-line approach is CBT. There is some evidence for internet-based self-help CBT programmes, which may become more readily available. CBT has been shown to be as effective as drug treatments in mild-to-moderate depression.

Talking therapies are broadly split into two groups: variations on psychodynamic psychotherapy and CBT. Psychodynamic psychotherapy is based on the theory that subconscious ideas/conflicts can lead to emotional and interpersonal difficulties. During therapy, if these ideas can be identified and insight gained, then they can be addressed and interpretations made. Important concepts include transference, which is the feelings and attitude of the patient towards the therapist, and countertransference, which is the feelings and attitudes of the therapist towards the patient. Traditionally, a great deal of time is needed (up to five 50-minute sessions per week, continuing for 2–5 years). Psychodynamic psychotherapy is mainly used for personality and long-standing relationship difficulties. The NICE guidelines for depression do not currently include psychodynamic psychotherapy.

CBT employs a more structured approach, with a limited course of sessions. It is based on the theory that thoughts, beliefs, behaviours and emotions are linked. In the context of depression, negative thoughts (frequently relating to low self-esteem) are exacerbated by unhelpful behaviours, which compound the thoughts and lead to unpleasant emotions. Clear goals are set to challenge specific beliefs and modify behaviour in order to break the cycle and improve mood.

2. D – Electroconvulsive therapy

ECT is the administration of an electric shock to the head (under general anaesthesia) in order to induce a seizure. The indications are severe depressive illness, especially if there is life-threatening behaviour, puerperal depressive illness, mania and catatonic schizophrenia. The absolute contraindication is raised intracranial pressure. Relative contraindications include high anaesthetic risk and known cerebral aneurysm. Long-term side effects of ECT are unknown, but some patients have complained of long-term memory loss. Short-term side effects are headache, temporary confusion and some short-term memory loss, which is usually reversible.

3. E – Fluoxetine

The first drug treatment of depression should be a SSRI, typically fluoxetine, paroxetine or citalopram. These drugs enhance the effect of the neurotransmitter serotonin (5-hydroxytryptamine [5-HT]) by inhibiting the 5-HT transporter on the presynaptic membrane. There is typically a 2-week delay before an improvement is noted, and it is usually recommended that treatment be continued for 6 months after remission. The most common side effects are hyponatraemia, gastrointestinal disturbance (nausea, vomiting, diarrhoea or pain), insomnia, sexual dysfunction and agitation. Patients should be told that, although the drug does not lead to tolerance or craving, stopping abruptly can lead to withdrawal effects. This is the SSRI withdrawal syndrome (characterized by transient dizziness, lethargy, nausea and headache).

4. G – Lithium

The mechanism of action of lithium is unknown, but it possibly acts on neuronal second-messenger systems. Indications for lithium therapy are augmentation of antidepressants in resistant depression and treatment/prophylaxis of bipolar disorder. Side effects at therapeutic levels include fine tremor, dry mouth, a metallic taste, mild polyuria, nausea and weight gain. Fetal abnormalities can occur if lithium is given during pregnancy. It can also cause hypothyroidism and renal impairment. At toxic levels (which can occur in mild dehydration), there can be twitching, polyuric renal failure, seizures, coma and death. Patients must have a physical examination before treatment is initiated, along with blood tests for thyroid and renal function, and a baseline ECG. Lithium levels should be measured every week until stable and every 3 months thereafter. Tests for renal function and thyroid function and a full blood count should be repeated after 6 months.

5. A – Amitriptyline

Amitriptyline was the drug of choice in this case because it has more sedating effects than imipramine. Taken at night, it can help people with initial insomnia. Amitriptyline is an example of a tricyclic antidepressant (TCA). The mechanism of action of TCAs is similar to that of SSRIs – inhibition of serotonin reuptake at the presynaptic membrane – but there is also inhibition of the reuptake of noradrenaline, histamine and acetylcholine, and stabilization of the membrane. The extent of the effect on each receptor depends on the individual drug, which is why the side effects vary among them. TCAs are no longer first-line antidepressants, due to their side-effect profile, particularly in overdose. Their side effects can be categorized according to which receptor is inhibited.

- Anticholinergic: dry mouth, constipation, blurred vision, urinary retention
- Antihistamine: weight gain, drowsiness
- Membrane stabilization: reduced seizure threshold, cardiotoxicity

Other side effects include sexual dysfunction, postural hypotension and haematological dysfunction (agranulocytosis, leucopenia, eosinophils and thrombocytopenia). Routine checks such as blood pressure and ECG should be done before initiating treatment. In overdose, the patient may present with decreased conscious levels, tachycardia, dry skin and dilated pupils (there may also be a divergent squint). ECG changes include sinus tachycardia, but there may be a prolonged QRS interval with a risk of ventricular tachycardia. Some of these changes can happen late (more than 36 hours) following an overdose and ongoing monitoring is important. Prolonged monitoring is also required following a staggered overdose.

TCAs can be used in low doses for neuropathic pain. The anticholinergic effects can be made use of in the treatment of children with nocturnal enuresis.

Monoamine oxidase inhibitors (MAOIs) are occasionally used for depression. They prevent breakdown of the neurotransmitters serotonin, dopamine and acetylcholine. Indications include treatment-resistant depression in secondary care, particularly in women with features of atypical depression. Phenelzine is the most commonly prescribed MAOI. The enzyme monoamine oxidase (MAO) metabolizes tyramine, a substance found in many foods (cheese, Marmite, red wine, game, pickled herrings and broad beans). If a patient on an MAOI eats tyramine, this can cause a hypertensive crisis (the 'cheese reaction'). The features are headache, palpitations, fever, convulsions and coma. Moclobemide is a reversible inhibitor of MAO and is less strongly associated with the cheese reaction. Before starting MAOIs, it is important to 'wash out' any previously used antidepressants from the body (i.e. have an antidepressant-free period: 5 weeks for SSRIs and 2 weeks for TCAs). This is to avoid the risk of serotonin syndrome, which most commonly occurs when MAOIs are used in combination with other antidepressants. Signs include severe hypertension, tachycardia and high pyrexia. There may be shock and agitated delirium. Earlier signs are myoclonus, overactive reflexes and sweating.

Other antidepressant agents include tetracyclics (e.g. mianserin). These are less cardiotoxic than TCAs, but can cause more severe haematological and hepatic reactions. Serotonin–noradrenaline reuptake inhibitors (e.g. venlafaxine) are more effective than other antidepressants when given in high doses. The side-effect profile is similar to that of the SSRIs, but adverse effects occur less frequently. Other agents are selective noradrenaline reuptake inhibitors (e.g. reboxetine) and noradrenergic and specific serotoninergic antidepressants (e.g. the tetracyclic mirtazapine). Benzodiazepines are not recommended for the treatment of depression.

THEME 7: TRANSCULTURAL PSYCHIATRIC DISORDERS

There are some conditions that are described only within certain cultures. There are other conditions that have a higher incidence in certain cultures; for example, there is a nine-fold increase in schizophrenia in second-generation African–Caribbean immigrants in Britain. Dissociative disorders are more common in developing countries. Depressive disorders associated with guilt are higher in Christian cultures. Presentations of similar underlying pathology may also differ between cultures. For example, non-western immigrants in Britain are more likely to complain of abdominal pain or erectile dysfunction instead of low mood when the underlying diagnosis is depression.

1. A – Amok

Amok is seen in south-east Asia, usually in Malaysian men. The features are acquisition of a weapon followed by a series of frenzied attacks, killing or seriously injuring anyone within reach. The attacks can last several hours and are frequently terminated only by the attacker being killed by someone else or himself. If he is not killed, amok is followed by a stupor/sleep lasting 1 day, followed by amnesia of the event. It is thought to be a form of dissociative disorder.

> Amok, from Malay *amuk* = mad with rage. It is the origin of the phrase 'to run amok'.

2. E – Koro

Koro is seen in Asian men, especially in Chinese cultures. It is the fear that the penis is retracting into the abdomen. Some have a secondary worry that full retraction will lead to death. Koro is more common in people who have limited access to education.

> Koro, from Malay *koro* = turtle head – retraction of the turtle's head is seen as similar to koro.

3. G – Piblokto

Piblokto is described in Inuit women living within the Arctic Circle. There is sudden-onset hysteria (screaming, crying, etc.) and bizarre behaviour. This may include removal of clothes, coprophagia (ingestion of faeces) and violence. Attacks last a couple of hours and there is often amnesia after the event.

> Piblokto is the Inuktun word for madness or hysteria.

4. C – Dhat

Dhat occurs in young Indian males. It is associated with anxiety and a belief that semen is being lost in the urine. It often accompanies excessive guilt about masturbation. There may be a belief that semen is 'vital fluid', more so than blood, and that its loss leads to fatigue.

> Dhat, from Sanskrit *dhatu* = the elixir that constitutes the body.

5. F – Latah

Latah is a culture-bound condition found in women in North Africa and the Far East (especially Malaysia). There is an exaggerated startle response, in which women sometimes start repeating the words of another person (echolalia) or obeying their commands. There is frequently amnesia after the event.

Susto usually occurs in people living in South America. It is a severe depressive episode usually occurring after a traumatic event. There are often physical symptoms such as diarrhoea and nervous tics. It is thought (within the culture in which it exists) to be caused by separation of the soul from the body. It has some features in common with acute stress reaction. Windigo is recognized in native North American tribes. Affected people believe that their body is possessed by a spirit that craves human flesh. This results in obsessive thoughts and compulsions regarding violence and cannibalism.

Susto, from Spanish *susto* = fright.
Windigo, from Ojibwe (indigenous North American language) *wiindigoo* = cannibal, a giant man-eating monster.

THEME 8: PSYCHIATRIC SIGNS OF PHYSICAL ILLNESS

1. C – Hyperthyroidism

Thyroid disease is one of the most common endocrine disorders. Thyroid dysfunction results in systemic symptoms. Psychological symptoms of hyperthyroidism include irritability, behaviour changes, restlessness, loss of libido, weight loss despite an increased appetite and, in extreme cases, psychosis (mania). Psychological symptoms of hypothyroidism include depression, tiredness, reduced libido, cognitive impairment and occasionally psychosis or coma. The accompanying physical symptoms of tremor, weight loss and atrial fibrillation in this case confirm hyperthyroidism. Investigations should proceed with measurement of thyroid hormones, expecting to find a raised thyroxine (T_4) with low levels of thyroid-stimulating hormone.

2. J – Systemic lupus erythematosus

Systemic lupus erythematosus is an autoimmune connective tissue disease. There is a very broad range of physical signs and symptoms. It can also cause depression, seizures and psychosis. A few of the possible physical manifestations mentioned in this case are malar (butterfly) rash, arthralgia and shortness of breath, which could be caused by lung fibrosis or several other pulmonary conditions.

3. I – Space-occupying lesion

Cerebral tumours should be considered as a differential diagnosis of psychiatric illness. Such space-occupying lesions present with headache that is worse in the morning and exacerbated by bending, straining and coughing. Possible psychological and psychiatric manifestations include impaired consciousness, irritability, apathy, hallucinations, seizures, neuroses and psychosis.

4. B – Delirium

This woman has a urinary tract infection causing delirium. Delirium is characterized by fluctuating impairment of consciousness, mood changes and abnormal perceptions. It affects 10%–25% of people aged over 65 years on medical wards. The patient may be obviously confused, with disruptive behaviour and expressing bizarre ideas, but it is important to recognize that delirium can also cause a decreased level of activity and speech. It develops over a short period of time and is due to an underlying physical condition. Common causes are infection, hypoxia, electrolyte disturbances, constipation, drugs and CNS disease. The main principle of management is to investigate and treat the cause, and to concurrently help relieve distress to the patient by optimizing their ability to orientate themselves. There should be a calm environment with adequate lighting, even at night. Patients should be wearing their glasses and hearing aids (if applicable), have continuity of staff contact where possible and ideally have family members or familiar belongings around them. In some circumstances, oral or intramuscular haloperidol or benzodiazepines can be used to relieve severe agitation, but these should be avoided where possible. The average duration of delirium is 7 days. Around 40% of patients with delirium die of the underlying condition and 5% go on to develop dementia.

5. A – Cushing's syndrome

The features of Cushing's syndrome are caused by raised levels of glucocorticoids from any sources. Causes include steroid use, ectopic adrenocorticotropic hormone secretion and a pituitary tumour (Cushing's disease). In addition to the physical features (hirsutism, striae, acne, plethora, bruising, thin skin and cataracts), psychological features include depression, insomnia, reduced libido and occasionally psychosis.

Multiple sclerosis is a disorder of the myelin-producing oligodendrocytes in the CNS. Psychological disturbance can occur, including depression, abnormal affect and occasionally disinhibition, aphasia and psychosis.

Neurosyphilis is an infection of the CNS by the sexually transmitted parasite *Treponema pallidum*. Before the advent of antibiotics, it occurred in 25%–30% of those infected. Features of neurosyphilis are cranial nerve palsies, meningitis and eventually tabes dorsalis. Another late manifestation is general paralysis of the insane, which causes chronic cognitive impairment and personality change, depression, psychosis and mania. Death usually occurs within 3 years.

Punch-drunk syndrome (also known as posttraumatic dementia or boxing encephalopathy) occurs after repeated blows to the head. Brain atrophy is a feature. Clinical features are cognitive impairment and personality deterioration, with cerebellar, extrapyramidal and pyramidal signs. Occasionally, pathological jealousy and rage reactions are associated.

Pellagra is a disorder caused by niacin (vitamin B$_3$) deficiency. It is most common in South America, where maize forms the staple diet. The main physical features are weakness, dermatitis and diarrhoea. There can also be personality change progressing to dementia. Treatment is with niacin. Death can occur within a few years if untreated.

THEME 9: THE MENTAL HEALTH ACT

These are all sections from Part II of the Mental Health Act for England and Wales 2007. They relate to compulsory detention in hospital of patients with a psychiatric disorder that requires treatment. The majority of psychiatric admissions to hospital are on a voluntary (informal) basis. Patients and their nearest relatives have the right to appeal against their section which is reviewed by either Mental Health Act managers or a mental health review tribunal, who have the authority to discharge patients.

1. L – Section 136

Sections 135 describes powers conferred by a magistrate to enter a private property of a person who is deemed at risk to himself or others by the nature of his or her mental illness. A registered medical officer, preferably a Section 12-approved doctor, has to be present with the police at the time of attempting entry to the property. Section 136 allows police to take someone from the community to a hospital or another safe place and does not require authorization by a magistrate. The detention lasts 72 hours.

2. A – Section 2

Section 2 is compulsory detention for assessment, when the exact diagnosis and response to treatment are unknown. Its duration is 28 days. It must be agreed by two doctors (one of whom must be Section 12 approved). To become approved under Section 12(2), one has to attend a specific Section 12 training course and be recommended to do so by two psychiatry consultants. Before attending training, doctors must usually hold membership of the Royal College of Psychiatrists or have at least 3 years' experience in psychiatry.

3. E – Section 5(4)

Section 5(4) is a nurse's holding power. This allows detention of informal psychiatry inpatients by nurses if there is no doctor available. It lasts 6 hours, allowing time for a doctor to assess the patient for detention of up to 72 hours (under Section 5[2], or, for longer periods of detention, typically under Sections 2 or 3). Section 5(2) is a doctor's holding power. It allows the detention of a hospital inpatient (under any specialty) by the doctor responsible for their care. It lasts 72 hours (long enough to arrange a Section 2). Note that, in even more acute situations, patients can be stopped under common law for a short time if there is an immediate threat to their health.

4. B – Section 3

Section 3 allows compulsory detention for treatment when the diagnosis is already known and treatment is available at the place where the person is detained. It lasts for 6 months, but may be renewed if necessary. It must be agreed by two doctors (one of whom must be Section 12 approved).

5. C – Section 4

Section 4 allows an emergency admission to hospital when there is not enough time to organize a Section 2. Its duration is 72 hours and there is no right of appeal against it. It can be arranged by one doctor.

Sections 35–37 can be requested by a court on advice of a Section 12-approved doctor when a patient has been charged with an offence that may lead to imprisonment. Section 35 is for the purpose of producing a medical report on the psychiatric illness of the offender. The duration is 28 days. Section 36 allows treatment of the patient. It also lasts 28 days, but requires two doctors to agree on it. Section 37 is for the detention and treatment of a patient already convicted of an imprisonable offence. This also requires two doctors' agreement and lasts 6 months.

Section 17 allows for set periods of leave (with a responsible adult) to be granted by the responsible medical officer.

THEME 10: PERSONALITY DISORDERS

The International Classification of Diseases-10 definition of a personality disorder is 'a severe disturbance in the characterological constitution and behavioural tendencies of the individual, usually involving several areas of the personality, and nearly always associated with considerable personal and social disruption'. These often become apparent during childhood or adolescence, and continue into adulthood. The prevalence of personality disorders is probably under-reported. They are likely to affect around 10% of the population, but the prevalence is higher in psychiatric settings. There are several theories regarding personality and personality disorders; the dimensional approach suggests that people with personality disorders exhibit traits that feature as a spectrum in the population, but to an exaggerated degree.

1. B – Antisocial

Antisocial personalities often display little feeling towards others. There is a tendency to be aggressive, commit crimes and lack remorse. Affected persons have difficulty in forming intimate relationships, and the diagnosis is supported by a previous childhood conduct disorder.

2. D – Dependent

Dependent personality types are often passive, relying on others to make decisions. They fear abandonment and find it difficult to cope with daily chores. Such personalities may excessively give priority to the needs and wishes of others over their own in an attempt to maintain their close relationships.

3. E – Emotionally unstable (borderline type)

The emotionally unstable (borderline type) personality disorder is characterized by emotional instability, disturbed views of self-image, feelings of emptiness and intense, but easily broken, relationships. Self-harm is a common feature, often in an attempt to avoid abandonment. The emotionally unstable (impulsive type) personality disorder is similar, but a lack of self-control and violent outbursts are more prominent features.

4. I – Schizoid

Schizoid personalities have a preference for their own company over that of others. They lack emotional expression and may consequently be perceived by others as cold and disinterested. They may not gain pleasure from many activities and have little interest in forming sexual or confiding relationships. Thought disorders and psychoses, which are features of schizophrenia, are not present in schizoid personalities. However, schizoid personalities are not exempt from developing schizophrenia.

5. G – Histrionic

Histrionic individuals crave attention, are preoccupied with appearance and are inappropriately flirtatious. They may display theatrical expressions of emotions, from excessive excitement to unexpected, manipulative tantrums.

Histrionic, from Latin *histrionicus* = pertaining to an actor.

People with a paranoid personality disorder are often suspicious of others (including their own partners) and are very sensitive to rejection. They often bear grudges and misinterpret the actions of others as malicious. Anxious (avoidant) personality disorder is characterized by a tendency to worry, extreme anxiety, feelings of inferiority and a fear of criticism/disapproval to the point of avoiding people/situations where this might happen. People with anankastic personality disorder frequently display an inflexible preoccupation with rules, order and attention to detail. They may be very cautious and stubborn, and may try to enforce their ways with others.

In Diagnostic and Statistical Manual of Mental Disorders, 5th edition (DSM-5), two further personality disorders are categorized: the narcissistic personality (arrogant with a grandiose sense of self-importance, often lacking empathy for others) and the schizotypal personality (eccentric behaviours, thinking, speech and appearance, and lacking social confidence and close relationships).

Personality disorders may be categorized into clusters (according to the Diagnostic and Statistical Manual of Mental Disorders (DSM-IV-TR), American Psychiatric Association):

- Cluster A (paranoid, schizoid, schizotypal): odd or eccentric
- Cluster B (antisocial, borderline, histrionic, narcissistic): emotional or dramatic
- Cluster C (avoidant, dependent, anankastic): anxious or fearful

Narcissism, from the Creek legend *Narcissus*, who was cursed into falling in love with his own reflection after breaking the heart of the shy nymph Echo. (Incidentally, Echo loved the sound of her voice so much, she was herself cursed into only being able to repeat what others said.)

Anankastic, from Greek *Ananke*, the goddess of necessity.

Index

A